STRESSE

NP CERTIF

Here's everything you need to pass the exams

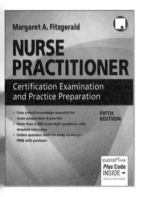

Nurse Practitioner
Certification Examination and Practice Preparation

Margaret A. Fitzgerald

Over 2,300 exam-prep questions representing every major clinical condition feature detailed rationales.

★ ★ ★ ★ ★

Family Practice and Adult-Gerontology Primary Care Nurse Practitioner
Certification Examination, 6th Edition

Jill E. Winland-Brown | Lynne M. Dunphy

Over 3,300 questions with detailed rationales parallel the domains and content areas of the FNP and AGNP exams.

★ ★ ★ ★ ★

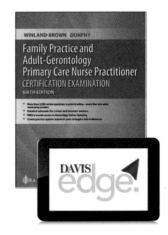

ADVANCED PRACTICE
NURSING
PROCEDURES

SECOND EDITION

Margaret R. Colyar, DSN, APRN, C-FNP
Family Nurse Practitioner
Hannibal Clinic
Hannibal, Missouri

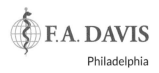

F.A. DAVIS

Philadelphia

F. A. Davis Company
1915 Arch Street
Philadelphia, PA 19103
www.fadavis.com

Printed in the United States of America
Last digit indicates print number: 10 9 8 7 6 5 4 3 2

Publisher: Susan R. Rhyner
Manager of Project and eProject Management: Catherine Carroll
Content Project Manager: Amanda Minutola
Design and Illustration Manager: Carolyn O'Brien

As new scientific information becomes available through basic and clinical research, recommended treatments and drug therapies undergo changes. The author(s) and publisher have done everything possible to make this book accurate, up to date, and in accord with accepted standards at the time of publication. The author(s), editors, and publisher are not responsible for errors or omissions or for consequences from application of the book, and make no warranty, expressed or implied, in regard to the contents of the book. Any practice described in this book should be applied by the reader in accordance with professional standards of care used in regard to the unique circumstances that may apply in each situation. The reader is advised always to check product information (package inserts) for changes and new information regarding dose and contraindications before administering any drug. Caution is especially urged when using new or infrequently ordered drugs.

Library of Congress Control Number 2014959076

ISBN: 978-0-8036-9813-0

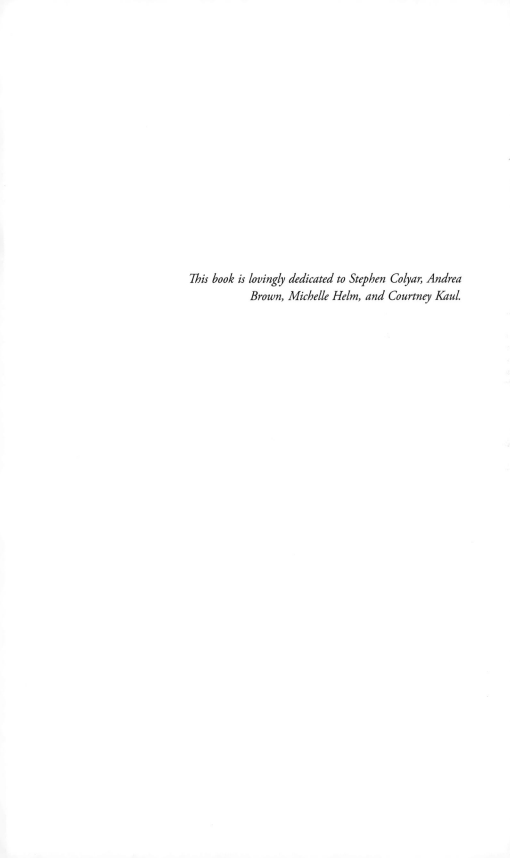

This book is lovingly dedicated to Stephen Colyar, Andrea Brown, Michelle Helm, and Courtney Kaul.

Preface

The new nurse practitioner and the practicing nurse practitioner in the ambulatory care setting must be prepared to perform an increasing array of skills competently to meet patient care needs. The inspiration for this book came when, on graduating from a nurse practitioner program, I found no procedural resources directed toward the needs of the nurse practitioner in ambulatory care. The need to perform many procedures—those not taught in my nurse practitioner program—was apparent. The physician I practiced with required a knowledge base in procedural skills greater than the one I possessed. Fortunately, this physician was willing to teach me the necessary procedures. This improved care to our patients and decreased the necessity to refer many patients for procedures easily performed in the ambulatory care (outpatient) setting.

This text was developed to assist in the many demands on the newly graduated nurse practitioner and the nurse practitioner currently in practice. We believe the procedures outlined will improve the marketability of the nurse practitioner and serve as a good reference tool for family and/or adult nurse practitioners in an ambulatory care setting. Prerequisites for this book are basic anatomy and physiology, microbiology, pharmacology, principles of aseptic technique, and basic nursing skills. This book would be an appropriate text for incorporation of procedural techniques throughout a family or an adult nurse practitioner curriculum. It also would be appropriate for an elective on minor surgery and diagnostic procedures and interpretation. Another potential use for this book would be as part of the protocol/guidelines in the nurse practitioner's practice.

Many procedures performed by primary care physicians are not currently appropriate for the nurse practitioner to perform. The procedures in this book were chosen based on a comprehensive study of types of procedures currently used in the nurse practitioner's practice. Many of the procedures can be used in any ambulatory setting.

Some of the procedures need specialized equipment, and some use equipment commonly found in any office. A few of the procedures—flexible chest tube insertion, colposcopy, endometrial biopsy, IUD insertion and removal, sigmoidoscopy, and thrombosed hemorrhoid removal—require additional training. They are included for reference only. Check with your state board of nursing if you are unsure whether or not a certain procedure may be performed by nurse practitioners in the state in which you practice.

The major theme of this book is clinical application of knowledge and clinical skills. There are seven sections in the book. These sections are based on body systems for ease of classification. Each major section begins with diagnostic procedures the nurse practitioner performs with the basis for their interpretation. Next in each section, listed in alphabetical order, are procedures performed in an ambulatory care setting.

Each procedure contains seven parts. First, an *Overview* is presented, outlining causes, incidence, and other specific information intrinsic to each procedure. The *Health Promotion/Prevention* section gives tips to the nurse practitioner to pass on to the client to help promote health or prevent the need for the procedure in the future. *Options* lists one to four methods of performing the procedure and gives a choice of how to perform the procedure. The *Rationale* section gives reasons to perform the procedure. *Indications* tell the nurse practitioner when the procedure should be performed, and *Contraindications* tells the nurse practitioner when not to perform the procedure. The *Procedure* section lists the necessary equipment and gives step-by-step instructions for performing each procedure listed under *Options*. *Client Instructions* assist the nurse practitioner with postprocedure instructions, listing what the client must and must not do to have an optimal recovery period. At the end of each is a bibliography for further information gathering.

We hope you will find this text to be a good learning tool and a great resource in your practice.

Acknowledgments

We acknowledge the following people for their contributions, assistance, and patience while compiling this book: Susan Rhyner, Publisher at F.A. Davis, for believing in the merits of this book, and Denise Melomo, artist, for her expertise in sketching the line drawings that guided the illustration team who created the artwork in the first edition of this text.

Many colleagues at Tri County Family Health Care in Madison, Florida, and Family Health Service in Ocala, Florida, were instrumental in this book. Colleagues at Rapides Regional Medical Center, Alexandria, Louisiana; Jackson Parish Hospital, Jonesboro, Louisiana; Hannibal Clinic, Hannibal, Missouri; and Stansbury Medical Center, Stansbury Park, Utah, posed for the photographs in the book. These models include Linda Alby, Steve Colyar, Hugh Gentry, Cindy Grappe, Aleene Hale, Lane Helm, Debra Lefler, Anne Martin, Mitzi Buckman, Cathy Taylor, and Shaneal Wright.

Contributors

Margaret Colyar, DSN, APRN, C-FNP
Hannibal Clinic
Hannibal, Missouri

Cynthia Ehrhardt, RN, ARNP, MSN, FNP-CS
Adjunct Faculty
University of Central Florida
Ocala, Florida

Contents

Section Two: MUSCULOSKELETAL PROCEDURES, 121

Diagnostic Testing

Procedures

Section Three: GENITOURINARY AND BREAST PROCEDURES, 199

Diagnostic Testing

Procedures

Section One

Dermatological Procedures

Chapter

Punch Biopsy
Margaret R. Colyar

CPT Code

21550	Biopsy of soft tissue of neck or thorax
21920	Biopsy of soft tissue of back or flank, superficial
23066	Biopsy of soft tissue of shoulder, superficial
24065	Biopsy of upper arm and elbow area
23066	Biopsy of soft tissue of forearm or wrist, superficial
27040	Biopsy of soft tissue of pelvis and hip area
27323	Biopsy of soft tissue of pelvis and hip area
27613	Biopsy of soft tissue of leg and ankle area
11100	Skin lesion—Depends on the site, technique, and if benign or malignant lesions

Biopsy is the removal of a small piece of tissue from the skin for microscopic examination. Partial or full thickness of skin over the lesion is removed for evaluation.

OVERVIEW

Punch biopsy is used for full and partial dermal lesions such as

- Basal cell carcinoma
- **Squamous cell carcinoma**
- **Actinic keratoses**
- **Seborrheic keratoses**
- **Lentigo (freckles)**
- Lipomas
- Melanomas
- Nevi
- Warts—**verruca vulgaris**

RATIONALE

- To confirm etiology of lesion for treatment
- To establish or confirm a diagnosis for treatment and/or intervention

INDICATIONS

- Partial- or full-dermal-thickness lesion not on the face, eye, lip, or penis

CONTRAINDICATIONS

- Lesion on eyelid, lip, or penis, REFER to a physician.
- Infection at the site of the biopsy.
- Bleeding disorder.
- Lesions that are deep or on the face, REFER to a physician.

▶ *Informed consent required*

PROCEDURE

Punch Biopsy

Equipment

- Antiseptic skin cleanser
- Drape—sterile
- Gloves—sterile
- Disposable biopsy punch (Fig. 1.1)
- Pickups—sterile
- Scissors—sharp for the fine tissue, sterile
- 3-mL syringe
- 27- to 30-gauge, ½-inch needle
- 1% lidocaine

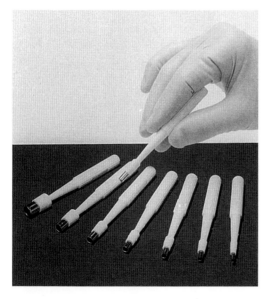

Figure 1.1 Disposable biopsy punches.

- Container with 10% **formalin**
- 4 × 4 gauze
- Nonstick dressing (Adaptic or Telfa)
- Kling bandage
- Tape
- **Steri-Strips** (if biopsy area will be greater than 4 mm) or **one suture**

Procedure

- Position the client so that the area to be biopsied is easily accessible.
- Cleanse the skin with antiseptic skin cleanser.
- Put on gloves.
- Drape the area to be biopsied.
- Anesthetize with 1% lidocaine.
- With the thumb and index finger, spread the skin to apply tension opposite natural skin tension lines. This allows a more elliptical-shaped wound for easy closure.
- Apply biopsy punch to skin, rotate per manufacturer's directions, and remove the punch (Fig. 1.2).
- With pickups, pull up loosened skin.
- Cut with scissors, and place tissue in tissue container of 10% formalin (Fig. 1.3).
- If less than 2 to 3 mm, apply nonstick dressing and pressure dressing.
- If greater than 4 mm, apply Steri-Strips and cover with 4 × 4 gauze.
- Apply Kling bandage and secure with tape.

Client Instructions

- Keep dressing clean, dry, and in place for 24 hours to decrease the chance of bleeding and oozing.
- Avoid touching or contaminating the area biopsied.
- To prevent the chance of infection, take cephalexin (Keflex) 500 mg three times per day or amoxicillin (Amoxil) 500 mg twice a day for 5 days.

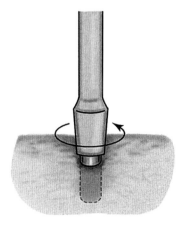

Figure 1.2 Apply biopsy punch to skin and rotate.

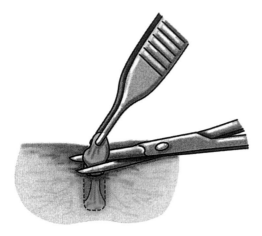

Figure 1.3 Cut with scissors.

- Some redness, swelling, and heat are normal. Return to the office if symptoms of infection occur, such as
  - Yellow or green drainage
  - Red streaks
  - Pain
  - Elevated temperature
- Take acetaminophen (Tylenol) or ibuprofen (Motrin) every 4 to 6 hours as needed for pain.

BIBLIOGRAPHY

De Vries HJ, Zeegelaar JE, Middelkoop E, et al. Reduced wound contraction and scar formation in punch biopsy wounds. Native collagen dermal substitutes. A clinical study. *Br J Dermatol.* 1995;132(5):690–697.

Nischal U, Nischal KC, Khopkar U. Techniques of skin biopsy and practical considerations. *J Cutan Aesthet Surg.* 2008;1(2):107–111.

Zuber TJ. Ingrown toenail removal. *Am Fam Physician.* 2002;65(12):2547–2550.

Chapter **2**

Skin Biopsy
Margaret R. Colyar

CPT Code

11300–03	Shaving of epidermal or dermal lesion; single lesion—trunk, arms, or legs
11305–08	Shaving of epidermal or dermal lesion; single lesion—scalp, neck, hands, feet, or genitalia
11400–06	Excision benign lesions—trunk, arms, or legs
11420–26	Excision benign lesions—scalp, neck, hands, feet, or genitalia
11600–06	Excision malignant lesions—trunk, arms, or legs
11620–26	Excision malignant lesions—scalp, neck, hands, feet, or genitalia

---

Skin **biopsy** is the excision of a small piece of living tissue for microscopic examination. The two major categories of skin biopsy are
* Partial dermal thickness—shave and **curettage**
* Full dermal thickness—punch and elliptical excision

HEALTH PROMOTION/PREVENTION
* Inspect the skin periodically for lesions.
* Note lesions that change size or color, are irregular, or are painful.

OPTIONS
* Method 1—Shave biopsy
  * Use for elevated skin lesions such as
    * Skin tags
    * Benign **nevi** (interdermal)
    * Epithelial tags
    * Small **basal cell carcinomas**
    * **Condyloma acuminatum**
    * Cherry **angiomas**
    * **Actinic keratoses**
    * **Seborrheic keratoses**
    * **Lentigo (freckles)**
    * **Verruca vulgaris** (warts)
* Method 2—Curettage biopsy
  * Use for
    * Seborrheic keratoses
    * Superficial basal cell carcinomas
    * Crusting actinic keratoses

- Method 3—Elliptical excisional biopsy
  - Use for full-dermal-thickness lesions such as
    - Basal cell carcinoma
    - **Squamous cell carcinoma**
    - Actinic keratoses
    - Seborrheic keratoses
    - Lentigo
    - Lipomas
    - **Melanomas**
    - Nevi
    - Verruca vulgaris (warts)

RATIONALE

- To confirm or make a diagnosis of a skin lesion
- To determine definitive treatment of a skin lesion
- To remove a disfiguring or painful lesion

INDICATIONS

- Nonmalignant skin lesions not on the eyelid, lip, face, or penis
- Superficial skin lesions

CONTRAINDICATIONS

- Infection suspected at biopsy site
- Bleeding disorder
- If melanoma is suspected, do not use shave or curettage methods. Elliptical excision is preferred.
- If on eyelid, lip, face, or penis, REFER to a physician.
- If deep lesions, REFER to a physician.
- ▶ *Informed consent required*

PROCEDURE

Skin Biopsy

Equipment

- Methods 1, 2, and 3
  - Antiseptic skin cleanser
  - Drape—sterile
  - Gloves—nonsterile
  - 3-mL syringe
  - 27- to 30-gauge, ½-inch needle
  - 1% lidocaine
  - Container of 10% **formalin**
  - Cautery or topical hemostatic agent such as Monsel's solution
  - Pickups—sterile (optional)
- Method 1 only
  - No. 15 scalpel or sterile scissors

- Method 2 only
  - Dermal curette
- Method 3 only
  - Needle driver with scissors—sterile
  - Suture (See Chapter 23 for information on choosing the appropriate type and size of suture.)
  - Tape
  - Nonstick dressing (Adaptic or Telfa)
  - 4 × 4 gauze
  - Topical antibiotic (Bactroban, Bacitracin, or Polysporin)

Procedure

METHOD 1—SHAVE BIOPSY

- Position the client for comfort with the area of the skin lesion easily accessible.
- Cleanse the skin lesion and a 3-inch-diameter circle around the lesion.
- Drape the area.
- Put on gloves.
- Inject 1% lidocaine under the lesion using a 27- to 30-gauge needle to create a wheal.
- Incise lesion parallel to the skin (Fig. 2.1).
- Place the tissue in a container of 10% formalin.
- Cauterize the base of the wound or apply topical hemostatic agent such as Monsel's solution to retard bleeding.

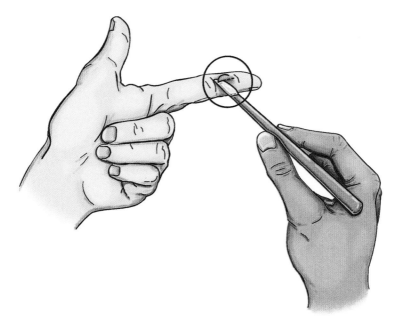

Figure 2.1 Shave biopsy. Incise parallel to the skin.

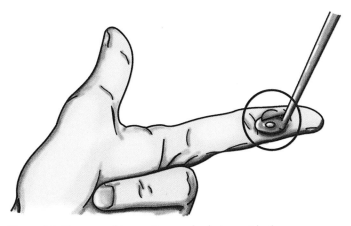

Figure 2.2 Curettage biopsy. Scrape the lesion with the curette.

METHOD 2—CURETTAGE BIOPSY

- Position the patient for comfort with the area of the skin lesion easily accessible.
- Cleanse the skin lesion and a 3-inch-diameter area around the lesion.
- Drape the area.
- Put on gloves.
- Inject 1% lidocaine under the lesion using a 27- to 30-gauge needle to create a wheal.
- Scrape the lesion with the curette (Fig. 2.2).
- Place the tissue in a container of 10% formalin.
- Cauterize the base of the wound or apply topical hemostatic agent such as Monsel's solution to retard bleeding.

METHOD 3—ELLIPTICAL EXCISIONAL BIOPSY (FULL DERMAL THICKNESS)

- Position the patient for comfort with the area of the skin lesion easily accessible.
- Draw an outline of the expected incision in the direction of the skin tension lines. The outline should be three times longer than it is wide.
- Cleanse the skin lesion and a 3-inch-diameter area around the lesion.
- Put on gloves.
- Inject 1% lidocaine under the lesion using a 27- to 30-gauge needle to create a wheal that covers the entire area of the proposed incision.
- Drape the area.
- Incise around the outline with the scalpel (Fig. 2.3).
- Pull up a corner of skin with pickups.
- Pull tissue as you excise just below full thickness of the tissue.
- Start at one corner and work to the center.
- Go to the other corner and work toward the center.
- Put all excised tissue in a container of 10% formalin.

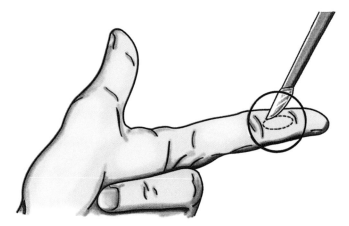

Figure 2.3 Elliptical excisional biopsy. Incise around the outline with the scalpel.

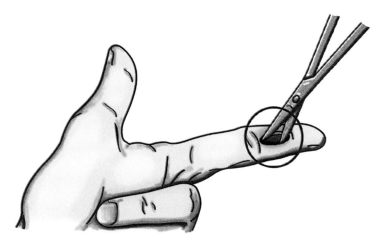

Figure 2.4 Undermine the edges of the wound to release tension.

- Closure
  - If a small lesion, simple single-layer closure with nylon suture is appropriate (see Chapter 22).
  - If lesion is larger with tension,
    - Undermine the edges of the wound to release the tension (Fig. 2.4).
    - Incise the subcutaneous tissue the entire length of each side of the wound with the scalpel.
    - Spread the incised subcutaneous tissue with scissors (Fig. 2.5).
    - Suture using the simple single-layer technique.
  - If a larger, deeper lesion with tension,
    - Undermine the subcutaneous tissue as just described.

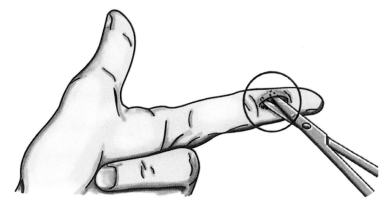

Figure 2.5 Spread the incised subcutaneous tissue with scissors.

- Close subcutaneous tissue with absorbable suture and **inverted** knot (see Chapter 22).
- Close skin using simple closure technique.
- Apply topical antibiotic, nonstick dressing, cover with 4 × 4 gauze, and secure with tape.

Client Instructions

- Some inflammation (redness, swelling, and pain) is normal.
- To prevent infection, keep the dressing in place for 24 hours, then remove the dressing and keep the area clean and dry. After the second day, you may wash the area gently with soap and water. Monitor for signs of infection, such as
  - Yellow and green drainage
  - Red streaks
  - Excessive pain
  - Elevated temperature
- Return to the office immediately if infection occurs.
- Some bleeding and oozing are normal for the first 24 to 48 hours. If your bandage becomes soaked with blood, reapply dry gauze and apply pressure for 2 minutes. If the bleeding does not stop, notify your practitioner.
- Avoid tension to the wound area by limiting movement. Tension may cause the wound to pull apart. If the wound does pull apart, notify the practitioner.
- Take Tylenol No. 3 (acetaminophen with codeine) every 4 to 6 hours as needed for pain. When the pain lessens, take Tylenol or ibuprofen (Motrin) every 4 to 6 hours as needed.
- Return to the office (in _____) for stitch removal (depends on site sutured; see Table 22.1).

BIBLIOGRAPHY

Nischal U, Nischal KC, Khopkar U. Techniques of skin biopsy and practical considerations. *J Cutan Aesthet Surg.* 2008;1(2):107–111.

Pfenninger JL, Fowler GC. *Procedures for Primary Care Physicians.* St. Louis, MO: Mosby; 2019.

Surajachar MD. Principles of skin biopsies for the family physician. *Am Fam Physician.* 1996;54(8):2411–2418.

Walters GK. Managing soft tissue wounds. *Adv Nurse Pract.* 1996;4(3):37–40, 54.

Zuber TJ, Dewitt DE. The fusiform excision. *Am Fam Physician.* 1994;49(2):371–376.

Chapter **3**

Wood's Light Examination

Margaret R. Colyar

CPT Code
None

The **Wood's light** is a useful and inexpensive tool in clinical practice. It is powered by alternating or direct current that converts ultraviolet light into visible light, and it usually has an accompanying magnification lens. It provides a simple diagnostic method in the evaluation of

* Many dermatological problems
* **Fluorescein**-staining evaluation of eye injuries

OVERVIEW

* Most common dermatological lesions that fluoresce are listed in Table 3.1.
* Detection of chemicals applied to the skin. Affected areas are a different color from that of the surrounding skin.
   * Prior cleansing of the area to be examined causes false-negative result.
   * Certain skin lesions do not fluoresce.
   * Systemic antibiotic therapy, such as with tetracyclines, can cause fluorescence in some lesions.
   * Cosmetics present on the skin interfere with fluorescence.
* Detection of eye injuries with fluorescein. When applied to the eye, fluorescein has a higher concentration of uptake in areas in which there has been disruption of the cornea or sclera. Under a Wood's light, the injured area fluoresces as a bright yellow-green.
* Detection of porphyrins in the urine. These appear bright red.

Table 3·1	Fluorescence of Lesions and Parasites With the Wood's Light
LESION	**FLUORESCENCE**
Erythrasma	
Corynebacterium minutissimum	Varying shades of pink to coral red
Tinea Capitis (Three Varieties)	
Microsporum audouinii	Brilliant green
Microsporum canis	Brilliant green
Trichophyton schoenleinii	Pale green
Tinea Versicolor	Yellow to deep green
Pseudomonas aeruginosa	Blue green to green
Pigmentation Alterations	
Albinism	Cold bright white
Ash-leaf spot of tuberous sclerosis	Blue-white
Depigmentation	Cold bright white
Hypopigmentation	Blue-white
Hyperpigmentation	Purple-brown
Leprosy	Blue-white
Vitiligo	Blue-white
Squamous cell carcinoma*	Bright red
Common Parasitic Infestations	
Scabies	Magnification of track and/or mite
Pediculosis *(capitis, corporis, pubis)*	Visualization of louse

* The diagnosis of this dermatological disorder should be made by pathological assessment.

RATIONALE

- Skin—To allow the clinician to differentiate dermatological presentation of types of bacterial, fungal, and pigmented lesions found on the skin
- Eye—To allow the visual assessment of injuries to the cornea and conjunctiva with fluorescein staining
- Urine—To screen for **porphyria**, a rare metabolic disorder
- Clinical evaluation of dermatitis, the eye, or urine by the unaided eye alone may result in an inappropriate assessment and render an unsuccessful treatment regimen.

INDICATIONS

- Skin or hair lesions
- Corneal abrasion
- Suspicion of porphyria

CONTRAINDICATIONS

- None

PROCEDURE
Wood's Light—Skin

Equipment
* Wood's light
* Darkened room

Procedure
* Have the client position himself or herself comfortably.
* Explain to the client that the Wood's light has the same characteristics as a typical black light; the room will be darkened, and the black light will be turned on to examine for fluorescence of the lesion in question.
* Have all lights turned off.
* Hold the Wood's light approximately 6 to 8 inches from the lesion in question, and observe the characteristics of the fluorescence of the lesion.

BIBLIOGRAPHY ▆▆▆▆▆▆▆▆▆▆▆▆▆▆▆▆▆▆▆▆▆▆

Driscoll C, Bope ET. *The Family Practice Desk Reference.* 4th ed. St. Louis, MO: Mosby; 2002.
Habif T. *Clinical Dermatology: A Color Guide to Diagnosis and Therapy.* 6th ed. St. Louis, MO: Mosby; 2015.
Murtagh J. *Practice Tips.* 5th ed. New York, NY: McGraw-Hill; 2008.
Pfenninger JL, Fowler GC. *Procedures for Primary Care Physicians.* St. Louis, MO: Mosby; 2019.

Chapter 4

Abscesses—Incision and Drainage
Furuncle, Felon, Paronychia, Pilonidal Cyst, Perianal Cyst

Margaret R. Colyar

CPT Code
10060   Incision and drainage of abscess
10080   Incision and drainage of pilonidal cyst; simple
10081   Incision and drainage of pilonidal cyst; complicated
10140   Incision and drainage of hematoma or seroma or fluid collection

An **abscess** is a localized collection of pus surrounded by inflamed tissue in any part of the body. Types of abscess included in this chapter are
- **Furuncle** (boil)—an abscess of the hair follicle or sweat gland
- **Felon**—an abscess of the soft tissue of the terminal joint of the finger
- **Paronychia**—an abscess or cellulitis of the nail folds, usually the proximal and lateral edges
- **Pilonidal cyst**—an abscess located in the gluteal fold close to the anus, caused by an ingrown hair. One or more sinus openings may exist. Males are more prone than females to develop pilonidal cysts. Younger people have pilonidal cysts more often than do the elderly.
- **Perianal cyst**—an abscess around or close to the anus

OVERVIEW
- Causative organisms of most abscesses
  - *Staphylococcus aureus*
  - *Streptococcus* species
- Areas of most frequent occurrence of abscesses
  - Extremities
  - Under the breasts
  - Axillae
  - Buttocks
  - Hair follicles

HEALTH PROMOTION/PREVENTION
- Cleanse skin daily with an antiseptic soap such as unscented Dial soap.
- Do not squeeze face lesions.
- Do not shave closely.
- Discourage nail-biting and finger sucking.

RATIONALE
- To diminish pain
- To promote healing

INDICATIONS
- Collection of pus causing pain and/or not resolved by use of an antibiotic
- Small abscesses
- Small abscesses that enlarge
- Large abscesses

CONTRAINDICATIONS
- Abscesses on the face in the triangle of the bridge of the nose and corners of the mouth
  - Use conservative measures to decrease or prevent the chances for septic phlebitis and intracranial extension.

- Observe carefully and obtain a culture of the abscess from people with
  - Debilitating disease
  - Compromised immune system
▶ *Informed consent required*

PROCEDURE

Incision and Drainage—Furuncle

Equipment

- Antiseptic skin cleanser
- Topical anesthetic—ethyl chloride or verruca freeze kit
- 1% to 2% lidocaine with or without epinephrine
- 3- to 10-mL syringe
- 27- to 30-gauge, ½-inch needle
- 4 × 4 gauze—sterile
- Tube gauze—optional for use on fingers
- No. 11 scalpel
- Drape—sterile
- Gloves—sterile
- Curved **hemostats**—sterile
- **Iodoform** gauze—¼ to ½ inch
- Culture swab
- Scissors—sterile
- Tape

Procedure

- Position the client with the abscess easily accessible.
- Cleanse the abscess and a 3-inch-diameter area surrounding the abscess with antiseptic skin cleanser.
- Drape the abscess with a sterile drape.
- Put on gloves.
- Perform a field block by anesthetizing the perimeter around the abscess with 1% or 2% lidocaine with or without epinephrine. Do *not* inject lidocaine into the abscess because it does not work well in an acidic medium. If the client cannot tolerate a field block, topical anesthesia can be used to freeze the top of the abscess if desired.
- Using the No. 11 scalpel, incise the abscess deeply enough and long enough to allow easy drainage of the purulent material and to prevent premature closure of the wound (Fig. 4.1).
- Obtain a culture (Fig. 4.2) by inserting the culturette deeply into the wound cavity or by withdrawing purulent drainage with a syringe and 18-gauge needle. In case of a breast abscess that is not subareolar, a biopsy should be done.
- Explore the abscess cavity. Break down any sacs or **septa** using curved hemostats (Fig. 4.3).

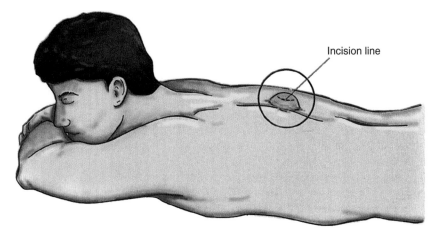

Incision line

Figure 4.1 Incise the abscess deep and wide to allow easy drainage and to prevent premature closure.

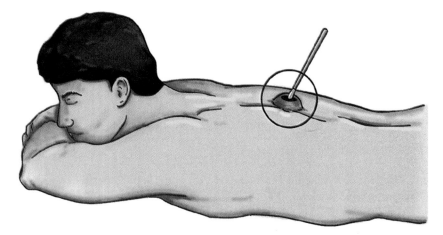

Figure 4.2 Obtain a culture from deep inside the wound cavity.

- After expressing all purulent material, pack with iodoform gauze, leaving a small amount protruding from the wound (Fig. 4.4).
- Dress with sterile gauze.

Incision and Drainage of Abscess—Paronychia

Additional Equipment for Paronychia

- 1% to 2% lidocaine without epinephrine
- If **subungual**, sterile paperclip or cautery tip

Procedure

- Position client with the abscess easily accessible.
- Cleanse the abscess and a 3-inch-diameter area around the abscess with antiseptic skin cleanser.

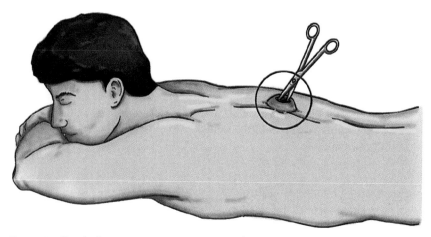

Figure 4.3 Break down any sacs or septa using hemostats.

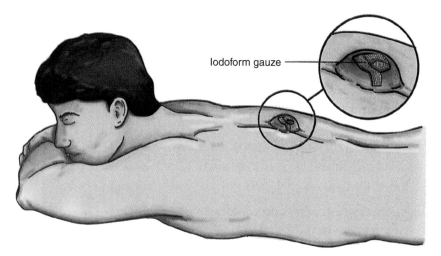

Iodoform gauze

Figure 4.4 Pack the wound with iodoform gauze, leaving a small amount protruding from the wound.

- Drape the abscess with a sterile drape.
- Put on gloves.
- Perform a field block by anesthetizing the perimeter around the abscess with 1% or 2% lidocaine without epinephrine. Do *not* inject lidocaine into the abscess because it does not work well in an acidic medium. If the client cannot tolerate a field block, topical anesthesia can be used to freeze the top of the abscess if desired.
- If the matrix is involved and an abscess has formed a subungual (under the fingernail) tract, use a hot paperclip or cautery tip to bore through the nail to drain pus and blood.
  - Partial removal of nail plate may be needed (see Chapter 10).

- Lift the proximal nail fold. If purulent material is not released freely, incise the skin at the point of highest tension using the no. 11 scalpel.
- Obtain a culture by inserting the culturette deeply into the wound cavity or by withdrawing purulent drainage with a syringe and 18-gauge needle.
- Explore the abscess cavity. Break down any sacs or septa using curved hemostats.
- After expressing all purulent material, pack with iodoform gauze, leaving a small amount protruding from the wound.
- Dress with sterile gauze.
- Cover with tube gauze.

Incision and Drainage—Pilonidal Cyst

Additional Equipment for Pilonidal Cyst

- Cotton-tipped applicator

Procedure

- Same as incision and drainage of furuncle except
  - Position patient in left lateral or lithotomy position.
  - Leave wound open to drain and heal by secondary intention (delayed closure 8 to 12 weeks).
  - Probe sinus tracts with cotton-tipped applicator. If deep, REFER to a surgeon.
  - Perform elliptical excision for pilonidal sinus if superficial (less than 5 mm).

Incision and Drainage—Perianal Abscess

Can be done if perianal or **ischiorectal**; if **supralevator** or **intersphincteric**, REFER to a surgeon.

Additional Equipment for Perianal Abscess

- 0.9% sodium chloride
- Peri-pads

Procedure

- Position patient in left lateral or lithotomy position.
- Perform a digital examination and/or anoscopy (see Chapter 104) to look for internal opening (i.e., fistula; usually 50% incidence).
- If a fistula is not present
  - Drape the abscess with sterile drapes.
  - Cleanse the area with an antiseptic skin cleanser.
  - Use topical anesthetic to freeze the top of the abscess. Local anesthetic is not practical because an acidic environment does not respond well to anesthesia.
  - Using the no. 11 scalpel, incise over the area of greatest tension.
  - Obtain a culture by inserting the culturette deeply into the wound cavity or by withdrawing purulent drainage with a syringe and 18-gauge needle.

- After expressing all purulent material, irrigate with 0.9% sodium chloride.
- Pack with iodoform gauze, leaving a small amount hanging from the wound.
- Dress with sterile gauze or peri-pad.
- To relieve pain when fistula is present, insert a 16- to 18-gauge needle into the abscess and withdraw purulent material. REFER to a surgeon.

Client Instructions

- Return to the office in 2 days to have dressing changed.
- Observe for signs and symptoms of infection, such as
  - Yellow or green drainage
  - Red streaks
  - Increasing pain
  - Elevated temperature
- If symptoms of infection occur, return to the office.
- Prevent recurrence of the abscess by taking an antibiotic—dicloxacillin 250 mg four times a day, cefadroxil 500 mg twice a day, or cephalexin 500 mg three times a day.
- Contrary to popular belief, incised abscesses are painful and usually require narcotic analgesia for the first 24 hours. For pain relief, take Tylenol No. 3 every 4 to 6 hours for the first 24 hours, then take ibuprofen.
- If you had a pilonidal or perianal cyst drained, take a sitz bath with warm water three or four times per day. You may cleanse the area by using the shower or irrigating the area with a squeeze bottle.
- If the abscess recurs, return to the office for evaluation.
- If the abscess was in an extremity, observe for cellulitis and/or gangrene.

BIBLIOGRAPHY

Armstrong JH, Barcia PJ. Pilonidal sinus disease. The conservative approach. *Arch Surg.* 1994;129:914–917.

Johnson RA. Cyst removal. Punch, push, pull. *Skin.* 1995;1(1):14–15.

Miller LG, Eisenberg DF, Liu H, et al. Incidence of skin and soft tissue infections in ambulatory and inpatient settings, 2005–2010. *BMC Infect Dis.* 2015;15:362.

Pfenninger JL, Fowler GC. *Procedures for Primary Care Physicians.* St. Louis, MO: Mosby; 2019.

Stevens DL, Bisno AL, Chambers HF, et al. Practice guidelines for the diagnosis and management of skin and soft tissue infections: 2014 update by the Infectious Diseases Society of America. *Clin Infect Dis.* 2014;59(2):e10–52.

5 Chapter

Bites
Ants, Arthropods (Spiders), Bees, and Wasps
Cynthia Ehrhardt

CPT Code
None—part of office visit.

Bites are puncture wounds and tears in the skin, with injection of a **proteolytic,** a venomous chemical, by an insect. Treatment of a bite depends on the type of offending organism, depth of the puncture, and extent of the tear in the skin.

OVERVIEW

- Incidence—In the southeastern United States, at least 60% of the population has been stung by these insects.
- **Hemolysis** and **cutaneous** infarct lead to necrosis of tissue at the site over a period of hours to days. Extent of the hemolysis and cutaneous infarct determines treatment regimen.
- Severe reactions present with symptoms such as
  - Generalized urticaria
  - Angioedema
  - Respiratory difficulty
  - Change in level of consciousness
- Clinical manifestations of insect bites (Table 5.1)
- Identification of type of spider (Table 5.2)
- Medications used with insect bites (Table 5.3)

HEALTH PROMOTION/PREVENTION

- Use natural organic and pesticide chemical controls.
- Observe for and avoid anthills.
- Avoid going barefoot in grassy areas.
- Thoroughly check all stored clothing for spiders.
- Before entering bed, inspect bedding for spiders.
- Avoid bright colors, perfumes, and scented products that can attract and agitate bees and wasps.

Table 5·1 Clinical Manifestations of Insect Bites

Fire Ant and Harvester Ant Bite

- Reactions of a mild to moderate nature will present as a localized response (urticaria wheal, localized induration, and erythema) and initially be painful, but decrease over time.
- Have small whitish pustule, central core with minimal erythema after the first 24 hours. After 48 hours, the white pustule remains but erythema subsides.

Brown Recluse and Black Widow

- Brown recluse bites
  - Painful
  - Blue cyanotic center surrounded by pallor and erythema
  - Necrotic ulcers within hours to days
- Black widow bites
  - Sharp stinging
  - Easy to overlook—white center with trace erythema
  - Necrotic ulcers within hours to days

Table 5·2 Identification of Type of Spider

Brown Recluse Spiders

- Rarely exceed 5 mm in size
- Fiddle shape on back—0.5 to 2 cm in length
- Hairy

Black Widow Spiders

- Black to dark brown with a characteristic "red hourglass" on the ventral surface of the body

Table 5·3 Overview of Medications Used With Insect Bites

Antibiotic Therapy

Topical or oral antibiotics have not been found to be effective with fire ant, spider, bee, or wasp bites unless evidence of secondary infection is present.

Antihistamines

May be of benefit in fire ant, bee, and wasp bites. Use of antihistamines such as diphenhydramine (Benadryl) appears to reduce localized reactions and pruritus. Use with brown recluse and black widow bites has not been of benefit.

Oral Steroids

Have been occasionally beneficial with brown recluse and black widow bites in reducing localized inflammation if greater than 2 cm in diameter. Use in lesions greater than 14 cm is recommended. Dosage: 1 mg/kg body weight. Oral dapsone 50 to 100 mg/day has been effective in reducing the incidence of **latrodectism** (abdominal rectus spasm) and hemolytic anemia resulting from black widow bites.

- Carry "bee-sting kit" if there is a known history of moderate-to-severe reaction to bee and wasp stings when out in known environmental habitat of these insects.

RATIONALE

- To prevent infection
- To diminish inflammation
- To diminish discomfort

INDICATIONS

- Bite by ant, spider, bee, or wasp

CONTRAINDICATIONS

- None

PROCEDURE

Bites

Equipment

- Basin—sterile
- Povidone-iodine (Betadine) soak or antibacterial soap
- Gloves—sterile
- Meat tenderizer paste—1 part water mixed with 1 part meat tenderizer
- Epinephrine 1:1,000 vial(s)
- 1-mL syringe (tuberculin) with needle
- Ice pack
- Magnifying lens—optional
- Adhesive bandage (Band-Aid) or dressing if indicated

Procedure

- Inspect area for puncture wound. (In early spider bites, it is possible to visualize the two-fang puncture bite.)
- Avoid warm compresses to the bite area. Heat causes vasodilation, allowing bite venom to be circulated more quickly.

BEE OR WASP STINGS

- If bite has occurred within 5 minutes, apply a paste of meat tenderizer (which is a proteolytic agent).

FIRE ANT AND SPIDER BITES

- Gently clean the bite area and soak in cool, soapy water for 10 to 15 minutes.
- Gently dry.
- No dressing is required unless it is an open, exudative, and gaping wound.
- Apply an ice pack for 12 to 24 hours.

Client Instructions

- Keep the wound clean and dry.
- Apply cool compresses to the bite for 12 to 24 hours to lessen localized inflammation.
- Antibiotics are not required.
- Observe for signs and symptoms of infection, such as
  - Increase in pain after 24 hours
  - Increase in temperature
  - Redness or swelling
  - Yellow or greenish drainage
  - Foul odor
- If any of the signs and symptoms of infection are found, return to the office.
- To relieve pain
  - Acetaminophen may be taken every 4 to 6 hours as needed for mild pain for first 24 hours.
  - Ibuprofen or other NSAIDs should be avoided for the first 24 hours to lessen bleeding.
  - After 24 hours, alternating NSAIDs with acetaminophen may be beneficial.
  - Tylenol No. 3 may be used for severe pain.
- Wound cleaning—The primary goal is to prevent secondary infection. Topical antibiotic ointment has not shown benefit or harm when applied to the bite.
  - Use hydrogen peroxide to remove any crusts.
  - Wash gently with soapy water and blot area dry.
  - Unless the wound is oozing, do not cover.
- Return to the office in 2 days for moderately severe brown recluse and black widow spider bites. If bite is mild, return to the office in 5 to 7 days.

BIBLIOGRAPHY

Habif T. *Clinical Dermatology: A Color Guide to Diagnosis and Therapy.* 6th ed. St. Louis, MO: Mosby; 2015.

Matzen R, Lang R. *Clinical Preventive Medicine.* St. Louis, MO: Mosby; 2004.

Miller T. Latrodectism. Bite of black widow spider. *Am Fam Physician.* 1992;45(1):45–56.

Murtagh J. *Practice Tips.* 5th ed. New York, NY: McGraw-Hill; 2011.

Pfenninger JL, Fowler GC. *Procedures for Primary Care Physicians.* St. Louis, MO: Mosby; 2019.

Ryan NM, Buckley NA, Graudins A. Treatments for latrodectism—a systemic review on their clinical effectiveness. *Toxin (Basel).* 2017;9(4):148.

6 Chapter

Bites
Cats, Dogs, and Humans

Margaret R. Colyar

CPT Code
12001–07 Simple repair of superficial wounds of scalp, neck, axillae, external genitalia, trunk, or extremities
12031–37 Layer closure of wounds of scalp, axillae, trunk, or extremities (not hands or feet)
12041–47 Layer closure of wounds of neck, hands, feet, or external genitalia

---

Bites include punctures, tearing wounds, crush injuries, or lacerations into the skin caused by the teeth of animals or humans. Children aged 5 to 14 years account for 30% to 50% of victims of all mammalian bites.

OVERVIEW
- Incidence—1% of all emergency department visits
  - Cat and dog bites—0.5 to 1 million per year
  - Human bites—incidence unknown
- Complicating factors
  - Cat and dog bites—Saliva contains gram-negative bacteria—*Pasteurella multocida.*
  - Human bites—Saliva contains 10 bacteria per milliliter, including the gram-positive bacteria *Staphylococcus aureus* (3% are resistant to antibiotics) and streptococci and the gram-negative bacteria *Proteus* species, *Escherichia coli, Pseudomonas* species, *Neisseria* species, and *Klebsiella* species.

HEALTH PROMOTION/PREVENTION
- Teach appropriate behavior around animals.
- Do *not* provoke attacks.

RATIONALE
- To prevent bacterial infection in the wound
- To promote wound healing

INDICATIONS
- Necrosis

CONTRAINDICATIONS

- Bite on the face, REFER to plastic surgeon or emergency department.
- Blood supply has been disrupted, REFER to emergency department.
▶ *Informed consent required*
  Determine the following.
- Origin of the bite
- Patient (If younger than 4 years old and older than 50 years, there is a greater risk of infection.)
- Severity
- Location
- Size
- Depth
- Amount of contamination (puncture wound has greatest risk of infection) and amount of time that has elapsed between the bite and treatment. Keep in mind that an area of poor vascularity is at greater risk for infection and poor healing. Do a culture and Gram stain of the wound.

PROCEDURE

Bites

Equipment

- Basin—sterile
- Povidone-iodine (Betadine) soak—povidone-iodine solution and 0.9% sterile sodium chloride mixed 50/50
- Gloves—sterile
- Syringe—20 to 60 mL
- Two needles—27 to 30 gauge and 18 to 20 gauge
- 1% lidocaine
- Scissors—sterile
- Curved hemostats—sterile
- Forceps—sterile
- Suture—No. 3-0 to 5-0 nylon
- 4 × 4 gauze—sterile
- Culture swab
- Topical antibiotic—Bactroban or Polysporin
- Iodoform gauze—¼ to ½ inch

Procedure

- Culture the wound if the bite is 72 hours old. If the client has an elevated temperature, get a complete blood count, erythrocyte sedimentation rate, and possibly blood cultures.
- If area of bite was on hands or feet, soak in povidone-iodine soak (50% povidone-iodine and 50% 0.9% sodium chloride) for 10 to 15 minutes. If unable to soak, irrigate with 250 to 500 mL of povidone-iodine/sodium chloride solution.

- Anesthetize wound with 1% lidocaine.
- Position the patient for comfort with the injured part easily accessible.
- Cleanse the skin with antiseptic skin cleanser.
- Irrigate the wound with 100 to 500 mL of sterile sodium chloride vigorously, using the syringe and 18-gauge needle.
- Put on gloves.
- Remove any devitalized tissue or foreign objects.
- Insert iodoform gauze snugly with a ½ inch protruding from the wound.
- Suture if the wound is clean and not a puncture.
- Apply topical antibiotic.
- Apply gauze dressing.

Client Instructions

- To prevent infection, abscess, cellulitis, septicemia, or osteomyelitis, take oral antibiotics (penicillin, amoxicillin/clavulanate [Augmentin], or erythromycin as prescribed) for 5 to 7 days.
- Observe for signs and symptoms of infection, such as
  - Increase in pain after 24 hours
  - Increase in temperature
  - Redness or swelling
  - Yellow or greenish drainage
  - Foul odor
- If any of these symptoms develop, return to the office immediately.
- To relieve pain
  - Take Tylenol No. 3 every 4 to 6 hours for 24 hours, then acetaminophen or ibuprofen every 4 to 6 hours for mild pain relief.
  - If fingers or toes are involved, exercise (wiggle) them frequently.
  - Elevate the wounded part above the heart for 48 hours or as long as possible.
  - Immobilize the wounded part for 48 hours.
  - Apply ice pack intermittently for the first 24 hours.
- Rabies—Consider rabies prophylaxis if the bite was from an animal.
- Tetanus—Tetanus prophylaxis (Tdap) is needed if not received within 10 years.
- Return to the office in 2 days for a recheck.

BIBLIOGRAPHY ■

Brandenberg MA, Hawkins L, Quick G. Hand injuries: Assessing the damage, closing the wound, preventing infection. *Consultant.* December 1995;1777–1786.

Ellis R, Ellis C. Dog and cat bites. *Am Fam Physician.* 2014;90(4):239–243.

Lewis KT, Stiles M. Management of cat and dog bites. *Am Fam Physician.* 1995;52(2):479–485.

Chapter **7**

Burns
Debridement
Cynthia R. Ehrhardt

CPT Code
16000 Initial treatment of first-degree burn when no more than local treatment is required
16010 Dressing and/or debridement, initial or subsequent, under anesthesia
16015 Dressing and/or major debridement, initial or subsequent, under anesthesia—medium or large area
16020 Dressing and/or debridement, without anesthesia, of a small area
16025 Dressing and/or debridement, without anesthesia, of a medium area (whole extremity)
16030 Dressing and/or debridement, without anesthesia, of a large area (more than one extremity)

A burn is trauma to skin from exposure to heat, flame, radiation, chemicals (acid or alkali), or other agent that results in a loss of skin integrity. Burns can be described in two ways:

- The extent of body surface area (BSA) involved (Fig. 7.1)
- The depth or amount of tissue destroyed (Table 7.1)

OVERVIEW

- Incidence
  - An estimated 2 million burns occur per year, with 25% of these requiring medical attention.
  - An estimated 100,000 burn patients require hospitalization, and 10,000 die of their burn injuries each year.
- Complications
  - Death
  - Temporary or permanent disfigurement
  - Temporary or permanent loss of function
  - Temporary or permanent disability
  - Psychosocial trauma
- Common causes are exposure to
  - Hot liquids
  - Steam
  - Flames

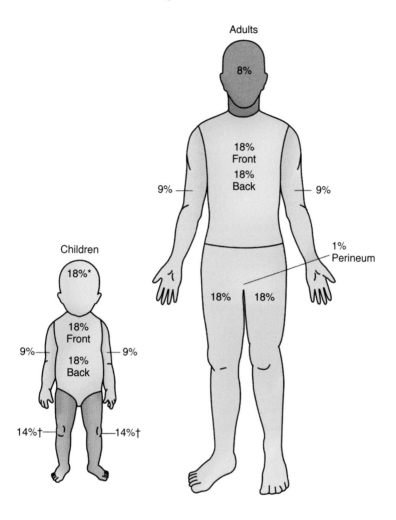

* Subtract 1% from head for each year over age one.
† Add 1/2% to each leg for each year over age one.

Figure 7.1 Rule of nines.

- Flash electricity
- Radiation, including sunlight
- Hot solid materials
- Caustic chemicals
- Explosions resulting from chemical mixtures
- Severe cold
- Burn assessment includes systemic and skin systems
  - Documentation of location and percentage of BSA involvement using rule of nines (Fig. 7.1)

Table 7·1	**Depth of Burn Injury**

- First degree
  - Superficial injection and redness of skin that blanches with pressure and has intact sensation
  - Varying depth of involvement of the epidermal and dermal layers of skin with intact dermal appendages such as hair and sweat and sebaceous glands
- Second degree
  - Superficial partial-thickness burn
    - Varying depth, but more involvement of dermal layer
    - Intact dermal appendages such as hair and sweat and sebaceous glands
    - Vascular dilation with accompanying blisters and bullae common
  - Deep partial-thickness burn
    - Some vasodilation of deep blood vessels
    - Wet or dry and red or waxy-appearing skin that has decreased sensation
    - Vasodilation of the blood vessels resulting in red, weepy, and painful skin that can be easily wiped away
    - Painful sensation with or without pressure to the tissue
- Third degree
  - Loss of all anatomical structures of skin
  - Thrombosis and coagulation of blood vessels with or without involvement of deeper anatomical structures of muscle, ligament, and bone
  - White and charred tissue with absence of blanching
  - Sensation intact only to deep pressure

- Observation for evidence of respiratory distress
  - Nasal flaring **intercostal** retractions
  - Dyspnea
  - Chest pain
  - Pale and/or **cyanotic**
  - Evaluation of cardiovascular status (blood pressure and pulse)

HEALTH PROMOTION/PREVENTION

Health promotion is focused on eliminating situations that can result in injury to the skin. These measures include

- Promotion of safety habits
- Use of protective clothing when working with agents that can traumatize skin
- Promotion of a safe environment

Prevention includes

- Avoiding sunburn by use of sunscreens, generally skin protection factor (SPF) 15 or greater

- Maintaining hot water heater temperature at lower than 120°F
- Keeping cooking pot handles pointed away from stove edge so that children cannot reach up and pull hot liquids onto themselves
- Keeping curling irons, clothes irons, and hair dryers out of reach of children
- Using stove guards, automatic coffeemakers, and fireproof portable heaters
- Using full-glove pot holders
- Temperature-testing all food
- Wearing gloves and goggles when mixing and using household chemicals
- Keeping all chemicals and caustic agents (e.g., batteries) stored in an elevated location and locked away from children
- Disposing of oily rags properly
- Storing flammables, including cigarette lighters and matches, properly and not smoking around flammable items or in bed
- Ensuring that protective equipment is selected, maintained, and used properly when working around chemical and/or caustic agents
- Using electrical outlet covers and ground-fault interrupter plugs to protect children from electrical shock
- Installing smoke detectors
- Having a planned fire evacuation route for home and work
- Having access to fire extinguishers and knowing how to use them
- Being cautious when using chemicals

OPTIONS

- First-degree burns—Treat in the office with
  - Analgesics
  - Antipyretics
  - Skin lubricants
- Second-degree burns—superficial—Treat in the office with
  - Thorough cleansing
  - Removal of blisters
  - Topical antibiotics
  - Observation for secondary infection
- Second-degree burns—deep partial thickness—REFER to emergency department of nearest hospital.
- Third-degree burns—Stabilize and transport patient to an emergency facility.

Emergency Treatment for Stabilization and Transportation

- If symptoms of hypovolemia are present, establish two IV lines using large-bore angiocaths (16 gauge preferred in adults and 18 gauge in children) with an IV solution of Ringer's lactate. Rate is based on the following formula: (2 to 4 mL of Ringer's lactate per kilogram of body weight) × (percentage of BSA burned) = the amount of fluid replacement in the first 24 hours (2 mL × 70 kg × 50 BSA = 7,000 mL); 50% of the solution should be given over the first 8 hours.
- Insert nasogastric tube and Foley catheter.

- Keep client warm.
- Apply sterile or clean sheets over the burned area.

Hospitalization is required based on burn center referral criteria.

- Second-degree to third-degree burns, more than 10% of BSA burned if the patient is younger than age 10 years or older than age 50
- Second-degree to third-degree burns with more than 20% of BSA damaged
- Second-degree to third-degree burns with a serious possibility of functional or cosmetic impairment (face, hands, feet, genitalia, perineum, major joints)
- Third-degree burns over greater than 5% of BSA
- Inhalation, electrical burns, and chemical burns that impair function or cause cosmetic damage

RATIONALE

- To minimize scarring and contractures
- To prevent infection
- To provide pain relief
- To decrease the extent of the burn
- To diminish the complications caused by the burn
- To promote optimal healing

INDICATIONS

- First-degree burns
- Second-degree superficial partial-thickness burns over less than 20% of BSA

CONTRAINDICATIONS

- Suspected deep second-degree or third-degree burn
- Suspected tendon, muscle, or bone involvement
- Meets criteria for hospitalization
  - Circumferential burns of the neck, trunk, arms, or legs
  - All but minimal burns of the eyes, ears, feet, perineum, genitalia, or hands
  - Presence of other trauma unless minor
  - Presence of any condition that may compromise wound healing, such as diabetes mellitus, cardiovascular disease, or immunodeficiency disorders
  - Wounds for which the estimated time for closure is greater than 3 weeks
  - Poor social situations, such as child abuse or poor compliance with wound care instructions
  - Younger than 2 years of age or extremely elderly (frail elderly)
  - Suspected inhalation exposure

PROCEDURE

Burn—Debridement

Equipment

- Towels or sheets—sterile
- Gloves—sterile
- 3-mL syringe

Table 7·2	**Topical Antimicrobials**	
NAME	**SPECTRUM**	**COST**
Silver sulfadiazine (Silvadene)	Good broad spectrum; covers *Staphylococcus*	Expensive
Furacin	Good broad bactericidal; covers *Pseudomonas* and Enterobacteriaceae	Expensive
Povidone-iodine (Betadine)	Superficial; can easily become skin irritant; cannot be mixed with silver sulfadiazine	Reasonable
Silver nitrate	Poor penetration; used primarily when sensitive to other therapy agents; prone to stain skin	Reasonable

- 25- or 27-gauge, ½-inch needle
- 30- to 60-mL irrigation syringe
- 1% or 2% lidocaine without epinephrine
- 0.09% sodium chloride—sterile
- 4 × 4 gauze—sterile
- Gauze wrap—sterile
- Tape
- Topical antimicrobial cream, ointment, or medicated gauze (Table 7.2)
- Sterile suture set (prepackaged or self-made) should include
  - Curved and straight hemostats
  - Needle holders (4½ and 6 inch)
  - Forceps with teeth
  - Scalpel (No. 11 or 15 blade)
  - Iris scissors
  - Cup to hold sterile sodium chloride solution

Procedure

- Put on gloves.
- Anesthetize the wound by local or digital block.
- Irrigate the wound sufficiently with 0.09% sodium chloride (usually 150 mL) to clean any cellular debris or residue.
- Blot the wound dry with sterile 4 × 4 gauze.
- Remove excess tissue, and drain any bullae or blisters present using iris scissors or scalpel blade.
- Apply liberal amount of antimicrobial ointment to the wound.
- Cover with 4 × 4 and dressing gauze wrap without restriction of range of motion or function.

Client Instructions

- Observe for signs of infection including
  - Increased redness and warmth at the site
  - Red streaks
  - Swelling with yellow or green drainage

- Keep the area as clean as possible.
- Topical antimicrobials, cream or ointment, usually are recommended for the first 7 days of treatment. Oral antibiotic therapy is required if secondary infection has occurred.
- Change the dressing twice a day for the first 7 days, then every 24 hours.
  - When redressing the wound, if the dressing adheres to the wound, saturate the dressing with 0.09% sodium chloride and remove.
- If an arm, leg, hand, or foot is involved
  - Keep elevated above the heart for 24 to 48 hours to reduce swelling
  - Perform range of motion exercises three to four times per day
- Pain medication
  - Avoid nonsteroidal drug usage because these drugs tend to retard healing.
  - Take Tylenol No. 3 every 4 hours as needed initially, then acetaminophen.
- The deeper the burn, the greater the risk of permanent skin color changes.
- Receive a tetanus injection if none has been given in the past 5 years.
- Avoid sunburn to the burned area for 6 months to 1 year because of increased risk of reinjury.
- Return to the office in 2 days for recheck, then weekly.

BIBLIOGRAPHY

Lloyd EC, Rodgers BC, Michener M, Williams MS. Outpatient burns: Prevention and care. *Am Fam Physician.* 2012; 85(1):25–32.

Pfenninger JL, Fowler GC. *Procedures for Primary Care Physicians.* St. Louis, MO: Mosby; 2019.

Trott A. *Wounds and Lacerations: Emergency Care and Closure.* St. Louis, MO: Mosby; 2012.

Chapter **8**

Digital Nerve Block

Margaret R. Colyar

CPT Code
01460   Anesthesia for all procedures on integumentary system of lower leg, ankle, and foot
01800   Anesthesia for all procedures on integumentary system of the forearm, wrist, and hand

Digital nerve blocks produce sensory anesthesia to selected toes and fingers before surgical repair, suture application, dislocation reduction, and nail procedures.

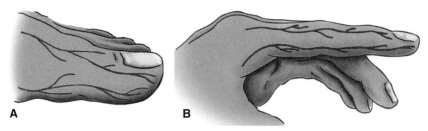

Figure 8.1 Neuroanatomy of the toe (A) and finger (B).

OVERVIEW

- Understanding of the neuroanatomy of the digit is necessary to perform the digital block correctly (Fig. 8.1).

RATIONALE

- To diminish pain during invasive procedures

INDICATIONS

- Nail removal
- Ingrown toenail procedures
- Felon
- **Paronychia**
- Sutures to fingers or toes
- Dislocation reduction
- Removal of foreign body from fingers or toes

CONTRAINDICATIONS

- None

▶ *Informed consent required*

PROCEDURE

Digital Nerve Block

Equipment

- Antiseptic skin cleanser
- Gloves—nonsterile
- 3-mL syringe
- 27- to 30-gauge, ½- to 1-inch needle
- 1% lidocaine—2 to 3 mL—*No* epinephrine should be used on digits.
- 4 × 4 gauze—sterile

Procedure

- Position the client supine with digit easily accessible.
- Cleanse the hand or foot with topical antiseptic skin cleanser.
- Put on gloves.

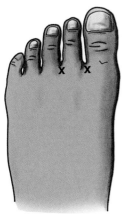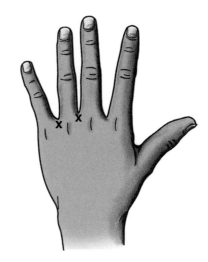

Figure 8.2 Injection sites.

FINGERS

- Insert needle at 45-degree angle.
  - Along the palmar crease on either side of the digit
  - On anterior surface of the digit close to the bone (Fig. 8.2)

TOES

- Insert the needle toward the plantar surface on both sides of the toe.
- Injection sites are below the nail on the outer edges of the toe. Be careful not to pierce the plantar skin surface.
- Do not forget to aspirate the syringe before injecting lidocaine. If no blood returns in the syringe, lidocaine can be injected safely.
- Inject 1 to 2 mL of lidocaine while withdrawing the needle. Do not withdraw the needle from the skin.
- Redirect the needle across the extensor surface, and insert the needle farther. Inject 0.5 mL of lidocaine while withdrawing needle.
  - Repeat procedure on opposite side of the toe.
  - Massage gently.
- Wait 5 to 10 minutes.

Client Instructions

- Sensation to the finger or toe should return within 1 to 2 hours. If this does not occur, call the practitioner's office.

BIBLIOGRAPHY

Brandenberg MA, Hawkins L, Quick G. Hand injuries: Assessing the damage, closing the wound, preventing infection. *Consultant.* December 1995;1777–1786.

Kroop K, Trott A, Syverud S. Comparison of digital versus metacarpal blocks for repair of finger injuries. *Ann Emerg Med.* 1994;23(6):1296–1300.

Okur OM, Sener A, Kavakli HS, et al. Two injection digital block versus single
subcutaneous palmar injection block for finger lacerations. *Eur J Trauma Emerg Surg.*
2017;42(6):863–868.

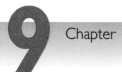

Chapter

Fishhook Removal

Margaret R. Colyar

CPT Code
10120   Incision and removal of foreign body, subcutaneous tissues;
        simple
10121   Incision and removal of foreign body, subcutaneous tissues;
        complicated

The removal of a fishhook from subcutaneous tissue can be accomplished using one
of three common methods or the angiocath method. The common methods include
(1) pull-through, (2) barb sheath, and (3) angler's string-yank.

OVERVIEW

- Incidence
  - Dependent on geographical location and season
  - Estimated at approximately 0.5 million to 1 million incidents per year
- Most common organisms found with secondary infection
  - Gram-positive: *Staphylococcus aureus,* streptococci
  - Gram-negative: *Klebsiella, Proteus, Pseudomonas* (salt water)

HEALTH PROMOTION/PREVENTION

- Use good fishing technique.
- Handle all fishhooks carefully.
- Store all fishhooks properly.
- Do not reach blindly into poorly lighted tackle boxes.
- Do not fish close to another person casting a line.

OPTIONS

To remove fishhook with minimal local trauma
- *Method 1*—Pull-through technique
  - Use with a single- or a multiple-barbed fishhook when the angle of
    penetration is such that the hook can be pushed through the skin.

- *Method 2*—Barb sheath method
  - Use with a single-barbed fishhook that is large but not too deep in the skin.
- *Method 3*—Angler's string-yank method
  - Use with a single-barbed fishhook that is embedded in such a way that it cannot be removed with the pull-through method.

RATIONALE

- To relieve pain and anxiety
- To diminish bacterial infection
- To promote healing

INDICATIONS

- Fishhook lodged in any subcutaneous tissue.
- Fishhook in or close to the eyes, REFER to a physician.
- Suspected ligament involvement, REFER to an orthopedic physician.
- Penetration into a large-bore artery, REFER to a surgeon.

▶ *Informed consent required*

PROCEDURE

Fishhook Removal

Equipment

- Methods 1, 2, and 3
  - Antiseptic skin cleanser
  - Gloves—nonsterile
  - 3-mL syringe
  - 27- to 30-gauge, ½-inch needle
  - 1% lidocaine
- Method 1 only
  - Wire cutter—from a hardware store
  - Pliers or **hemostats**—nonsterile
- Method 2 only
  - 18-gauge, 1½-inch needle
- Method 3 only
  - Silk suture or 2 to 3 feet of strong string or fishing line

Procedure

METHOD 1—PULL-THROUGH TECHNIQUE

- Position the client with fishhook easily accessible.
- Put on gloves.
- Cleanse skin around the fishhook with antiseptic.
- Inject 1% lidocaine using the 27- to 30-gauge needle at the point of the hook.
- Force the fishhook tip through the skin using pliers or hemostats.
- Cut off the eye of the fishhook close to the skin with wire cutters.
- Attach pliers or hemostats to the sharp end of the hook and pull the hook out (Fig. 9.1).

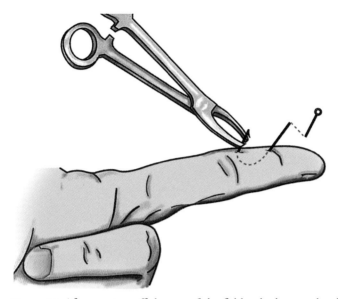

Figure 9.1 After cutting off the eye of the fishhook close to the skin, attach pliers or hemostats to the sharp end of the hook and pull the hook out.

METHOD 2—BARB SHEATH METHOD
- Position the client with fishhook easily accessible.
- Put on gloves.
- Cleanse the skin around the fishhook with antiseptic skin cleanser.
- Inject 1% lidocaine using the 27- to 30-gauge needle at the point of the hook.
- Insert the 18-gauge needle parallel to the hook with bevel toward the inside curve of the hook (Fig. 9.2). Attempt to cover the barb with the bevel of the needle.
- Back the hook and needle out as a unit.

METHOD 3—ANGLER'S STRING-YANK METHOD
- Position the client with fishhook easily accessible.
- Put on gloves.
- Cleanse the skin around the fishhook with antiseptic skin cleanser.
- Inject 1% lidocaine using the 27- to 30-gauge needle at the point of the hook.
- Tie the string or suture around the hook where it enters the skin.
- Push the hook farther into the skin with your finger, then lift the shank of the hook parallel to the skin (Fig. 9.3). The barb should be disengaged.
- Jerk the hook out quickly using the string or suture.

Client Instructions
- Tetanus prophylaxis is necessary if last tetanus injection was more than 5 years before the current incident.

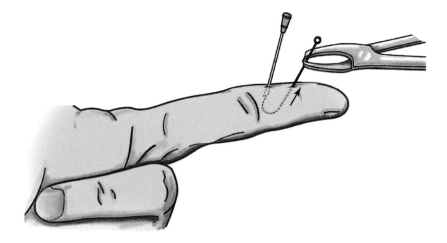

Figure 9.2 Cover the sharp end of the hook with an 18-gauge needle. Back the hook and needle out as a unit.

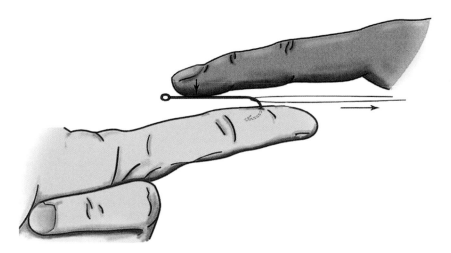

Figure 9.3 Push the fishhook downward with your finger. Using string or suture, quickly jerk the hook out.

- Observe for signs and symptoms of infection, such as
  - Increase in pain after 24 hours
  - Redness or swelling
  - Yellow or greenish drainage
  - Foul odor
- If any signs and symptoms of infection are found, return to the office.
- Take antibiotics as ordered for 5 days—cephalexin 500 mg three times per day or cefadroxil 500 mg twice per day—if infection is probable.

- Use pain medications as ordered. Take acetaminophen or ibuprofen every 4 to 6 hours as needed.
- Soak the affected part three times per day in warm salt water (1 teaspoon salt per 1 quart of water) for 2 days.
- Return to the office for a follow-up visit in 48 hours, then as needed.

BIBLIOGRAPHY

Brandenberg MA, Hawkins L, Quick GG. Hand injuries: Assessing the damage, closing the wound, preventing infection. *Consultant.* December 1995:1777–1786.
Pfenninger JL, Fowler GC. *Procedures for Primary Care Physicians.* St. Louis, MO: Mosby; 2019.
Stone DB, Scordino DJ. Foreign body removal. In: *Roberts and Hedges' Clinical Procedures in Emergency Medicine.* 6th ed. Philadelphia, PA: Elsevier Saunders; 2014.
Terrill P. Fishhook removal. *Am Fam Physician.* 1993;47(6):1372.

10 Chapter

Nail Removal

Margaret R. Colyar

CPT Code
11730–32	Nail removal, partial or complete
11750	Permanent nail removal, partial or complete
	No code for cotton wick insertion—Use 11730–32 if part of the nail was removed.

An ingrown toenail or onychocryptosis occurs when the nail edge grows into the soft tissues, causing inflammation, erythema, pain, and, possibly, abscess formation (Fig. 10.1). Many times there is an offending nail **spicule** (small needle-shaped body) that must be removed.

OVERVIEW

Causes

- Curved nails
- Congenital malformation of the great toenail, an autosomal dominant trait
- Nails cut too short
- Nail trimmed with round edges
- Poorly fitting or too-tight shoes
- High-heeled shoes
- Accumulation of debris under nail
- Poorly ventilated shoes
- Chronically wet feet

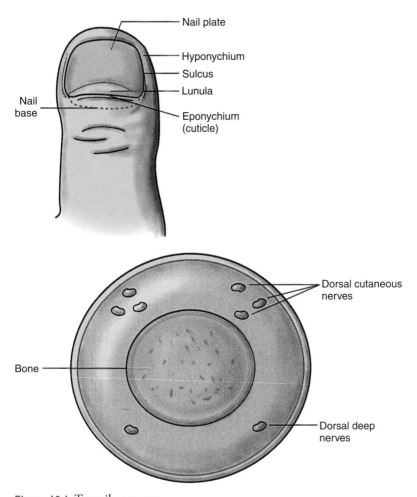

Figure 10.1 Toenail anatomy.

HEALTH PROMOTION/PREVENTION

- Cut nails straight across.
- Notch center of nail with a V.
- Wear absorbent socks.
- Wear shoes that allow proper ventilation.
- Wear shoes that fit properly.
- Avoid high-heeled shoes.
- Use good foot hygiene.

OPTIONS

- *Method 1*—Cotton wick insertion
  - A noninvasive technique to be used as the initial treatment. Six treatments may be required.

- *Method 2*—Partial avulsion with phenolization
  - For lesions lasting more than 2 months with significant infection and development of granulomatous tissue

RATIONALE

- To diminish pain
- To prevent or relieve abscess formation
- To promote healing
- To prevent toenail regrowth

INDICATIONS

- Ingrown toenail without complicating medical history (onychocryptosis)
- Chronic, recurrent inflammation of the nail fold **(paronychia)**

CONTRAINDICATIONS

- Diabetes mellitus
- Peripheral vascular disease
- Peripheral neuropathy
- Anticoagulant therapy
- Bleeding abnormalities
- Immunocompromised state
- Pregnancy because of need to use phenol
- Allergy to local anesthetics

PROCEDURE

Nail Removal

Equipment

- Method 1 only
  - Antiseptic skin cleanser
  - Nail file or emery board
  - Cotton: 3-mm (⅛-inch) thick by 2.5-cm (1-inch) long
  - Gloves—nonsterile
  - Splinter forceps—sterile
  - Tincture of iodine
  - Silver nitrate stick
  - 4 × 4 gauze—sterile
  - Tape
- Method 2 only—Digital nerve block
  - 5-mL syringe
  - 25- to 27-gauge, ½- to 1-inch needle
  - 1% lidocaine without epinephrine
- Method 2—Avulsion
  - Tourniquet
  - Gloves—sterile
  - Drape—sterile

- **Hemostat**—sterile
- Surgical scissors—sterile
- Small straight hemostat—sterile
- Cotton swabs—sterile
- Silver nitrate stick
- 80% or 88% phenol
- Alcohol swabs
- Alcohol
- Antibiotic ointment (Bactroban, Bacitracin, or Polysporin)
- Nonadherent dressing—Telfa or Adaptic
- Bandage roll (tube gauze)

Procedure

METHOD 1—COTTON WICK INSERTION

- Have the client lie supine with knees flexed and feet flat.
- Cleanse affected toe with antiseptic cleanser.
- File middle third of nail on the affected side with a nail file or emery board as illustrated (Fig. 10.2).
- Roll cotton to form a wick.
- Gently push the cotton wick under the distal portion of the lateral nail groove on the affected side using splinter forceps (Fig. 10.3).
- Identify the offending spicule and remove it.
- Continue to insert cotton wick to separate the nail from the nail groove (1 cm of cotton wick should remain free).
- Apply tincture of iodine to the cotton wick.
- Cauterize granulomatous tissue with silver nitrate stick.
- Bandage the toe.

Client Instructions

- Change bandage daily, and apply tincture of iodine every other day.
- Return to the office weekly for cotton wick replacement.

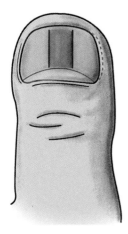

Figure 10.2 File the middle third of the nail.

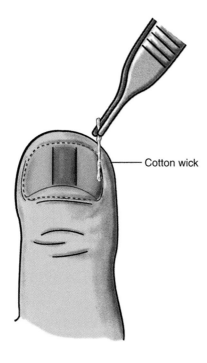

Cotton wick

Figure 10.3 Gently push a cotton wick under the lateral nail groove.

METHOD 2—PARTIAL AVULSION WITH PHENOLIZATION

▶ *Informed consent required*

- Have the client lie supine with knees flexed and feet flat.
- For digital nerve block, prepare 3 to 5 mL of lidocaine without epinephrine to anesthetize the affected area.
- To anesthetize the nerves innervating the proximal phalanx on the extensor surface, insert the needle toward the plantar surface on the affected side.
- Injection sites are below the nail on the outer edges of the toe (Fig. 10.4). Be careful not to pierce the plantar skin surface.
- Inject 1 to 2 mL of lidocaine while withdrawing the needle. Do not withdraw the needle from the skin.
- Redirect the needle across the extensor surface, and insert the needle farther. Inject 1 mL of lidocaine while withdrawing the needle.
- Repeat procedure on opposite side of the digit.
- Allow 5 minutes for lidocaine to take effect before beginning procedure.
- Scrub the toe with antiseptic, rinse, dry, and drape with sterile drapes.
- Place the tourniquet around the base of the toe. Perform procedure in 15 minutes or less to avoid ischemia.
- Insert a single blade of a small hemostat between the nailbed and the toe to open a tract (Fig. 10.5). Remove hemostat.
- Place the blade of the scissors in the tract, and cut the nail plate from distal edge to the proximal nail base (Fig. 10.6).
- Remove the nail with a small hemostat, using gentle rotation toward the affected nail (Fig. 10.7).

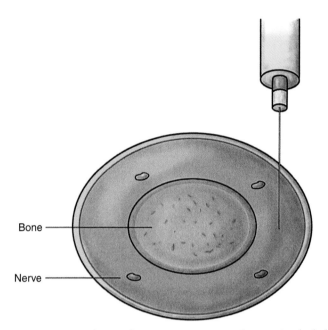

Bone

Nerve

Figure 10.4 Anesthetize the nerve innervating the proximal phalanx. Inject the toe on the outer edges just below the nail.

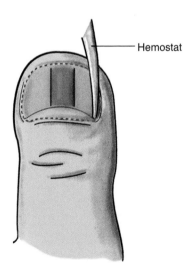

Hemostat

Figure 10.5 Insert a single blade of a hemostat between the nailbed and the toe to open a tract.

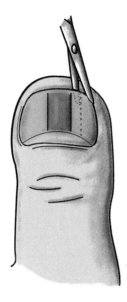

Figure 10.6 Cut the nail plate from distal edge to proximal nail base.

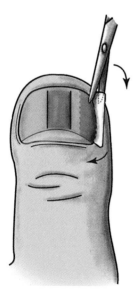

Figure 10.7 Remove the nail using gentle outward rotation toward the affected nail.

- Using a hemostat, inspect the nail groove for spicules.
- Dry the newly exposed nailbed.
- Rub cotton swab saturated with phenol on germinal matrix beneath the cuticle for 2 minutes.
- Cauterize granulomas with silver nitrate stick.
- Remove tourniquet and elevate foot for 15 minutes.
- Place a dressing in the toe.

Client Instructions

- Avoid ischemia of toe by loosening the bandage and hanging foot down.
- Notify the practitioner if pain or swelling increases or green or yellow discharge is present.
- If toes become cold and pale
  - Elevate foot above heart level.
  - Flex the toes.
  - Check circulation by pressing on the toe and watching for return of redness when pressure is released.
  - Call the practitioner if symptoms do not subside within 2 hours.
- Use pain medications as ordered. Take Tylenol No. 3 every 4 to 6 hours for the first 24 hours; then take an NSAID such as ibuprofen.
- Take ordered antibiotics for 5 days (cephalexin, tetracycline, trimethoprim-sulfamethoxazole, amoxicillin).
- Return to the office for follow-up visit in 2 days.

BIBLIOGRAPHY

Heidelbaugh JJ, Lee H. Management of the ingrown toenail. *Am Fam Physician.* 2009;79(4):303–308.

Park DH, Singh D. The management of ingrowing toenails. *BMJ*, 2012; 344:e2089.

Pfenninger JL, Fowler GC. *Procedures for Primary Care Physicians*. St. Louis, MO: Mosby; 2019.

Zuber TJ. Ingrown toenail removal. *Am Fam Physician.* 2002;65(12):2547–2550.

Chapter

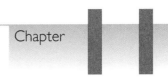

Ring Removal

Cynthia R. Ehrhardt

CPT Code
20670 Superficial removal of constricting metal band
20680 Deep removal of constricting metal band

Occasionally, a ring must be removed from a digit. Whenever possible, a nondestructive method is preferred. Only when conservative methods have been exhausted should a ring cutter be used.

OVERVIEW

- Complicating factors
  - Swelling or **edema** to the digit
  - Increased pain and sensitivity to area
  - Embedding of metal filings into digit

General Principles

- Minimize the amount of pain.
- Smooth technique minimizes further trauma to area.
- Anesthesia may be necessary with severe pain.
- If skin integrity is compromised, treat as a puncture wound.
- Verify no ligamentous involvement.
- After ring is removed, reevaluate vascular and motor functions.

HEALTH PROMOTION/PREVENTION

- Removal on a regular basis allows the wearer to be aware of ring size changes.
- Routinely remove the ring from the digit when working with hands.
- When trauma has occurred and the ring does not appear embedded, attempt to remove the ring immediately.
- If swelling has occurred, do not attempt removal without proper equipment.

OPTIONS

- *Method 1*—Lubricant removal method
  - Used if
    - No skin breakdown
    - Minimal edema to digit
    - No history of peripheral vascular disease
- *Method 2*—String-wrap method without tape anchor
  - Used if
    - No skin breakdown
    - Minimal edema to digit
    - No suspected fracture or ligament damage
- *Method 3*—Circular-blade ring cutter method
  - Used if
    - Suspected fracture or ligament injury
    - Ring embedded in the digit
    - Moderate-to-severe edema
    - Preservation of the ring not necessary

RATIONALE

- To prevent circulatory and nerve impairment to the digit

INDICATIONS

- Voluntary request for removal of the constricting ring
- Involuntary removal required because of circulatory compromise

CONTRAINDICATIONS

- Lack of patient cooperation.
- Suspected open or closed fracture of the digit, REFER to orthopedic surgeon.
- Deep laceration with potential ligament involvement, REFER to orthopedic surgeon.
- Deeply embedded ring, REFER to orthopedic hand surgeon.

PROCEDURE

Ring Removal

Equipment

- Method 1 only
  - Liquid dishwashing soap or lubricant jelly
  - Windex—optional
  - Gloves—nonsterile
- Methods 2 and 3
  - Paper clips
  - Tape
  - Dental floss or 4–0 silk suture material
  - 1% lidocaine (no epinephrine)
  - 3-mL syringe
  - 27-gauge, ½-inch needle
  - Needle-nose forceps or Kelly clamps—nonsterile
  - Topical antibiotic (Bactroban, Bacitracin, or Polysporin)
  - Elastic bandages (Band-Aids) or suitable dressing material
  - Gloves—nonsterile
- Method 3 only
  - Antiseptic skin cleanser
  - 0.9% sodium chloride
  - 20- to 30-mL syringe
  - Circular-blade ring cutter
  - Cool water

Procedure

METHOD 1—LUBRICANT REMOVAL METHOD

- Position the client comfortably.
- Soak affected digit in cool water for approximately 5 minutes with extremity elevated above the heart to decrease swelling.
- Apply a liberal coating of dishwashing liquid or lubricant jelly over the affected digit. If this fails, try spraying ring and finger with Windex.
- Rotate ring until ring slides off.

METHOD 2—STRING-WRAP METHOD WITHOUT TAPE ANCHOR

- Position the patient comfortably.
- If the patient is in moderate pain, consider anesthesia with lidocaine to the affected digit.

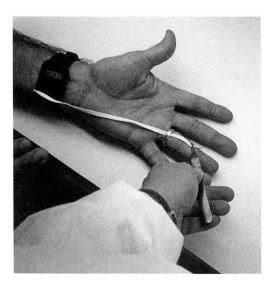

Figure 11.1 Method 2—String wrap method.

- Advance the ring to the narrowest part of the digit.
- Insert the thread (dental floss or 4–0 suture) under the ring using one of the following methods:
  - *Straight thread technique*—Using forceps, slide the thread under the ring and pull through (Fig. 11.1).
  - *Paper-clip technique*—Bend paper clip to an approximately 45-degree angle.
- Insert the threaded paper clip between ring and digit; gently pull through with fingers or forceps and remove the paper clip (Fig. 11.2A).
- Apply a liberal coat of lubricant to distal part of digit.
- Wind thread with some tension around finger, beginning close to ring and continuing distally until six or eight single-layer wraps have been made (Fig. 11.2B).
- Holding distal part of thread firmly, begin pulling proximal end parallel to digit, causing the thread to unwind and removing the ring successfully (Fig. 11.2C).

Method 3—Circular-Blade Ring Cutter Method
- Position the client comfortably, palm up.
- If the client is in moderate pain, consider the use of digital block anesthesia with lidocaine.
- If possible, advance the ring to the narrowest part of the digit.
- Cleanse the area with antiseptic skin cleanser.
- Slip the small hook guide of the ring cutter.
- Position the ring cutter beneath the ring.
- When it is positioned, grip the saw handle and begin to apply a squeezing pressure to the ring while turning the circular blade until the cut is complete (Fig. 11.3).

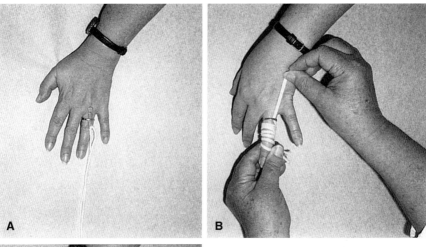

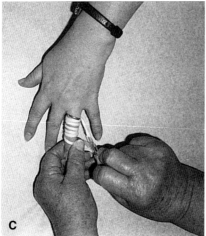

Figure 11.2 Method 2. (A) Insert the threaded paper clip between the finger and the ring. (B) Wind the thread around the finger. (C) Pull the proximal end of the thread parallel to the digit.

- Release pressure, and remove the circular saw.
- Use needle-nose forceps or Kelly clamps to pull ring apart and remove ring.
- Use large syringe and flush area vigorously with 50 to 100 mL of 0.9% sodium chloride to remove any metal filings.
- Apply dressing as needed.

Client Instructions

- Observe for signs and symptoms of infection, such as
  - Increase in pain after 24 hours
  - Increase in temperature
  - Redness or swelling
  - Yellow or greenish drainage
  - Foul odor

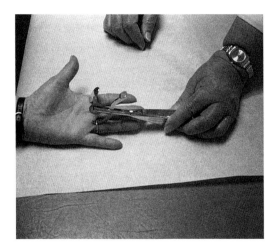

Figure 11.3 Method 3—Circular-blade ring cutter method.

- If any signs and symptoms of infection are found, return to the office.
- *Superficial skin abrasions*—Cleanse the abrasions with soapy water three times a day. Optional use of topical triple antibiotic (if no allergy).
- *To prevent infection*—Take oral antibiotics as prescribed for 7 to 10 days (cephalexin).
- *Pain and swelling*—Cool compresses to area for 5 to 10 minutes per hour for the first 24 hours. After 24 hours, apply heat for 5 to 10 minutes four to six times per day for 2 to 3 days.
  - Tylenol No. 3 one or two tablets every 4 to 6 hours for 24 hours for severe pain; then use plain or extra-strength acetaminophen.
- *Tetanus*—Tetanus prophylaxis is needed if skin is broken and the patient has not had a booster in the past 5 years.
- Return to the office in 48 hours for recheck if there was a break in the skin, difficult removal, or moderate amount of edema to the finger; then return as needed.

BIBLIOGRAPHY

Huss CD. Removing a ring from a swollen finger. In: Driscoll CE, Rakel RE, eds. *Patient Care: Procedures for Your Practice*. Oradell, NJ: Medical Economics; 1988.

Kates SL. A novel method of ring removal from the aging finger. *Geriatr Orthop Surg Rehabil*. 2010;1(2):78–79.

Murtagh J. *Practice Tips*. 5th ed. New York, NY: McGraw-Hill; 2017.

Pfenninger JL, Fowler GC. *Procedures for Primary Care Physicians*. St. Louis, MO: Mosby; 2019.

Chapter

12

Sebaceous Cyst Removal

Margaret R. Colyar

CPT Code

11400	Excision, benign lesion except skin tag, trunk, arms, or legs; lesion diameter 0.5 cm or less
11401–06	Differing lesion diameters
11420	Excision, benign lesion except skin tag, scalp, neck, hands, feet, genitalia; lesion diameter 0.5 cm or less
11421–26	Differing lesion diameters

A **sebaceous cyst** is not really an abscess by definition. A sebaceous cyst is a small, mobile, superficial sac containing sebum or keratin. Sebaceous cysts are found frequently on the scalp, back, neck, or face. Other names commonly used to describe a sebaceous cyst are *wen* and *epidermal cyst.*

OVERVIEW

* Areas of most frequent occurrence
  * Hair follicles
  * Back

OPTIONS

* *Method 1*
  * Used when the cyst sac is identified and pulled easily through the incision
* *Method 2*
  * Used when the cyst sac is not identified or pulled easily through the incision

RATIONALE

* To diminish pain
* To remove unsightly masses
* To prevent secondary infection

INDICATIONS

* Cosmetic
* Recurrent infection

CONTRAINDICATIONS

* Cyst is on the face.
* Client has bleeding disorder.

- Proceed cautiously with clients who are diabetic or immunocompromised.
- Cyst is currently infected.

▶ *Informed consent required*

PROCEDURE

Sebaceous Cyst Removal

Equipment

- Methods 1 and 2
  - Antiseptic skin cleanser
  - Gloves—sterile
  - Drape—sterile
  - 1% to 2% lidocaine
  - 2 syringes—3 and 10 mL
  - 27- to 30-gauge, ½-inch needle—for anesthesia
  - 18-gauge, 1½-inch needle—for irrigation
  - No. 11 scalpel
  - Curved hemostats—sterile
  - 0.9% sodium chloride—sterile
  - **Iodoform gauze** ¼- to ½-inch
  - Container with 10% **formalin**
  - 4 × 4 gauze—sterile
  - Scissors—sterile
  - Tape

Procedure

METHOD 1—SEBACEOUS CYST REMOVAL

- Position the client with the cyst easily accessible.
- Cleanse the area and 3 inches surrounding with antiseptic skin cleanser.
- Drape the cyst with the sterile drape.
- Put on gloves.
- Perform a **field block** by anesthetizing the perimeter around the abscess with 1% or 2% lidocaine without epinephrine. Do not inject lidocaine into the abscess because it does not work well in an acidic medium.
- Using the no. 11 scalpel, incise the cyst lengthwise to allow easy extraction of the cyst material and sac.
- With curved **hemostats**, pull sac out onto the surface of the skin (Fig. 12.1).
- Using the no. 11 scalpel, cut the elastic tissue around the outer edges of the sac until released.
- Irrigate with 0.9% sodium chloride.
- Close wound with sutures.
- Apply a pressure dressing.

METHOD 2—SEBACEOUS CYST REMOVAL

- Position the client with the cyst easily accessible.
- Cleanse the area and 3 inches surrounding with antiseptic skin cleanser.

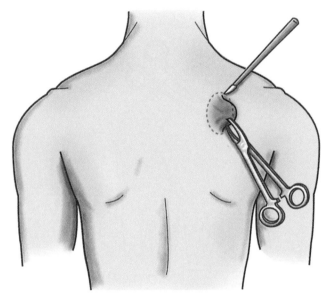

Figure 12.1 Cut the elastic tissue around the outer edges of the sac until released.

- Drape the cyst with the sterile drape.
- Put on gloves.
- Perform a field block by anesthetizing the perimeter around the abscess with 1% or 2% lidocaine without epinephrine. Do not inject lidocaine into the abscess because it does not work well in an acidic medium.
- Using the no. 11 scalpel, incise the cyst lengthwise to allow easy extraction of the cyst material and sac.
- Express cyst contents and put into a jar containing 10% formalin, then send to the pathology laboratory.
- Explore the cavity with curved hemostats (Fig. 12.2).
- Break down any sacs or septa using curved hemostats.
- After expressing all purulent material, pack the wound with iodoform gauze, leaving a small amount protruding from the wound. Advance the iodoform gauze daily for approximately 10 to 14 days until all is removed (Fig. 12.3).
- Cover with 4 × 4 gauze and tape. If the cyst is on the head, do not pack with iodoform gauze. Instead, roll 4 × 4 gauze into a gauze roll. Suture incision in two places, leaving room for drainage (Fig. 12.4). Leave ends of sutures 2 to 3 inches long. Place gauze roll on top of the incision, and tie tightly in place with the ends of the suture to form a pressure dressing. Remove the gauze roll in 7 days.

Client Instructions

- Observe for signs and symptoms of infection, such as
  - Increase in pain after 24 hours
  - Increase in temperature

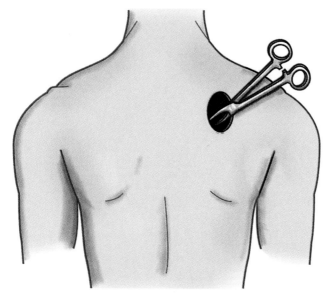

Figure 12.2 After expressing the contents of the cyst, explore the cavity with hemostats.

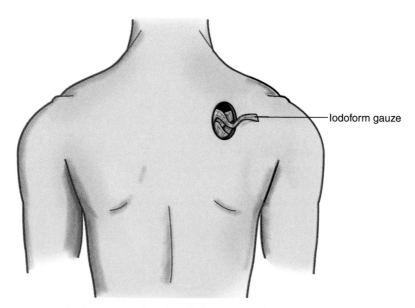

Figure 12.3 Pack the wound with iodoform gauze, leaving a small amount protruding from the wound.

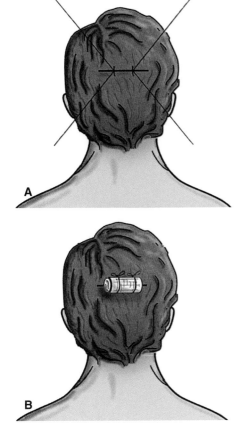

Figure 12.4 Head wounds. (A) Suture the incision in two places, leaving the ends of the suture long. (B) Place a gauze roll on top of the incision and tie tightly in place with the long ends of the suture.

- Redness or swelling
- Yellow or greenish drainage
- Foul odor
- If any signs and symptoms of infection are found, return to the office.
- *Pain and swelling*—Apply cool compresses to the area for 5 to 10 minutes per hour for the first 24 hours. After 24 hours, apply heat for 5 to 10 minutes four to six times per day for 2 to 3 days.
- Take Tylenol No. 3 one or two tablets every 4 to 6 hours for 24 hours for severe pain, then use plain or extra-strength acetaminophen.
- Return to the office in 48 hours for recheck.

BIBLIOGRAPHY

Pfenninger JL, Fowler GC. *Procedures for Primary Care Physicians.* St. Louis, MO: Mosby; 2019.

Zuber TJ. Minimal excision technique for epidermoid (sebaceous) cysts. *Am Fam Physician.* 2002;65(7):1409–1412.

13 Chapter

Skin Closure
Dermabond Application

Cynthia R. Ehrhardt

CPT Code
12001–07 Simple repair of wounds

Skin closure using **Dermabond** (tissue adhesive) in combination with Steri-Strips is less invasive than, has a shorter time of application than, and results in outcomes similar to suturing for smaller lacerations that do not have jagged edges and approximate well. Only about one-third of wounds meet criteria for tissue adhesive closure.

OVERVIEW

• Complicating factors of secondary infection similar to suturing

General Principles

• More efficient and less invasive method of wound repair
• Generally does not require anesthesia
• Lower incidence of irritation than with traditional suturing
• Equal to or better than cosmetic response with traditional suturing
• Within 2.5 minutes, bonding strength equivalent to 7 days of tissue healing by traditional suture closure
• Torso and extremity applications do better with subcutaneous suturing before application.
• High-tension locations and joints require splinting.

INDICATIONS

• Tissue adhesives such as Dermabond should be considered in place of 5–0 or smaller diameter sutures.
• Small wound repair
• Facial wounds

CONTRAINDICATIONS

• Adhesive sensitivity
• Jagged or irregular lacerations
• Mucosa or moist surface
• Contaminated wounds

- Bites or punctured wounds
- Highly movable sites of hands and feet that cannot be splinted
- Crushed wounds
- Axillae and perineum areas
- Evidence of or potential for purulent exudate from the wound
- Wound greater than 5 cm

PROCEDURE

Skin Closure—Dermabond Application

Equipment

- Dermabond
- Povidone-iodine
- Alcohol prep pads
- Petroleum jelly
- Gloves—nonsterile
- Optional—topical anesthetic
- Optional—Steri-Strips

Procedure

- Assess the wound and irrigate with saline as needed.
- Apply povidone-iodine to the wound beginning at the wound edges and expanding out in a circular pattern.
  - Allow to dry.
  - Remove with alcohol prep pad before application of Dermabond.
  - Put on gloves.
- If needed, apply topical anesthetic.
- Oppose the wound edges with good approximation.
- Crush the Dermabond vial and invert. You have only a few minutes to use this vial before polymerization results in sealing of the applicator orifice. Excessive pressure to the vial results in dripping.
- When the adhesive is at the tip of the applicator, apply to the approximated wound edges with a gentle brushing motion to the edges. This method of application avoids tissue adhesive oozing into the wound.
- Hold wound edges in place for 30 seconds.
- If edges are not approximated, you have 10 seconds to make any corrections before the wound is "glued." If an error is made, wipe as much of the adhesive off and apply liberal petroleum jelly to the exterior site for 30 minutes to neutralize the adhesive.
- Apply a total of three layers of adhesive. The layer must be dry before the next can be applied. Blowing on or fanning the area does not accelerate drying time.
- *Optional*—Steri-Strips may be applied only if over high-tension areas.

Client Instructions

- No bandage is required for adults. In active children, a bandage may be used to prevent the child from picking at the wound.

- You may shower within 6 hours after the application.
  - Avoid prolonged water exposure.
  - Dry area immediately after showering.
- Do not use topical antibiotics. They weaken the glue.
- Adhesive spontaneously peels in 5 to 10 days.
- Observe for signs and symptoms of infection, such as
  - Increase in pain after 24 hours
  - Increase in temperature
  - Redness or swelling
  - Yellow or greenish drainage
  - Foul odor
- If any signs and symptoms of infection are found, return to the office.
- Return to the office in 48 hours for wound recheck.

BIBLIOGRAPHY

Bruns T, Worthington J. Using tissue adhesive for wound repair: A practical guide to Dermabond. *Am Fam Physician.* 2000;61(5):1382–1388.
Forsch RT. Essentials of skin laceration repair. *Am Fam Physician.* 2008;78(8):945–951.
King M, Kinney A. Tissue adhesives: a new method of wound repair. *Nurse Pract.* 1999;24(10):66, 69–70, 73–74.
Knott PD, Zins JE, Banbury J, Djohan R, Yetman RJ, Papay F. A comparison of Dermabond tissue adhesive and sutures in the primary repair of the congenital cleft lip. *Ann Plast Surg.* 2007;58(2):121–125.

Chapter **14**

Skin Lesion Removal
Cautery and Cryosurgery
Margaret R. Colyar

CPT Code

17000	Destruction, any method, including laser, with or without surgical curettement, all benign lesions/premalignant lesions any location or benign lesions other than cutaneous vascular proliferative lesions, including local anesthesia; one lesion.
17003	Multiple lesions
17110	Destruction, any method, flat warts or molluscum contagiosum, milia; up to 14
17260	Destruction, malignant lesion, any method, trunk, arms, or legs; lesion diameter 0.5 cm or less
17261–66	Differing lesion diameters
17270	Destruction, malignant lesion, any method, scalp, neck, hands, feet, genitalia; 0.5 cm or less
17271–76	Differing lesion diameters

Two methods of removing skin lesions are **cautery** and **cryosurgery**. Another method, minor surgery (elliptical excision biopsy), is discussed in Chapter 2. Cautery is the destruction of tissue by the use of electricity, freezing, heat, or corrosive materials. Thermocautery is the process of tissue removal or destruction by the use of red-hot or white-hot heat.

Cryosurgery is a technique of exposing tissues to extreme cold to produce cell injury and destruction. This technique is safe and easy. Lesions heal with minimal or no scarring. No injections of local anesthetics or sutures are involved. Cryosurgery feels like an ice cube stuck to the skin. Temperatures that destroy tissues

- −10°C to −20°C
- Temperatures to −50°C ensures malignant cells are completely destroyed.

OVERVIEW

- Freeze time guidelines for cryosurgery are recommended for different types of lesions (Table 14.1).

Table 14·1	**FreezeTime Guidelines for Skin Lesions**
TYPE OF SKIN LESION	**FREEZE TIME, SEC**
Full thickness (benign)	60–90
Plantar warts (after debridement)	30–40
Condylomata	45
Verrucae	60–90
Seborrheic keratoses (2 mm)	30
Actinic keratoses (2 mm)	90

OPTIONS

- *Method 1*—Cautery
- *Method 2*—Cryosurgery
  - Superficial lesions—seborrheic keratoses
    - Freeze for 30 to 40 seconds or until a 2- to 3-mm ice ball forms beyond the lesion.
    - −89°C
  - Benign or premalignant lesions—actinic keratoses
    - Freeze 1 to 1.5 minutes or until a greater than 3-mm ice ball forms beyond the lesion (freeze, thaw, refreeze).
    - −89°C
  - Malignant lesions—basal cell carcinoma
    - Freeze for 1.5 minutes or until a greater than 5- to 8-mm ice ball forms beyond the lesion (freeze, thaw, refreeze).
    - Activate rapid thaw.
  - Large or irregular lesions
    - Same as malignant lesions except
      - Start on one side and progress to the opposite side.
      - Refreeze overlapping first freeze zone by 50% (Fig. 14.1).
  - Keloids or hypertrophic scars
    - See Chapter 15.

RATIONALE

- To remove lesions for cosmetic reasons
- To remove cancerous lesions
- To prevent further tissue destruction caused by spread of malignant lesions

INDICATIONS

- Skin tags
- Basal cell carcinoma
- **Condyloma acuminatum**
- Actinic keratoses
- Seborrheic keratoses

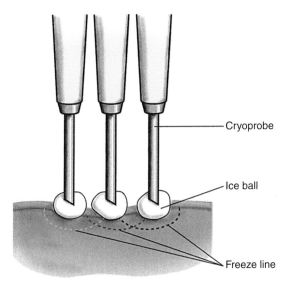

Figure 14.1 For large or irregular lesions—refreeze, overlapping first freeze zone by 50%.

- **Lentigo** (freckles)
- Benign **nevi**—papular or acquired
- **Telangiectasias**—small
- Warts—**verruca vulgaris** and plantaris

CONTRAINDICATIONS

- Face lesions
- Dark skin due to pigment changes
- Area that is hairy because freezing destroys hair follicles
- **Melanoma**
- Compromised circulation
- Areas in which biopsy is required
- Clients with high levels of cryoglobulins (abnormal proteins that precipitate when cooled and dissolve when reheated to body temperature)
  - Endocarditis
  - Syphilis
  - Epstein-Barr virus
  - Cytomegalovirus
  - Hepatitis B—chronic
  - On high-dose steroid treatment
- Collagen disease
- Active ulcerative colitis
- Glomerulonephritis
- Recurrent basal cell carcinoma
- ▶ *Informed consent required*

PROCEDURE

Skin Lesion Removal

Equipment

- Methods 1 and 2
  - Antiseptic skin cleanser
  - Gloves—nonsterile
  - Tape
  - Topical antibiotic (Bactroban, Bacitracin, or Polysporin)
- Method 1 only
  - Drape—sterile
  - 3-mL syringe
  - 27- to 30-gauge, ½-inch needle
  - 1% lidocaine
  - 4 × 4 gauze—sterile
  - Disposable cautery pen
- Method 2 only
  - Verruca Freeze Kit or nitrous oxide cryosurgery unit (Fig. 14.2)
  - Cotton-tipped applicators
  - Water-soluble lubricant (K-Y jelly)
  - 4 × 4 gauze soaked with water

Procedure

METHOD 1—CAUTERY

- Position the client so that the lesion is easily accessible.
- Cleanse the area and a 3-inch-diameter space around the lesion with antiseptic skin cleanser.

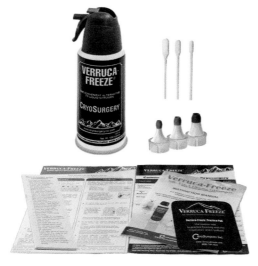

Figure 14.2 Verruca Freeze Kit (from CryoSurgery, Inc., Nashville, TN).

- Inject the tissue under the lesion with 1% lidocaine. If a large lesion (greater than 3 mm), then perform a **field block**.
- Drape the lesion.
- Put on gloves.
- Cauterize the lesion with the disposable cautery pen.
- Wipe off the burned area.
- Apply topical antibiotic.
- Cover with 4 × 4 gauze and tape.

METHOD 2—CRYOSURGERY
- Position the client so that the lesion is easily accessible.
- Cleanse the area and a 3-inch-diameter space around the lesion with antiseptic skin cleanser.
- Apply water-soaked gauze for 5 to 10 minutes.
- Drape the lesion.
- Put on gloves.
- Apply K-Y jelly with a cotton-tipped applicator to the lesion.
- Choose the tip desired (Fig. 14.3).
- Freeze the lesion for the appropriate amount of time (see Options section).
- Apply topical antibiotic.
- Cover with 4 × 4 gauze and tape.

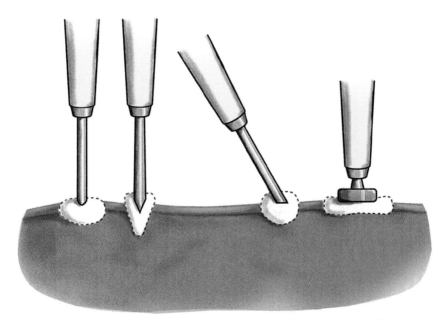

Figure 14.3 The shape of the cryoprobe affects depth and extent of the freeze. By applying pressure, a deeper freeze can be achieved.

Client Instructions—Methods 1 and 2

- Although infection is unlikely, observe for signs and symptoms of infection, such as
  - Increase in pain after 24 hours
  - Increase in temperature
  - Redness or swelling
  - Yellow or greenish drainage
  - Foul odor
- If any signs and symptoms of infection are found, return to the office.
- The following are considered normal reactions:
  - Redness—immediate response
  - Swelling and blisters form—within 24 to 48 hours—and decrease within 72 hours
  - Within 72 hours, crusts form and slowly wither over 1 week
  - Heals from outer margin toward the center
  - Skin may be lighter color and less hair may be present at the site.
  - Not much scar formation
  - Wound weeping up to 8 weeks
  - Sensitive skin—wear sunscreen
- Return to the office in 1 week for recheck.

BIBLIOGRAPHY ▰▰▰▰▰▰▰▰▰▰▰▰▰

Andrews MD. Cryosurgery for common skin conditions. *Am Fam Physician.* 2004;69(10):2365–2372.

Basco MT, Aruny JE, Cheng S, Sumpio BE. Cryosurgery: A review. *Int J Angiol.* 2007; 16(1):1–6.

Habif T. *Clinical Dermatology: A Color Guide to Diagnosis and Therapy.* 6th ed. St. Louis, MO: Mosby; 2015.

Hocutt J. Skin cryosurgery for the family practice physician. *Am Fam Physician.* 1993;48(3):445–447.

Pfenninger JL, Fowler GC. *Procedures for Primary Care Physicians.* St. Louis, MO: Mosby; 2019.

Chapter **15**

Skin Lesion Removal
Keloids, Moles, Corns, Calluses

Margaret R. Colyar

CPT Code

11050	Paring or curettement of benign hyperkeratotic skin lesion with or without chemical cauterization (verrucae, callus, corns), single lesion
11056	Two to four lesions
11057	Greater than four lesions
11300–33	Shaving of epidermal or dermal lesion, single lesion; trunk, arms, or legs
11305–38	Shaving of epidermal or dermal lesion, single lesion; scalp, neck, hands, feet, genitalia

---

Skin lesions such as **keloids**, moles, corns, and calluses are removed easily. Keloids are benign, hard, fibrous proliferations of collagen that expand beyond the original size and shape of the wound, sometimes 20 times normal size. They invade surrounding soft tissue in a clawlike fashion. Moles, or **nevi**, are discolorations of circumscribed areas of the skin resulting from pigmentation. They can be congenital or acquired. Acquired nevi usually appear first in childhood and in sun-exposed areas. These nevi extend into the dermis and epidermis (Fig. 15.1) by late adolescence and intradermis by late adulthood. Nevi always should be assessed for

- Asymmetry
- Border irregularities
- Color variation
- Diameter greater than 6 mm
- Elevation above the skin surface

Corns, or keratomas, are hyperkeratotic lesions or horny indurations with thickening and nucleation of the skin, usually on the toes. Hard corns are located on the dorsal aspect of the toes. Soft corns are located between the digits, usually the fourth interdigital space.

Calluses are hypertrophied, hyperkeratotic thickenings of the stratum corneum, usually located around the heel of the foot, great toe, metatarsal heel, and distal aspect of the first three digits of the dominant hand or palmar aspect of the metacarpal head. There is no underlying nucleus (core).

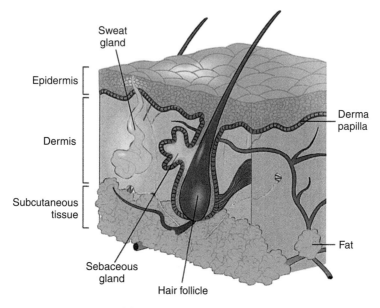

Sweat gland

Epidermis

Dermis

Subcutaneous tissue

Derma papilla

Fat

Sebaceous gland

Hair follicle

Figure 15.1 Anatomy and layers of skin.

OVERVIEW

- Incidence—keloids
  - 15 to 20 times greater in dark-skinned people. They develop more frequently in areas of motion or high skin tension, such as
    - Shoulders
    - Back
    - Presternum
    - Earlobe
    - Face
- Incidence—moles, corns, and calluses—unknown
- Causes
  - Moles
  - Congenital
    - Acquired
  - Corns
    - Pressure from poorly fitting shoes
  - Calluses
    - Continuous friction
    - Pressure from poorly fitting shoes
    - Pencil and pen use
    - Physical labor using the unprotected hand

HEALTH PROMOTION/PREVENTION

Corns

- Wear properly fitting shoes.
- Use moleskin or felt spacer to relieve pressure of bony prominences.

OPTIONS

Keloids

- Method 1—**Cryotherapy**—earlobe and all areas
- Method 2—Corticosteroid injection—early, small, narrow, or softened lesions or to soften and/or flatten
- Method 3—Surgical excision—any keloid

RATIONALE

- To remove unsightly skin lesions
- To relieve pain

INDICATIONS

- Cosmetic
- Pressure and pain
- Limitation of use
- Suspicion of malignancy

CONTRAINDICATIONS

- Poor circulation to the area
- Diabetic
- Immunocompromised

▶ *Informed consent required*

PROCEDURE

Keloid Removal

Equipment

- Methods 1, 2, and 3
  - Antiseptic skin cleanser
  - Gloves—nonsterile
- Methods 2 and 3
  - 10-mL syringe
  - 25- to 27-gauge, 1½-inch needle (very small needles usually are unable to penetrate the lesions adequately)
  - 1% lidocaine
  - Corticosteroid of choice
- Method 1 only
  - Water-soluble lubricant (K-Y jelly)
  - Cotton-tipped applicators
  - Liquid nitrogen (−89°C, −129.2°F)

- Method 3 only
  - 6–0 nylon suture
  - Needle driver—sterile
  - Scissors—sterile
  - No. 15 scalpel

Procedure

METHOD 1—CRYOTHERAPY
- Position the client with the lesion easily accessible.
- Cleanse the area and a 3-inch-diameter space around the keloid with antiseptic skin cleanser.
- Apply water-soaked gauze for 5 to 10 minutes to soften the lesion.
- Apply K-Y jelly for 5 to 10 minutes.
- Using a cryotip narrower than the lesion
  - Freeze for 10 to 15 seconds at −189°C (−308°F), then
  - Freeze for 30 to 45 seconds at −89°C (−129.2°F).
- Wait 15 to 30 minutes for tissue edema to develop.
- Inject the keloid with corticosteroids (see Corticosteroid Injection, next).

METHOD 2—CORTICOSTEROID INJECTION
- Position the client with the keloid easily accessible.
- Cleanse the area and a 3-inch-diameter space around the keloid with antiseptic skin cleanser.
- Draw 2.5 mL of 1% lidocaine and 0.5 mL of corticosteroid into the syringe.
- Inject the medication into the lesion. The keloid will blanche. Do not inject the medication under or around the lesion.

METHOD 3—SURGICAL EXCISION
- See Chapter 2 (Method 3—Elliptical Excisional Biopsy).

Mole Removal

Equipment
- Antiseptic skin cleanser
- Gloves—sterile
- 10-mL syringe
- 25- to 27-gauge, 1½-inch needle (very small needles usually are unable to penetrate the lesions adequately)
- 1% lidocaine
- Corticosteroid of choice
- 6–0 nylon suture
- Needle driver—sterile
- Scissors—sterile
- No. 15 scalpel

Procedure

Same as for cryosurgery, surgical excision, punch biopsy, and shave biopsy.

Corn Removal

Equipment

- Wash basin—nonsterile
- Warm water—tap
- Antiseptic skin cleanser
- Drape—nonsterile
- Gloves—nonsterile
- No. 15 scalpel
- 1% lidocaine
- 3-mL syringe
- 27- to 30-gauge needle
- Self-adherent web spacer
- Topical antibiotic (Bactroban, Bacitracin, or Polysporin)
- 4 × 4 gauze—sterile
- Tape

Procedure

- Soak the foot for 15 to 20 minutes in warm water.
- Cleanse the skin around the corn with antiseptic skin cleanser.
- Anesthetize under the corn with 1% lidocaine.
- Drape the area.
- Put on gloves.
- Pare with No. 15 scalpel and remove core.
- Apply antibiotic, cover with 4 × 4 gauze, and tape.

Callus Removal

Equipment

- Pumice stone or file
- Wash basin—nonsterile
- Warm water
- Antiseptic skin cleanser
- Gloves—nonsterile
- No. 15 scalpel

Procedure

- Soak the foot for 15 to 20 minutes in warm water.
- Cleanse the foot with antiseptic skin cleanser.
- Put on gloves.
- Pare thick callous layers with No. 15 scalpel.
- File down with file or pumice stone.

Client Instructions

KELOIDS, MOLES, AND CORNS

- Apply antibiotic ointment, cover with 4 × 4 gauze, and tape or apply Band-Aid for 2 days; then leave open to air.

- Observe for signs of infections, such as
  - Green or yellow drainage
  - Red streaks
  - Increase in pain after 24 hours
  - Elevated temperature
  - Foul odor from wound
- If infection occurs, return to the office.
- Take acetaminophen or ibuprofen every 4 to 6 hours as needed for pain.
- Return to the office in 1 week for recheck.

CALLUSES

- Perform the following procedure weekly after bathing
  - Pare thick callous layers.
- File down with file or pumice stone.
- Apply felt spacers or moleskin.
- Take acetaminophen or ibuprofen every 4 to 6 hours as needed for pain.
- Return to the office in 1 month, unless condition worsens.

BIBLIOGRAPHY

Berman B, Bieley HC. Adjunct therapies to surgical management of keloids. *Dermatol Surg.* 1996;22(79):126–130.

Juckett G. Management of keloids and hypertrophic scars. *Am Fam Physician.* 2009;80(3):253–260.

Pfenninger JL, Fowler GC. *Procedures for Primary Care Physicians.* St. Louis, MO: Mosby; 2019.

Schneider M, Meites E, Daane SP. Keloids: Which treatment is best for your patient? *J Fam Pract.* 2013, May;62(5):227–233.

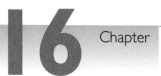

Chapter

Skin Tag (Acrochordon) Removal

Margaret R. Colyar

CPT Code

11200   Removal of skin tags, multiple fibrocutaneous tags, any area; up to and including 15 lesions

11201   Removal of skin tags, multiple fibrocutaneous tags, any area; each additional 10 lesions

---

Skin tags, or **acrochordons**, are benign skin lesions that can be removed by scissoring, any sharp method, or chemical or electrocauterization of the wound. Local anesthesia may or may not be used. Removal usually is done because of irritation of the lesion or for cosmetic reasons.

HEALTH PROMOTION/PREVENTION

- Avoid chronic irritation to the skinfolds of the body.
- Examine the body regularly for changes in color and size of skin lesions.

OPTIONS

- *Method 1*—Snips technique
  - Use with small skin tags.
- *Method 2*—Cryogenic technique
  - Use with large skin tags.

RATIONALE

- To reduce the possibility of inflammation and infection caused by local irritation
- To promote cosmetic enhancement

INDICATIONS

- Unsightly skin tags
- Skin tags irritated by clothing

CONTRAINDICATIONS

- Any lesion that is suspect for malignancy
- High-dose steroid therapy
- Individuals with underlying medical diseases, such as
  - Active severe collagen vascular diseases
  - Acute poststreptococcal glomerulonephritis
  - Acute severe subacute bacterial endocarditis
  - Acute cytomegalovirus infection
  - Acute Epstein-Barr virus infection
  - Acute syphilis infection
  - Chronic severe hepatitis B
  - **Cryoglobulinemia**
  - Diabetes with history of poor healing

▶ *Informed consent required*

PROCEDURE

Skin Tag Removal

Equipment

- Methods 1 and 2
  - Antiseptic skin cleanser
  - Water-soluble lubricant (K-Y Jelly)
  - Cotton-tipped applicators—sterile
  - Topical antibiotic (Bactroban, Bacitracin, or Polysporin)—optional

- Band-Aids
- Drape—sterile
- Goggles—optional
- Tape—optional
- Method 1 only
  - Gloves—sterile
  - Sterile surgical kit that includes
  - 2 × 2 or 4 × 4 gauze
  - Forceps with teeth
  - Iris scissors
  - No. 11 or 15 scalpel
  - 1% lidocaine
  - 5-mL syringe
  - 27-gauge, ½- to 1-inch needle
  - Hemostatic agent—aluminum chloride or ferrous subsulfate
  - Container with 10% **formalin**
- Method 2 only
  - Nitrous oxide cryosurgery unit or cryogun
  - Timer
  - Gloves—nonsterile

Procedure

METHOD 1—SNIPS TECHNIQUE

- Position the client for comfort.
- Put on gloves.
- Apply antiseptic skin cleanser to the skin tag and surrounding area.
- Infiltrate the base of the skin tag with 1% lidocaine (Fig. 16.1).
- Grasp the skin tag at the largest part (Fig. 16.2).

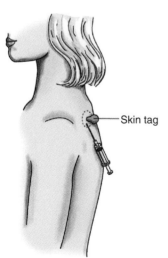

Skin tag

Figure 16.1 Infiltrate the base of the skin tag with lidocaine.

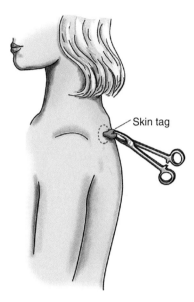

Figure 16.2 Grasp the skin tag at the largest part with hemostats.

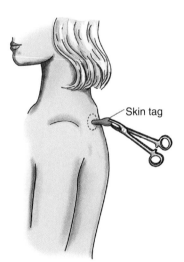

Figure 16.3 Pull the skin tag until the stalk base is visible.

- Gently pull the skin tag until the stalk base is visible (Fig. 16.3).
- Using the iris scissors or scalpel, cut or slice the stalk as close to the base of the stalk as possible (Fig. 16.4).
- Apply a hemostatic agent (ferrous subsulfate or aluminum chloride) with cotton-tipped applicator. Hold on the area until the bleeding stops.
- Place the skin tags in the container with 10% formalin for laboratory pathology.
- Apply topical antibiotic—optional.
- Apply a Band-Aid.

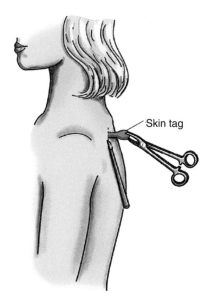

Figure 16.4 Cut the stalk of the skin tag as close as possible to the base of the stalk.

METHOD 2—CRYOGENIC TECHNIQUE
See Chapter 14.
- Position the client so that the lesion is easily accessible.
- Cleanse the area and a 3-inch-diameter space surrounding with antiseptic skin cleanser.
- Drape the lesion.
- Put on gloves.
- Prepare equipment as manufacturer recommends.
- Select the appropriate-size device to match the size of the lesion.
- Anesthetize the site—optional.
- Use a cotton-tipped applicator to apply enough K-Y jelly to cover the skin tag but not beyond the tag.
- Apply the selected probe to the site and penetrate approximately halfway into the jelly.
- Squeeze the cryogun trigger to release the nitrogen oxide. The jelly is transformed into an ice ball.
- If area of skin is thin, when the jelly is frozen, pull up slightly on the skin to lessen depth of the tissue freezing.
- Application time is usually 30 seconds. Larger skin tags may require 45 seconds.
- Release the trigger.
- Allow the jelly to thaw before removing the probe from the site of the cryosurgery.
- Depending on the response of the lesion, a repeat freeze-thaw may be required for an additional 30 seconds.
- Do not apply any dressing until lesion becomes irritated and/or is bleeding.

- Topical antibiotic ointment is not recommended.
- Apply a Band-Aid to be removed when the client gets home.

Client Instructions

- On completion of treatment of the skin tag, the area appears erythematous and indurated (hard). A red ring may be visible around the site 2 weeks after removal. This is a normal response.
- Retreatment may be required if the entire lesion does not **slough** off.
- Keep the wound clean and dry.
- A Band-Aid is not required usually after 1 hour.
- Antibiotics are not required.
- Observe for signs and symptoms of infection, such as
  - Increase in pain after 24 hours
  - Increase in temperature
  - Redness or swelling
  - Yellow or greenish drainage
  - Foul odor
- If any signs and symptoms of infection are found, return to the office.
- Pain—acetaminophen every 4 hours as needed for mild pain for the first 24 hours. After 24 hours, ibuprofen or naproxen may be used.
  - Acetaminophen with codeine rarely is used for severe pain because most skin lesions have few nerve endings. If discomfort continues and infection has been excluded, use Tylenol No. 3 every 4 to 6 hours as needed.
- Bathing is permitted 48 hours after the procedure.
- If the cryogenic technique was used
  - First 24 to 48 hours, a blister may form; if it does, apply a small, nonstick Band-Aid until the weeping has stopped.
- Ideally, leave the wound exposed for more rapid healing.
- Redness to the site is common and lessens with time.
- The pain should lessen within 24 hours.
- A cotton swab with hydrogen peroxide may be used if the site becomes crusty.
- No topical antibiotic should be applied.
- Nonaspirin pain reliever is suggested.
- Rarely, painful and large blisters can occur. If they do, contact the practitioner to determine course of management. (Usually, these blisters are drained.)
- If infection is suspected, contact health-care provider.
- Within 7 to 10 days, a scab should form. Do not pick it. Let it fall off naturally.
  - Most redness and decreased skin coloration resolve within 3 to 6 months.
  - Some lesions may require retreatment.
- Remove the Band-Aid. Keep the area covered only if it is being irritated constantly. Continuous covering of the wound increases risk of infection.

BIBLIOGRAPHY

Habif T. *Clinical Dermatology: A Color Guide to Diagnosis and Therapy.* 6th ed. St. Louis, MO: Mosby; 2015.

Matzen R, Lang R. *Clinical Preventive Medicine.* St. Louis, MO: Mosby; 1993.
Murtagh J. *Practice Tips.* 5th ed. New York, NY: McGraw-Hill; 2017.
Pfenninger JL, Fowler GC. *Procedures for Primary Care Physicians.* St. Louis, MO: Mosby; 2019.

Chapter 17

Soft Tissue Aspiration

Margaret R. Colyar

CPT Code

20600 Arthrocentesis, aspiration, or injection: small joint, bursa, or ganglionic cyst (e.g., fingers or toes)
20605 Arthrocentesis, aspiration, or injection: intermediate joint, bursa, or ganglionic cyst (e.g., temporomandibular; acromioclavicular; wrist, elbow, or ankle; olecranon bursa)
20610 Arthrocentesis, aspiration, or injection: major joint or bursa (e.g., shoulder, hip, knee joint, subacromial bursa)

Soft tissue aspiration is the removal of fluid or exudate in an area of soft tissue for comfort and evaluation.

RATIONALE

* To diagnose
  * Infection
  * Rheumatoid disease
  * Crystals
  * Bursitis
  * Chondritis
* To provide symptomatic relief

INDICATIONS

* Pain and/or swelling in soft tissue
* Hematoma from trauma

CONTRAINDICATIONS

* Severe coagulation problems
* Swelling on the face
* Cellulitis or broken skin at the site
* Joint prosthesis
* *Informed consent required*

PROCEDURE
Soft Tissue Aspiration

Equipment

- Antiseptic skin cleanser
- Drape—sterile
- Gloves—sterile
- **Hemostats**—sterile
- 6- to 10-mL syringe
- 18- to 20-gauge, 1-inch needle
- Container with 10% **formalin**, specimen tube, or microscope slide
- Ace wrap
- 4 × 4 gauze—sterile
- Tape

Procedure

- Position the client for comfort with the affected area easily accessible.
- Cleanse the area with antiseptic skin cleanser.
- Drape the area.
- Put on gloves.
- Insert 18- to 20-gauge needle into the area of soft tissue swelling and withdraw fluid.
- If the syringe becomes full (Fig. 17.1)
  - Stabilize the needle with hemostats.
  - Remove the full syringe.
  - Attach a new syringe.
  - Withdraw the remaining fluid.

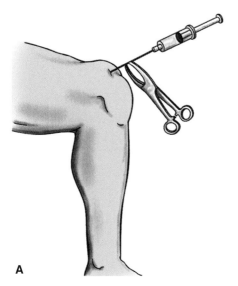

A

Figure 17.1 When the syringe becomes full, stabilize the needle with hemostats. (A) Remove the full syringe. (B) Attach a new syringe. (C) Withdraw the remaining fluid.

Continued

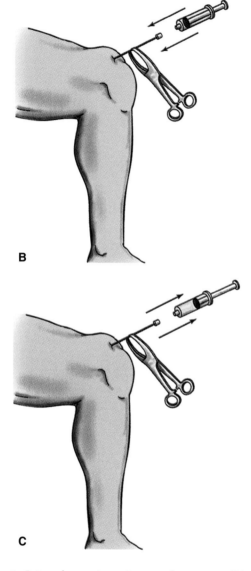

B

C

Figure 17.1 cont'd

- Inject the specimen into a tube or on a slide and send to the laboratory for evaluation.
- Apply a pressure dressing and tape.
- Apply the Ace wrap.

Client Instructions

- Keep the pressure dressing in place for 24 hours; then remove it.
- Observe for signs of infection, such as
  - Increase in pain and heat at the site
  - Red streaks

- Yellow or green drainage
- Chills and fever
- Foul odor from wound
- Soft tissue swelling may recur. If this happens, return to the office.

BIBLIOGRAPHY ▰▰▰▰▰▰▰▰▰▰▰▰▰▰

Cardone DA, Tallia AF. Joint and soft tissue injection. *Am Fam Physician.* 2002;66(2):283–289.
Pfenninger JL, Fowler GC. *Procedures for Primary Care Physicians.* St. Louis, MO: Mosby; 2019.

Chapter **18**

Staple Insertion

Margaret R. Colyar

CPT Code
12001–07 Simple repair of superficial wounds of scalp, neck, axillae, external genitalia, trunk, or extremities (including hands and feet); based on length

Simple wound closure with the use of stapling devices can be done easily by the nurse practitioner.

OVERVIEW

- Types of staple material available
  - Ethicon
  - 3M
  - Deknatel

RATIONALE

- For rapid insertion
- To reduce skin allergies
- To prevent unsightly wound healing
- To promote accelerated wound healing

INDICATIONS

- Long, linear lacerations
- Scalp wounds
- Wounds in area of less cosmetic importance

CONTRAINDICATIONS

- Crush wounds
- Ischemic wounds
- Highly contaminated wounds

▶ *Informed consent required*

PROCEDURE

Staple Insertion

Equipment

- Antiseptic skin cleanser
- 0.9% sodium chloride—250 to 500 mL
- Drape—sterile
- Gloves—nonsterile
- Stapling device
- Staples
- 1% or 2% lidocaine with epinephrine if the area to be anesthetized is not on a digit, nose, ear, or penis
- 3-mL syringe
- 27- to 30-gauge, 1-inch needle
- 18-gauge, 1½-inch needle
- Cotton-tipped applicator—sterile
- Topical antibiotic ointment (Bactroban, Bacitracin, or Polysporin)
- Nonstick dressing such as Telfa
- 4 × 4 gauze—sterile
- Tape

Procedure

- Position the client for comfort with laceration easily accessible.
- Irrigate vigorously with 0.9% sodium chloride using 10-mL syringe and 18-gauge needle.
- Cleanse a 3-inch-diameter area around the laceration with antiseptic skin cleanser.
- Put on gloves.
- Infiltrate wound with 1% or 2% lidocaine. Epinephrine may be used if the wound is not on a digit, ear, nose, or penis.
- **Approximate** the skin edges.
- Start in the center of the laceration and work outward to prevent puckering.
- Place the stapling device perpendicular to the skin and depress the top handle.
- Insert staples perpendicular to the skin at ¼-inch intervals.
- Apply topical antibiotic ointment.
- Apply nonstick dressing.
- Cover with 4 × 4 gauze.
- Secure with tape.

Client Instructions

- Remove the dressing in 48 hours.
- Keep the wound clean and dry.
- Observe for signs and symptoms of infection, such as
  - Increase in pain after 24 hours
  - Increase in temperature
  - Redness or swelling
  - Yellow or greenish drainage
  - Foul odor
- If any of the signs and symptoms of infection are found, return to the office.
- Return to the office in _____ days for staple removal.

BIBLIOGRAPHY

Forsch RT. Essentials of skin laceration repair. *Am Fam Physician.* 2008;78(8): 945–951.
Lipsett S. Closure of minor skin wounds with staples. UpToDate. September 15, 2017. https://www.uptodate.com/contents/closure-of-minor-skin-wounds-with-staples.

Chapter **19**

Staple Removal

Margaret R. Colyar

CPT Code
None. Included as part of staple insertion.

Removal of staples after initial healing has occurred should be done within a specified time frame. The suggested times for removing staples are

- Face, neck—3 to 5 days
- Ear, scalp—5 to 7 days
- Arm, leg, hand, foot—7 to 10 or more days
- Chest, back, abdomen—7 to 10 or more days

OVERVIEW

- Incidence unknown

OPTIONS

- *Method 1*—Staple removal (complete)
  - Used for wounds that are
    - Small
    - Well approximated
    - Not oozing
- *Method 2*—Staple removal (partial)
  - Used for wounds that are
    - Large
    - Healing poorly
    - Have a possibility of evisceration

RATIONALE

- To prevent scarring and infection from retained staples

INDICATIONS

- Staples in place for appropriate healing period.
- Wound does not need extra stability of staples.
- Allergic reaction to staples.

CONTRAINDICATIONS

- Wound has not healed well.

PROCEDURE

Method 1—Staple Removal (Complete)

Equipment

- Alcohol
- Staple remover—sterile
- Gloves—nonsterile
- Steri-Strips (method 2)
- Benzoin (method 2)
- Cotton-tipped applicators (method 2)
- Alcohol prep pads (method 2)

Procedure

- Position the client for comfort with laceration easily accessible.
- Put on gloves.
- Insert the bottom prongs of staple remover under a staple and depress the top handle.
  - Edges of the staple will rise (Fig. 19.1).
- Rock the staple gently from side to side, if needed, to remove edges of the staple from the skin.
- Continue with each staple until all staples are removed.
- Cleanse incision with alcohol prep pads.

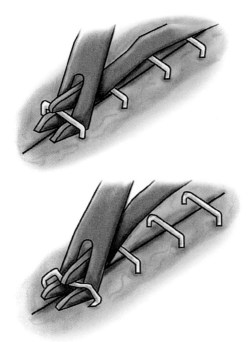

Figure 19.1 Insert the bottom prongs of the staple remover under a staple and depress the top handle.

Method 2—Staple Removal (Partial)

Procedure

- Position the client for comfort with laceration easily accessible.
- Put on gloves.
- Insert the bottom prongs of staple remover under a staple and depress the top handle.
  - Edges of the staple will rise.
- Rock the staple gently from side to side, if needed, to remove edges from skin.
- Continue with *alternate staples* until all staples are removed.
- Apply benzoin in spaces where staples have been removed. Start at wound edge and spread benzoin away from wound approximately 1½ inches (see Chapter 20).
- When benzoin is tacky, apply Steri-Strips between every remaining staple.
- Cleanse the incision with alcohol prep pads.

Client Instructions

- Observe for signs and symptoms of infection, such as
  - Increase in pain after 24 hours
  - Increase in temperature
  - Redness or swelling
  - Yellow or greenish drainage

- Foul odor
- Wound separation
- If any signs and symptoms of infection are found, return to the office.

BIBLIOGRAPHY ▬▬▬▬▬▬▬▬▬▬▬▬▬▬▬▬▬

Forsch RT. Essentials of skin laceration repair. *Am Fam Physician.* 2008;78(8):945–951.
Lipsett S. Closure of minor skin wounds with staples. https://www.uptodate.com/contents/
closure-of-minor-skin-wounds-with-staples. UpToDate. September 15, 2017.

20 Chapter

Steri-Strip Application
Margaret R. Colyar

CPT Code
None. Included in evaluation and management charge (office visit charge).

Steri-Strips are noninvasive skin closure devices. They are used when sutures are not necessary, but approximation of the wound is needed to promote healing. Steri-Strips should be used with minimal wound trauma. Advantages include more resistance to wound infections. Disadvantages include poor wound eversion and more difficult wound edge approximation.

RATIONALE
- To provide wound stability while healing process takes place

INDICATIONS
- Small, superficial wounds
- Wounds under little tension
- Stapled or sutured wounds that need extra support

CONTRAINDICATIONS
- Large, deep wounds
- Wounds that are under tension

PROCEDURE

Steri-Strip Application

Equipment

- Antiseptic skin cleanser
- Skin adhesive, such as **benzoin**
- Steri-Strips—⅛ to ½ inch
- Cotton-tipped applicators—sterile
- 4 × 4 gauze—sterile
- Tape

Procedure

- Position the client with area to be Steri-Stripped easily accessible.
- Cleanse skin 3 inches around the wound with antiseptic skin cleanser.
- Using cotton-tipped applicators, apply benzoin or other skin adhesive.
- Start next to the wound edges and extend outward approximately 1½ inches (Fig. 20.1).
- Allow the skin adhesive to become tacky.
- Apply Steri-Strips toward the wound, pulling one skin edge to the other (Fig. 20.2).
- Apply a sufficient number of Steri-Strips to ensure wound closure.
- A nonocclusive dressing using 4 × 4 gauze may be applied to keep the wound clean and dry and to absorb drainage that oozes from the wound for the first 24 hours.

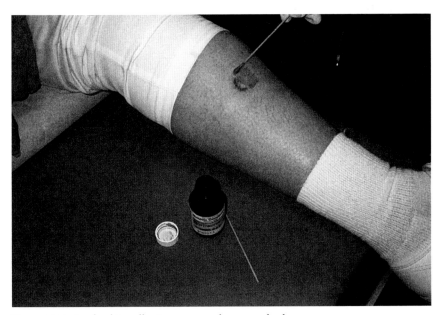

Figure 20.1 Apply skin adhesive next to the wound edges.

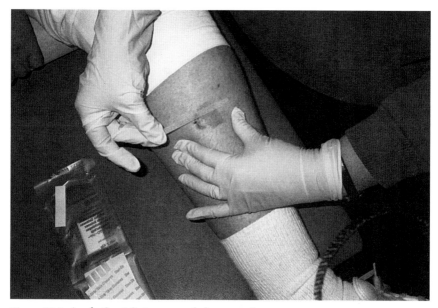

Figure 20.2 Apply Steri-Strips toward the wound.

Client Instructions

- If a dressing was applied over the Steri-Stripped area, remove it in 24 hours and leave the area open to air.
- Keep Steri-Strips clean and dry.
- If Steri-Strips become dislodged and the wound separates, return to clinic for reapplication of Steri-Strips.
- A small amount of redness around the wound is normal.
- Observe for signs and symptoms of infection, such as
  - Increase in pain after 24 hours
  - Increase in temperature
  - Redness or swelling
  - Yellow or greenish drainage
  - Foul odor
- If any signs and symptoms of infection are found, return to the office.
- Return to the office in 1 week for recheck and removal of the Steri-Strips.

BIBLIOGRAPHY

Smeltzer S, Bare BG. *Brunner and Suddarth's Textbook of Medical-Surgical Nursing.* Philadelphia, PA: Lippincott-Raven; 2010.

Subungual Hematoma Excision

Margaret R. Colyar

CPT Code
11740 Subungual hematoma evacuation

OVERVIEW

- Complicating factors
  - Temporary or permanent disfigurement to the nail
  - Temporary or permanent loss of the nail
  - Infection arising from the trauma or treatment
- Consider an x-ray if the subungual hematoma is greater than 25% of the nail.

General Principles

- Inspect the area for contraindications to the procedure.
- Palpate for tenderness beyond the nailbed.
- Determine the vascular and neurological status of the digit.
- Perform active and passive range of motion of the distal joint.
- Test for instability of the digit's joint.

HEALTH PROMOTION/PREVENTION

- Follow safety measures around all machinery.
- Avoid placing digits in the path of closing doors.
- Use hammers carefully.
- Do not use unfamiliar machinery without proper instruction.

OPTIONS

- *Method 1*—Cautery technique
- *Method 2*—Paper clip technique

RATIONALE

- To relieve pain
- To prevent possible infection

INDICATIONS

- Complaint of digit pain following trauma with the presence of a subungual hematoma less than 4 hours old

CONTRAINDICATIONS

- Presence of hematoma greater than 50% of the nail surface
- Crushed or fractured nail
- Known history of poor healing (physician referral)
- Suspected distal phalanx fracture

▶ *Informed consent required*

PROCEDURES

Subungual Hematoma Excision

Equipment

- Method 1 only
  - Battery-powered cautery device
  - Basin—sterile
  - Povidone-iodine soak or antibacterial soap
  - Gloves—sterile
  - Safety goggles and mask—optional
  - 0.9% sodium chloride—sterile
  - 4 × 4 gauze—sterile
- Method 2 only
  - Alcohol lamp, Bunsen burner, or cigarette lighter
  - Paper clip—medium or large
  - **Hemostat**—sterile
  - Safety goggles and mask—optional
  - Gloves—nonsterile

Procedure

METHOD 1—CAUTERY TECHNIQUE

- Soak the affected digit in lukewarm povidone-iodine or antibacterial soapy water for 5 to 10 minutes.
- Position the client for comfort.
- Drape the digit with the sterile 4 × 4 gauze to absorb the blood.
- If necessary, have someone hold the digit securely to prevent movement during the procedure.
- Put on gloves.
- Activate the cautery.
- When the cautery needle becomes red hot, apply the needle directly over the middle of the subungual hematoma at a 90-degree angle with firm, gentle pressure (Fig. 21.1).
- Be sure not to stand in the direct line of the hole because the release of the hematoma can result in the forceful splattering of blood.
- As the needle burns a hole (approximately 1 to 2 mm) through the nail, resistance can be felt.
- When resistance ceases, this indicates full penetration through the nail.
- Proceed to lift the cautery probe away from the nail, and allow blood to drain if clotting has not occurred (Fig. 21.2).

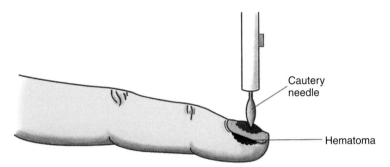

Figure 21.1 Apply the heated cautery needle over the middle of the hematoma at a 90-degree angle.

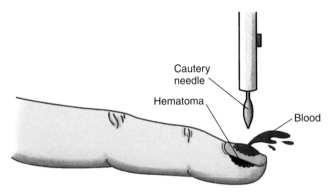

Figure 21.2 Remove the cautery probe and allow the blood to drain.

- Dab with the 4 × 4 gauze to facilitate drainage.
- Administer tetanus-diphtheria booster (Tdap) if immunization was more than 5 years ago.

METHOD 2—PAPER CLIP TECHNIQUE
- Soak the affected digit in lukewarm povidone-iodine or antibacterial soapy water for 5 to 10 minutes.
- Position the client for comfort.
- Drape the digit with the sterile 4 × 4 gauze to absorb the blood.
- If necessary, have someone hold the digit securely to prevent movement during the procedure.
- Straighten one end of a medium or large paper clip and clamp a hemostat to the opposite end.
- Light the alcohol lamp, Bunsen burner, or cigarette lighter.
- Put on gloves.
- Place the tip of the paper clip into the hottest part of the flame and heat until red hot.
- Using firm, gentle pressure, apply the paper clip to the nail surface at a 90-degree angle (Fig. 21.3).

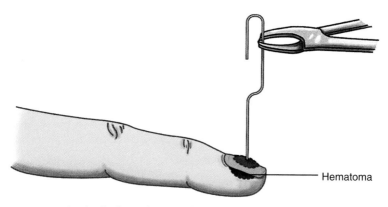

Hematoma

Figure 21.3 Apply the heated paper clip to the nail surface at a 90-degree angle.

- As the paper clip burns a hole (approximately 1 to 2 mm) through the nail, resistance can be felt.
- Resistance ceases with full penetration through the nail.
- Lift the paper clip away from the nail, and allow blood to drain if clotting has not occurred.
- Dab with the 4 × 4 gauze to facilitate drainage.
- Administer tetanus-diphtheria (Tdap) booster if immunization was more than 5 years ago.

Client Instructions

- Keep wound clean and dry.
- To lessen pain, apply cool compresses and elevate the hand above the heart.
- Antibiotics are not required.
- Observe for signs and symptoms of infection, such as
  - Increase in pain after 24 hours
  - Increase in temperature
  - Redness or swelling
  - Yellow or greenish drainage
  - Foul odor
- If any signs and symptoms of infection are found, return to the office.
- To relieve pain
  - Take acetaminophen every 4 to 6 hours as needed for mild pain for first 24 hours.
  - Ibuprofen, naproxen, and other NSAIDs should be avoided for the first 24 hours to lessen the risk of increased bleeding.
  - After 24 hours, alternating NSAIDs with acetaminophen may be beneficial.
  - Tylenol No. 3 is used rarely for severe pain.
- Return to the office if the nail appears to need removal.

BIBLIOGRAPHY

Habif T. *Clinical Dermatology: A Color Guide to Diagnosis and Therapy.* 6th ed. St. Louis, MO: Mosby; 2015.

Hoffman D, Schaffer T. Management of common finger injuries. *Am Fam Physician.* 1991;43(5):850–862.

Pfenninger JL, Fowler GC. *Procedures for Primary Care Physicians.* St. Louis, MO: Mosby; 2019.

Wang QC, Johnson BA. Fingertip injuries. *Am Fam Physician.* 2001;63(10):1961–1966.

Chapter **22**

Suture Insertion

Cynthia Ehrhardt

CPT Code

12001–07	Simple repair, superficial wounds; scalp, neck, axillae, external genitalia, trunk, or extremities
12011–18	Simple repair, superficial wounds; face, ears, eyelids, nose, lips, or mucous membranes
12020	Superficial dehiscence, simple
12031–37	Intermediate repair with layer closure; scalp, axillae, trunk, or extremities (not hands and feet)
12041–47	Intermediate repair with layer closure; neck, hands, feet, or external genitalia
12051–57	Intermediate repair with layer closure; face, ears, eyelids, nose, lips, or mucous membranes

Suturing is a procedure used to repair lacerations of the skin. The length of time sutures are left in depends on location. Leaving sutures in too long or removing them too soon increases the risk of unnecessary scarring (Table 22.1). Do not close grossly contaminated wounds, bites, gunshot or fragmentation wounds, or wounds greater than 12 hours old. If delayed primary closure is necessary, it should be done at day 5 postinjury and after debridement of dead tissue. Delayed closure allows for the wound to pass the period of greatest risk of infection and will heal equally as fast as normal primary closure.

OVERVIEW

- Complicating factors of secondary infection are usually the result of
  - Gram-positive bacteria
    - *Staphylococcus aureus* (3% resistance)
    - Streptococci
  - Gram-negative bacteria
    - *Proteus*
    - *Klebsiella*
    - Pseudomonas

Table 22·1 Suggested Length of Time Sutures Should Be Left in Place	
BODY PART	**LENGTH OF TIME (DAYS)**
Face	3–4
Neck	5
Scalp	6–7
Arms and back of hands	7
Chest and abdomen	7–10
Legs and top of feet	10
Back	10–12
Palms of hands, soles of feet	14

General Principles

- Minimize the amount of pain to the site with anesthesia.
- Irrigate all wounds with sterile 0.9% sodium chloride (60 to 120 mL) to ensure removal of foreign matter and to improve clean closure.
- Avoid infection and poor wound healing, minimize scarring, and obtain good cosmetic results by
  - Maintaining uniform tensile strength
  - Making precise approximation of skin edges
  - Closing all dead space in wound
  - Avoiding excessive suturing
- If laceration is located over a joint, it is recommended after suturing that the joint be splinted for the length of time the sutures are in place to prevent rupture of the suture line. It is permitted to remove the splint a minimum of four times a day for gentle active range of motion to prevent loss of joint mobility.
- If sutures are needed in a hairy area of the body, use a different color of suture material (e.g., blue filament in a person with black hair).
- Prophylactic antibiotic therapy no longer is recommended.
- Oral antibiotic therapy should be considered when the risk for infection is greater than side effects of medication.
  - Guidelines include
    - Wounds more than 6 hours old
    - Wounds caused by crushing mechanism with tissue compromise
    - Contaminated or soiled wounds that require extensive cleansing and/or debridement
    - Extensive lacerations to the hand
    - Immunocompromised and diabetic clients

Commonly Used Anesthetic Agents

- Lidocaine (Xylocaine) 1% to 2.5%—1 to 2 hours of relief
- Bupivacaine (Marcaine) 0.25% to 1.5%—6 to 8 hours of relief

RATIONALE

- To avoid infection
- To promote good wound healing
- To minimize scarring
- To obtain good cosmetic results
- To repair the loss of tissue integrity because of trauma

INDICATIONS

- Superficial or intermediate laceration to the skin without artery, bone, ligament, nerve, or tendon involvement

CONTRAINDICATIONS

- Complex laceration, REFER to a physician.
- Involvement of artery, bone, ligament, nerve, or tendon, REFER to a physician.
- More than 6 hours after the occurrence. *(Consultation with collaborative physician is strongly advised with delayed treatment of lacerations.)*

▶ *Informed consent required*

PROCEDURE

Suture Insertion

Equipment

- Povidone-iodine solution or swabs
- 1% lidocaine with or without epinephrine
  - Lidocaine with epinephrine generally is reserved for wounds that have considerable bleeding characteristics, such as wounds in the scalp and eyebrow areas.
  - *Lidocaine with epinephrine should never be used in digits and appendages of the body because of vasoconstriction.*
- Two syringes—5 and 30 mL
- Angiocath—16 or 18 gauge
- 25- to 27-gauge, 1- to 1½-inch needle
- Appropriately selected suturing material for the laceration
- Gloves—sterile
- 0.9% sodium chloride—sterile
- Sterile towels (fenestrated and nonfenestrated)
- Sterile suture kit (prepackaged or self-made) should include
  - Curved and straight **hemostats**
  - Needle holders (4½ and 6 inch)
  - Forceps with teeth
  - Iris scissors
  - Knife handle and blades (usually no. 11 blade)
  - Cups to hold povidone-iodine and sterile normal saline solution
  - 4×4 sterile gauze

Procedure

- Position client comfortably with area of laceration easily accessible.
- Apply povidone-iodine to the wound beginning at the wound edges and expanding out in a circular pattern.
- Put on gloves.
- Infiltrate wound with 1% lidocaine (5-mL syringe with 25- to 27-gauge needle).
- Insert the needle parallel along each side of the edge of the laceration to the farthest point, and begin to infiltrate the wound while slowly withdrawing the needle (Fig. 22.1). This procedure results in a more uniform anesthesia with fewer injections.
- Carefully explore the wound for foreign bodies and involvement of the joint capsule, tendons, and other related anatomical structures.
- If there are no anatomical contraindications to suturing, irrigate the wound with 60 to 100 mL of sterile normal saline. (Be sure to document this in your procedure note.)
- If wound edges are ragged, trim with iris scissors. Minimize the amount of debridement of epidermis (Fig. 22.2). Occasionally, undermining may be required to give good approximation of the edges (Fig. 22.3).
- Place suture needle in needle holder, using proper hand position.
- With the opposite hand, use forceps with teeth to grasp wound edge and evert the edges. Penetrate the wound edge with the suture needle

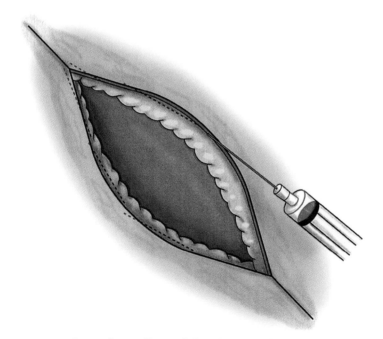

Figure 22.1 Insert the needle parallel to the edge of the laceration, and begin to infiltrate with lidocaine while withdrawing the needle.

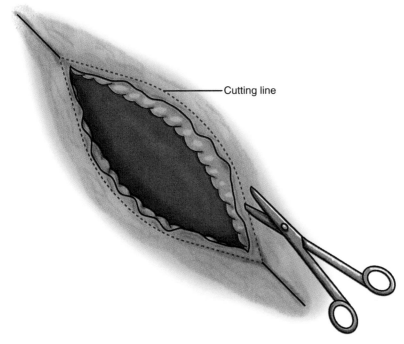

Figure 22.2 Trim ragged edges with scissors.

(Fig. 22.4), ensuring the suture is far enough from the wound edge to prevent tearing (generally 0.5 cm, but no greater than 1 cm from wound edge).

- Tie suture off as determined by chosen technique.
- Trim leftover suture to a length suitable for grasping with forceps for easy removal.
- When wound is completely sutured, cleanse area with 0.9% sodium chloride.
- Pat dry.
- Apply dressing. (If highly vascular, consider a pressure dressing for several hours.)
- Be precise and descriptive when documenting the procedure performed in the medical record. Include
  - Anesthetic used
  - Cleansing preparation performed
  - Whether irrigation occurred (amount of irrigation)
  - Type of suture material
  - Number of sutures
  - Outcome of the suturing
  - How the procedure was tolerated

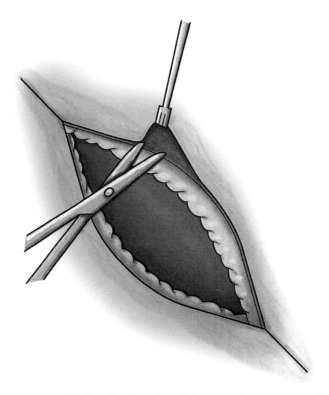

Figure 22.3 Undermine the edge of the wound to ensure good approximation of the wound.

Client Instructions

- Keep wound clean and dry.
- Do not wash area for 24 hours after the procedure. After 24 hours, dressing may be removed and site may be left open to air.
  - Continuous covering of wound increases risk of infection.
- Bathing 48 hours after the procedure is permitted.
- If crust develops over the sutured site
  - Cleanse with a cotton-tipped swab saturated with hydrogen peroxide.
  - Take the swab and gently roll over the wound site.
  - Gently rinse the area with warm water.
  - Blot dry with clean towel or cotton gauze.
- To decrease pain
  - Use Tylenol No. 3 for severe pain every 4 to 6 hours as needed for the first 24 hours.
  - Then use acetaminophen, ibuprofen, or naproxen every 4 hours for mild pain.

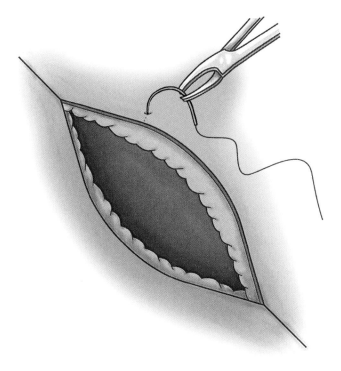

Figure 22.4 Penetrate the edge of the wound with the suture needle approximately 0.5 cm from the wound edge.

- Observe for signs and symptoms of infection, such as
  - Increase in pain after 24 hours
  - Increase in temperature
  - Redness or swelling
  - Yellow or greenish drainage
  - Foul odor
- If any of the signs and symptoms of infection are found, return to the office.
- Apply antibiotic ointment to the wound to lessen the development of scab formation.
- Return to the office in 48 hours for wound recheck.

BIBLIOGRAPHY

Forsch RT. Essentials of skin laceration repair. *Am Fam Physician.* 2008;78(8): 945–951.

Pfenninger J, Fowler G. *Procedures for Primary Care Physicians.* St. Louis, MO: Mosby; 2019.

Trott A. *Wounds and Lacerations: Emergency Care and Closure.* St. Louis, MO: Mosby; 2012.

23 Chapter

Suture Selection

Margaret R. Colyar

The ideal suture needle should be inexpensive, appropriate to the type of wound repair, and of maximum sharpness and strength to complete the task with the least amount of tissue injury. The ideal suture material should be inexpensive, strong, form secure knots, handle easily, stretch and recoil easily during wound healing, and cause minimal tissue inflammation. In order to reduce tissue trauma, sutures now come with the needles firmly attached.

SELECTION OF SUTURE NEEDLES

- Point types include
  - Cutting (conventional, reverse, or side [spatula])
  - Taper-point (round)
  - Beveled, conventional cutting edge
- For most superficial and intermediate suture repair, use a P-1 to P-3 (Ethicon) ⅜- to ½-inch cutting circle.
- Deep suturing or buried sutures may require PS-1 or PS-2 (Ethicon) needle.

SELECTION OF SUTURE MATERIAL

- The advantages and disadvantages of each suture material should be taken into consideration (Table 23.1).

GENERAL RECOMMENDATIONS FOR SUTURE USE

- The larger the number of the suture (e.g., 3-0 vs. 5-0), the smaller the filament thickness will be.
- Absorbable sutures elicit more inflammatory reactions than do nonabsorbable sutures.
- Monofilaments usually require more knots to prevent slippage.
- Braided sutures handle easily and knot easily, but may harbor bacteria.
- Fascia heals slowly—use bigger, stronger suture.
- Mucosa heals quickly—use small suture.

For Extremities

- External—4-0 or 5-0 polypropylene (Prolene) nonabsorbable
- Buried—3-0 or 4-0 mild chromic gut (Vicryl)

Table 23·1 | Suture Material

SUTURE MATERIAL	ADVANTAGES	DISADVANTAGES
Silk (nonabsorbable)	Natural product; easiest to handle of all suture materials; produces least amount of wound irritation	Lowest in tensile strength and breaks easily; high absorption capacity increases wound infections
Polypropylene (nonabsorbable) (Prolene, Surgilene)	Synthetic product; hydrolyzes slowly; high elasticity and tensile strength; minimal tissue reaction; inexpensive	Stiff; difficult to knot
Braided polyester (nonabsorbable) (Ethibond, Dacron)	Synthetic; low tissue adherence; stretches	Knots poorly; loose after tissue edema resolves; expensive
Nylon (nonabsorbable)	Synthetic; handles easily; good knot control	Uncoated—leads to increased tissue friction and drag; increases incidence of wound infection; expensive
Polybutester (nonabsorbable) (Novafil)	Elastic; accommodates change in wound edema; less stiffness and tissue drag	Moderately expensive
Treated catgut (absorbable) (mild chromic gut)	Natural product; inexpensive; good tensile strength for 4–5 days	Poor knot handling; moderate tissue inflammation
Polyglycolic (absorbable) (Dexon)	Synthetic; less tissue reactivity; prolonged tensile strength	Poor knot tying; stiff
Polyglactic acid (absorbable) (Vicryl)	Synthetic; easy to handle; prolonged tensile strength; decreased tissue reactivity	Dyed for visibility
Polyglyconate (absorbable) (Maxon)	Extended duration of tensile strength—80% after 2 weeks; easy to handle	Expensive; recent market introduction

For Trunk

- External—4-0 or 5-0 polypropylene nonabsorbable
- Buried—3-0 or 4-0 mild chromic gut

For Face

- External—5-0 to 6-0 nylon (Ethilon)
- Buried—4-0 or 5-0 absorbable

BIBLIOGRAPHY

Forsch RT, Little SH, Williams C. Laceration repair: A practical approach. *Am Fam Physician.* 2017;95(10):628-636.

Pfenninger J, Fowler G. *Procedures for Primary Care Physicians.* St. Louis, MO: Mosby; 2019.

Trott A. *Wounds and Lacerations: Emergency Care and Closure.* St. Louis, MO: Mosby; 2012.

24 | Chapter

Suture Removal

Margaret R. Colyar

CPT Code
99211 Simple removal—nurse

Suture removal is the withdrawal of artificially inserted polyfilament thread used to repair a laceration. Leaving foreign material in the body after healing increases inflammation and scarring to the site.

OVERVIEW

- Sutures should be removed in a timely manner to prevent scarring and inflammation (see Table 22.1).

OPTIONS

- *Method 1*—Standard suture removal technique
- *Method 2*—Running suture line technique
- *Method 3*—Small loop sutures, closed sutures, and difficult anatomical position sutures technique

RATIONALE

- To diminish the occurrence of inflammation and scarring

INDICATIONS

- Presence of suture material in superficial layers of the skin

CONTRAINDICATIONS

- Removal before recommended length of time for healing of the laceration

PROCEDURE

Suture Removal

Equipment

- Methods 1 and 2 only
  - Scissors—sterile
- **Forceps** without teeth—sterile
- Methods 1, 2, and 3
  - Gloves—sterile
  - Hydrogen peroxide

- Cotton-tipped applicators—clean or sterile
- 4 × 4 gauze—clean or sterile
- Steri-Strips or butterfly Band-Aids—optional
- Method 3 only
  - No. 11 scalpel

Procedure

METHOD 1—STANDARD SUTURE REMOVAL TECHNIQUE

- Position the client comfortably with sutured area easily accessible.
- Examine sutures to determine the type of suture technique that was used.
- Locate the end tie knot(s).
- If crust is present over suture site
  - Gently roll a cotton-tipped applicator saturated with hydrogen peroxide over the site to remove crust.
  - Rinse with cotton-tipped applicator saturated with 0.9% sodium chloride.
  - Blot the site dry.
- Grasp the tip of the suture (tail) with forceps and gently lift upward on the suture.
- Slide scissors under the suture (Fig. 24.1).
- Cut the suture.
- Gently remove the suture.
- Repeat this procedure until all sutures are removed.
- Blot the area dry as needed with 4 × 4 gauze.
- If the suture line appears slightly unstable, a Steri-Strip or butterfly Band-Aid may be used (see Chapter 20).

METHOD 2—RUNNING SUTURE LINE TECHNIQUE

- Position the client comfortably with sutured area easily accessible.
- Examine sutures to determine the type of suture technique that was used.

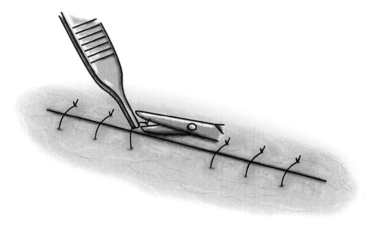

Figure 24.1 Pull the suture tail upward with forceps, slide the scissors under the suture, and cut.

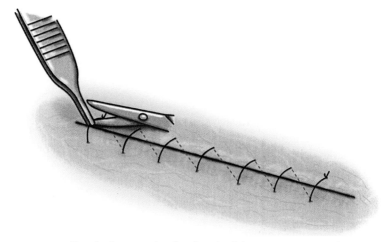

Figure 24.2 Cut the knot at the distal end of the running suture line, grasp the knot at the opposite end with forceps, and gently pull.

- Locate the end tie knot(s).
- If crust is present over suture site
  - Gently roll a cotton-tipped applicator saturated with hydrogen peroxide over the site to remove crust.
  - Rinse with cotton-tipped applicator saturated with 0.9% sodium chloride.
  - Blot the site dry.
- Cut the knot at the distal end of the suture line (Fig. 24.2).
- Grasp the opposite knot with forceps.
- Pull gently with a continuous steady motion until suture is removed.
- Blot the area dry as needed with 4 × 4 gauze.
- If the suture line appears slightly unstable, a Steri-Strip or butterfly Band-Aid may be used (see Chapter 20).

METHOD 3—SMALL LOOP SUTURES, CLOSED SUTURES, AND DIFFICULT ANATOMICAL POSITION SUTURES TECHNIQUE

- Position the client comfortably with sutured area easily accessible.
- Examine sutures to determine the type of suture technique that was used.
- Locate the end tie knot(s).
- If crust is present over suture site
  - Gently roll a cotton-tipped applicator saturated with hydrogen peroxide over the site to remove crust.
  - Rinse with cotton-tipped applicator saturated with 0.9% sodium chloride.
  - Blot the site dry.
- Take no. 11 scalpel and place flat on skin (Fig. 24.3).
- Slide the scalpel under the suture, and exert the sharp edge against suture.
- Use forceps to remove the suture.
- Blot the area dry as needed with 4 × 4 gauze.
- If the suture line appears slightly unstable, a Steri-Strip or butterfly Band-Aid may be used (see Chapter 20).

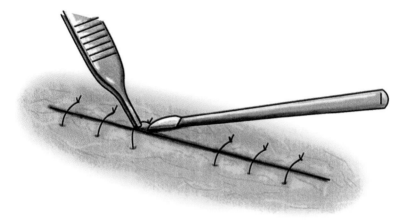

Figure 24.3 Pull the suture tail upward with forceps, slide the no. 11 scalpel under the suture, and cut.

BIBLIOGRAPHY

Forsch RT, Little SH, Williams C. Laceration repair: A practical approach. *Am Fam Physician.* 2017;95(10):628–636.
Pfenninger J, Fowler G. *Procedures for Primary Care Physicians.* St. Louis, MO: Mosby; 2019.
Trott A. *Wounds and Lacerations: Emergency Care and Closure.* St. Louis, MO: Saunders; 2012.

Chapter **25**

Tick Removal
Margaret R. Colyar

CPT Code
10120   Removal of superficial foreign body, skin
10121   Removal of foreign body, complex

Ticks are small, blood-sucking ectoparasites. Ticks burrow into the skin and may become buried, resulting in pain and infection.

OVERVIEW

- Incidence is unknown.
- Ascertain the following:
  - Length of time the tick has been embedded
  - What attempts have been made to remove it
  - Locale (camping, woods, contact with animals) where the tick may have been picked up
- Presence or absence of **erythema migrans**.
- If possible, attempt to identify the tick (dog tick versus deer tick).
  - If the tick has been removed, did the individual bring the tick to the office?
  - Is the tick intact (no missing parts)?
  - Knowledge of ticks indigenous to the geographical location where the individual had spent time
- Allergies to medication.
- History of immunosuppressive disorders or poor wound healing.

General Principles

- Avoid use of finger to "pull tick out."
- Use gloves to protect self from contamination.
- Avoid manipulating the tick because this increases the release of more irritant juices into the tissue.
- Avoid crushing the tick.
- Avoid tearing tissue on removal of the tick.
- Prevent residual parts of the tick from being left in tissue.
- Alcohol, nail polish, and burning tick off no longer are considered appropriate intervention therapies because these techniques increase the chance of the tick releasing juices and leaving body parts embedded in the skin.

Different types of ticks cause different diseases that are endemic to different areas (Table 25.1). Ticks are known vectors of the following diseases:

- Babesiosis
- Colorado tick fever
- Ehrlichiosis
- Lyme disease
- Q fever
- Relapsing fever
- Rocky Mountain spotted fever
- Tick fever
- Tularemia
- Typhus

Antibiotic therapy for tick infestations (especially Lyme disease) should not be initiated unless the clinical presentation includes erythema migrans and/or bacterial **cellulitis.**

Table 25·1	**Types of Ticks**	
TYPE AND SUBTYPE	**DISEASE CAUSES**	**ENDEMIC AREA**
Hard-Shelled Tick (Ixodidae)		
	Highest frequency in causing localized reaction; highest percentage vector of disease	Northeast United States, Wisconsin, Minnesota, California
Spirochete	Lyme disease (*Borrelia burgdorferi*)	Western United States
Soft-Shelled Ticks (*Ornithodoros, Dermacentor, Amblyomma*)		
Spirochete	Relapsing fever (*Borrelia* spp.)	Southeastern United States
Rickettsia	Q fever	Western United States
	Rocky Mountain spotted fever (*Rickettsia rickettsii*); Ehrlichiosis (*Ehrlichia chaffeensis*)	South-central United States
	Typhus (*Rickettsia* spp.)	South-central and southern Atlantic United States
Bacteria	Tularemia (*Francisella tularensis*)	Arkansas, Missouri, Oklahoma
Protozoa	Babesiosis (*Babesia* spp.)	Northeastern United States
Virus	Colorado tick fever (*Coltivirus* spp.)	Western United States
Toxin	Neurotoxin	Northwestern and southern United States

HEALTH PROMOTION/PREVENTION

Environmental

- Avoid areas that support tick populations.
- Avoid direct contact with mammals with a high population of ticks (especially deer and rodents).
- Avoid wooded areas and activities such as
  - Camping
  - Hunting

Physical

- When out in the woods, wear the following:
  - Light-colored clothing, which allows ticks to be spotted before they become embedded in the skin
  - Tight-fitting clothes around the wrists, neck, and ankles
  - Closed-toe shoes
- Inspect for tick infestations.
  - All sleeping bags
  - Tents
  - Body, especially crevices during and after outdoor exposure

- Prompt and proper technique in removal of the tick lessens the risk of transmission of the disease. *Most disease transmission (including Lyme disease) requires 24 to 48 hours of contact for vector transmission.*

Chemical

- Wear insect repellents such as
  - Natural repellents, including oil of citronella (Treo and Avon's Skin-So-Soft)
  - DEET (*N,N*-diethyl-meta-toluamide) on body and clothing to retard tick infestations
  - Permethrins in aerosols for clothing to retard tick infestations

Tetanus (Tdap)

- Give prophylactic injection if not received within the past 5 years.

OPTIONS

- *Method 1*—Forceps/tweezers technique
- *Method 2*—Thread technique
- *Method 3*—Punch biopsy technique
  - Use if the other two methods are unsuccessful.

RATIONALE

- Prompt and proper removal of an embedded tick reduces the incidence of disease transmission to the individual.

INDICATIONS

- Presence of embedded tick

CONTRAINDICATIONS

- Near eye
- Near artery

▶ *Informed consent required.*

PROCEDURE

Tick Removal

Equipment

- Methods 1, 2, and 3
  - Antiseptic skin cleanser
  - Gloves—nonsterile
  - 1% lidocaine
  - 3-mL syringe
  - 25- to 27-gauge, ½- to 1-inch needle
  - Magnifying lens—optional
  - Blunted curved forceps or tweezers—sterile
  - 4 × 4 gauze—sterile

- Band-Aids
  - 0.9% sodium chloride—sterile
- Method 2 only
  - Suture material (nylon), 4-0 or 5-0
- Method 3 only
  - Iris scissors—sterile
  - Punch biopsy

Procedure

METHOD 1—FORCEPS/TWEEZERS TECHNIQUE

- Position client comfortably with tick site easily accessible. Cleanse area with topical antiseptic cleanser.
- Put on gloves.
- Inject 1 mL of 1% lidocaine at the base of the embedded tick until a small wheal has formed, being careful not to inject the tick until the wheal has formed (Fig. 25.1).
- Grasp tick as close to the skin as possible (Fig. 25.2).
  - Use extra caution if the tick is buried in areas where there is hair.
- Pull on the tick using gentle and steady upward pressure for 2 to 4 minutes. This should permit the tick to back out of the site.
  - Do not twist or jerk the tick out because this may result in incomplete removal of the tick and tearing of the skin.
- Dispose of tick in a container to prevent reinfestation.
- Wash area gently with topical antiseptic cleanser.
- Rinse with 0.9% sodium chloride.

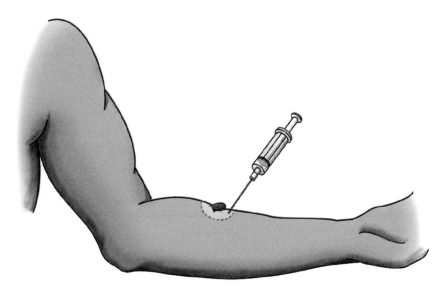

Figure 25.1 Inject lidocaine at the base of the embedded tick, but do not inject the tick.

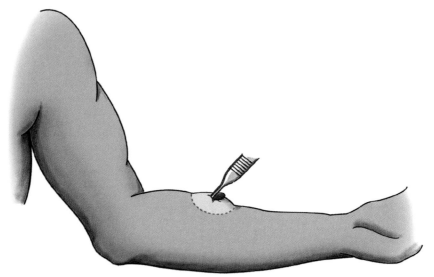

Figure 25.2 Method 1—Grasp the tick as close to the skin as possible and pull gently, allowing the tick to back out of the site.

- Topical antibiotic ointment is not recommended.
- Apply a Band-Aid. Instruct the client to remove the Band-Aid as soon as he or she arrives home. Exposure to air lessens risk of secondary infection.

METHOD 2—THREAD TECHNIQUE
- Position client comfortably with tick site easily accessible. Cleanse area with topical antiseptic cleanser.
- Put on gloves.
- Inject 1 mL of 1% lidocaine at the base of the embedded tick until a small wheal has formed, being careful not to inject the tick until the wheal has formed.
- Cut a 6-inch length of 4-0 or 5-0 polyfilament suture.
- Make a loop knot.
- Slide it over the embedded tick.
- Gently draw it tight over the smallest part of the tick as close to the skin as possible.
- Pull both ends of the suture firmly upward until the skin is lifted (Fig. 25.3).
- Hold tension on the tick for 3 to 4 minutes to allow the tick to back out.
- Dispose of the tick in a container to prevent reinfestation.
- Wash the area gently with antiseptic skin cleanser.
- Rinse with 0.9% sodium chloride.
- Topical antibiotic ointment is not recommended.
- Apply Band-Aid. Instruct the client to remove the Band-Aid as soon as he or she gets home. Exposure to air lessens risk of secondary infection.

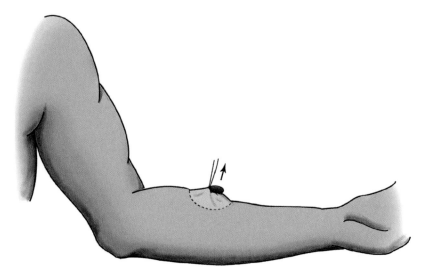

Figure 25.3 Method 2—Slide a loop of suture over the tick, and pull gently, allowing the tick to back out of the site.

METHOD 3—PUNCH BIOPSY TECHNIQUE

Used in situations in which other techniques have not been successful or body parts of the tick have been retained in the skin.

- Position client comfortably with tick site easily accessible. Cleanse area with topical antiseptic cleanser.
- Put on gloves.
- Inject 1 mL of 1% lidocaine at the base of the embedded tick until a small wheal has formed, being careful not to inject the tick until the wheal has formed.
- Follow the steps for punch biopsy technique in Chapter 1.
- Dispose of the tissue in a container to prevent reinfestation.
- Consider sending tissue for pathology to ensure all tick body parts have been removed.
- Irrigate wound with 0.9% sodium chloride (approximately 30 to 60 mL).
- Apply pressure to the site for 2 minutes.
- If persistent bleeding occurs despite pressure to site, use of coagulant agent (aluminum chloride, Gelfoam) or suture may be required.
- Apply 4 × 4 gauze dressing and tape in place.

Client Instructions

METHODS 1 AND 2

- Keep the wound clean and dry.
- After 24 hours, the dressing may be removed, and the site may be left open to air. Continuous covering of wounds increases the risk of infection.

- If crust develops over the bite site,
  - Cleanse by gently rolling a cotton-tipped swab saturated with hydrogen peroxide over the wound site.
  - Gently rinse the area with warm water.
  - Blot dry with clean towel or cotton gauze.
- Observe for signs and symptoms of infection, such as
  - Elevated temperature
  - Yellow or greenish drainage
  - Redness or swelling
  - Foul odor
  - Increase in pain after 24 hours
- If any signs and symptoms of infection are found, return to the office.
- Return to the office in 48 hours for wound recheck.

METHOD 3 ONLY

- Keep dressing clean, dry, and in place for 48 hours to decrease the chance of bleeding and oozing.
- Avoid touching or contaminating the area biopsied.
- To prevent the chance of infection, take cephalexin 500 mg three times per day or cefadroxil 500 mg twice per day for 5 days.
- Some redness, swelling, and heat are normal.
- Return to the office if symptoms of infection occur, such as
  - Elevated temperature
  - Yellow or greenish drainage
  - Redness or swelling
  - Foul odor
  - Increase in pain after 24 hours
- To decrease pain, use Tylenol No. 3 for severe pain every 4 to 6 hours as needed. After 24 hours, use acetaminophen, ibuprofen, or naproxen every 4 to 6 hours as needed for mild pain.

BIBLIOGRAPHY ▪▪▪▪▪▪▪▪▪▪▪▪▪▪▪▪▪▪▪▪▪▪▪▪▪▪

Habif T. *Clinical Dermatology: A Color Guide to Diagnosis and Therapy.* 6th ed. St. Louis, MO: Mosby; 2015.

Kimberlin DW, Brady MT, Jackson MA, Long SS, eds. *Red Book: 2018 Report of the Committee on Infectious Disease.* Elk Grove Village, IL: American Academy of Pediatrics; 2018.

Murtagh J. *Murtagh's Practice Tips.* 7th ed. New York, NY: McGraw-Hill; 2017.

Pfenninger JL, Fowler GC. *Procedures for Primary Care Physicians.* St. Louis, MO: Mosby; 2019.

Chapter **26**

Topical Hemostatic Agent Application

Margaret R. Colyar

CPT Code
    None

Application of a chemical agent ensures rapid hemostasis of capillaries and small blood vessels and is used frequently as an initial agent in situations in which rapid hemostasis or vasoconstriction to small areas of tissue is required and/or in which there is the lack of available electrocautery. It also commonly is used in dermatological situations.

OVERVIEW

- Complications
  - Rare hypopigmentation or hyperpigmentation of skin
  - Rare localized inflammation and scarring of skin
- Obtain the following information
  - Sensitivity to the agent being used
  - Medical contraindications to use of epinephrine (if used)
  - History of poor healing characteristics
  - History of exaggerated hypopigmentation or hyperpigmentation of the skin caused by chemical agents

RATIONALE

- To promote hemostasis without the use of electrocautery

INDICATIONS

- Skin lesions

CONTRAINDICATIONS

- With a distal digit or skin appendage, may cause ischemia and necrosis
- Cardiovascular diseases

PROCEDURE

Topical Hemostatic Agent Application

Equipment

- Gloves—nonsterile
- Cotton-tipped applicators—sterile
- Fenestrated drape—sterile
- 4 × 4 gauze—sterile
- Topical **hemostatic agent** of choice (Table 26.1)

Procedure

- Position the client with the area easily accessible.
- Put on gloves.
- Establish a clean field around lesion using fenestrated drape.
- Choose topical hemostatic agent.
- Prepare the topical applicator.
  - If solution, dip the cotton-tipped applicator to impregnate it with the solution. Caution should be taken not to spill or splash the solution.

Table 26·1   **Types of Common Topical Hemostatic Agents**
Monsel's Solution (Ferric Subsulfate)
• Allows rapid hemolysis
• Good agent with **seborrheic keratoses** and **basal cell carcinoma**
• Disadvantage: Can cause pigment changes and staining
Aluminum Chloride 30% (Drysol)
• Fast hemolysis, but not as fast as Monsel's solution
• Not as irritating to the skin
• Liquid application or cotton applicator
• Less incidence of pigment changes and staining
Silver Nitrate
• Fast hemolysis, equal to aluminum chloride
• Least expensive of topical hemostatic agents
• Usually in the form of impregnated cotton applicators
• Disadvantage: Sensitive to moisture exposure
• High incidence of pigment changes and staining
Epinephrine (Topical or Injectable Application). *Never use in digit applications.*
• Extremely potent vasoconstriction agent
• May be applied topically, intradermally, or subcutaneously
• Disadvantage: Use of large amount can result in tissue necrosis and sloughing.

- Using two digits, apply tension to the skin surrounding the lesion.
- Wipe excess blood off with sterile gauze.
- Apply the chemically impregnated cotton-tipped applicator to the desired site for approximately 15 seconds.
- Remove the cotton-tipped applicator and release the skin.
- Observe to determine whether successful hemolysis has occurred.
- May need to repeat the procedure twice for successful hemolysis.

Client Instructions

- Infection rarely is associated with this procedure. Observe for signs and symptoms of infection, such as
  - Increased redness and warmth at the site
  - Red streaks
  - Swelling with green or yellow drainage
- Skin may appear inflamed and reddened for 24 to 48 hours from normal chemical irritation of the hemostatic agent.
- Hyperpigmentation and hypopigmentation changes can occur and usually do not resolve.
- Pain is usually minimal and may be relieved with acetaminophen taken every 4 hours as needed.
- Tetanus injection is not indicated if the wound was surgically induced.
- Return to the office if rebleeding occurs.

BIBLIOGRAPHY

Habif T. *Clinical Dermatology: A Color Guide to Diagnosis and Therapy.* 6th ed. St. Louis, MO: Mosby; 2015.
Pfenninger JL, Fowler GC. *Procedures for Primary Care Physicians.* St. Louis, MO: Mosby; 2019.
Trott A. *Wounds and Lacerations: Emergency Care and Closure.* St. Louis, MO: Mosby; 2012.

Chapter **27**

Ulcer Debridement
Margaret R. Colyar

CPT Code
11040   Debridement: Skin, partial thickness
11041   Debridement: Skin, full thickness
11042   Debridement: Skin, and subcutaneous tissue

Table 27·1 Types of Debridement Materials	
TYPE OF DRESSING	**USED FOR**
Alginates (Kaltostat, Sorbsan)	Prevents maceration of surrounding skin from excess fluid.
Hydrogels (IntraSite, Elasto-Gel, ClearSite, Aquasorb)	Wounds with larger volumes of exudate.
Hydrocolloid wafers (DuoDERM, Comfeel, Tegasorb, Restore) • Promote autolysis, angiogenesis, and granulation.	To "seal" a wound that is otherwise clean in order to promote healing. Self-adhesive. Remain in place for 5–7 days. Can also be used to seal an underlying dressing in order to maintain a moist environment in which the wound can heal.
Thin films (OpSite, Tegaderm)	For skin at risk or Stage I pressure ulcers. Can also hold another type of absorbent dressing in place.
Cotton gauze	Covering the primary dressing. Rarely an appropriate dressing for a significant skin ulcer.

Debridement is the process of removing nonliving (necrotic) tissue from pressure ulcers, burns, and other wounds. There are four types of debridement: surgical (sharp), mechanical, autolytic, and enzymatic debridement. Sharp debridement uses scalpels, scissors, or other instruments to cut dead tissue from a wound and is the quickest and most efficient method. Mechanical debridement uses a saline-moistened dressing applied to the dead tissue; it is allowed to dry overnight and adhere to the dead tissue. It can be very painful. Autolytic and enzymatic debridement use synthetic dressings (see Table 27.1).

OVERVIEW—DOCUMENTATION REQUIREMENTS
• Indications for debridement
• Size
• Location
• Observed depth of ulcer(s)
• Specific depth/level of debridement

RATIONALE
• To remove necrotic tissue
• To preserve granulation tissue
• To speed the healing of pressure ulcers, burns, and other wounds

INDICATIONS
• Dry ulcers need moisture added through a hypotonic gel (donates water).
• Wet exudates require a hypertonic gel or foam to remove water.

CONTRAINDICATIONS

- Significant vascular compromise
- No healing potential
- Deep structures involve tendons, bones
- Clean, granulating wounds

Before performing debridement, consider the following:

- Inadequate blood flow
- Immunosuppressive therapies
- Poor nutrition
- Inadequate diabetes control
- High levels of anticoagulants

Complications

- Do not use cytotoxic fluids (Betadine) to cleanse area; it will kill granulation tissue.

▶ *Informed consent required*

PROCEDURE

Debridement of Ulcers

Equipment

- *Method 1*—Surgical (sharp) debridement
  - Scalpel
  - Scissors
  - Forceps
  - 4 × 4 gauze
  - Gloves
  - Saline solution for flushing
  - Topical anesthetic gel
  - Topical antibiotic
  - Nonadherent dressing material (Telfa)
  - Tape
- *Method 2*—Mechanical debridement
  - Gloves
  - Saline-moistened dressing
  - Dry topical dressing
  - Tape
- *Method 3*—Autolytic debridement
  - Gloves
  - Synthetic dressing such as hydrogel or hydrocolloid for mildly draining wounds
  - Synthetic dressing such as alginate for moderately to strongly draining wounds
  - DuoDerm

- *Method 4*—Enzymatic debridement (chemical debridement)
  - Gloves
  - Accuzyme, Panafil, Xenaderm, or Santyl
  - DuoDerm

Procedure

METHOD 1—SURGICAL DEBRIDEMENT

- Put on gloves.
- Cleanse area to be debrided with saline and 4 × 4 gauze.
- Apply topical anesthetic gel to edges of the wound.
- Using forceps, grip the necrotic tissue.
- Cut away the necrotic tissue bit by bit with scalpel or scissors.
- Apply topical antibiotic.
- Cover with nonadherent dressing (Telfa).
- Secure with tape.

METHOD 2—MECHANICAL DEBRIDEMENT

*Note: Mechanical debridement cannot select between good and bad tissue; therefore, it is an unacceptable debridement method for clean wounds in which a new layer of healing cells is already developing.

- Put on gloves.
- Cleanse area to be debrided with saline and 4 × 4 gauze.
- Saturate dressing for saline.
- Express excess water.
- Apply dressing to necrotic tissue only.
- Cover with dry dressing.
- Apply tape.
- Allow dressing to dry for 24 hours; then pull the dressing from the wound.

METHOD 3—AUTOLYTIC DEBRIDEMENT—CONTRAINDICATED WITH INFECTED WOUNDS

- Put on gloves.
- Cleanse area to be debrided with saline and 4 × 4 gauze.
- Apply dressing to necrotic tissue.
- Cover with DuoDerm.

METHOD 4—ENZYMATIC DEBRIDEMENT

Use when surgical debridement is not possible and wound is infected.

- Put on gloves.
- Cleanse area to be debrided with saline and 4 × 4 gauze.
- Apply dressing to necrotic tissue.
- Cover with DuoDerm.

Client Instructions

- Tylenol or Ibuprofen for pain

- Monitor for
  - Yellow or greenish drainage
  - Red streaks
  - Elevated temperature
- Keep follow-up appointment.

BIBLIOGRAPHY ▬▬▬▬▬▬▬▬▬▬▬▬▬▬▬▬▬▬▬▬▬

Dziedzic ME. *Fast Facts About Pressure Ulcer Care for Nurses: How to Prevent, Detect, and Resolve Them in a Nutshell.* New York, NY: Springer; 2013.

Prevention and Treatment of Pressure Ulcers: Clinical Practice Guidelines. https://www.ehob.com/media/2018/04/prevention-and-treatment-of-pressure-ulcers-clinical-practice-guidline.pdf.

von Gunten CF, Ferris F. Pressure ulcers: debridement and dressings. 2nd ed. *Fast Facts and Concepts.* August 2005;41. mywhatever.com/cifwriter/library/eperc/fastfact/ff41.html.

Musculoskeletal Procedures

Chapter **28**

Bone Marrow Aspiration and Biopsy

Cynthia R. Ehrhardt

CPT Code
85095   Bone marrow aspiration
85102   Bone marrow biopsy, needle or trocar

Bone marrow aspiration is one of the diagnostic tools used to assess the status of the hematopoietic system. It involves extracting small amounts of myeloid tissue from a bony cavity (e.g., the sternum or iliac crest). The posterior-superior spine portion of the iliac crest is considered the first choice site because there is a higher percentage of success in obtaining quantities of bone marrow sufficient for diagnostic testing.

Bone marrow aspiration provides accurate information on the relative number of stem cells and their development and morphological structure. A follow-up technique, bone marrow **biopsy**, provides a more specific morphology of the bone.

OVERVIEW

- Complications
  - Potentially painful
  - Potential hemorrhage at the site
  - Risk of introducing infection to the bone, which can lead to **osteomyelitis**
  - Retroperitoneal hemorrhage caused by penetration into the bowel cavity by too deep a penetration of the iliac crest
  - Unsuccessful biopsy (known as *dry tap*)

OPTIONS

- Bone marrow aspiration
- Bone marrow biopsy

RATIONALE

- To assess the hematopoietic system
- To evaluate hematopoietic abnormalities

INDICATIONS

- Unexplained anemia
- Unresolved neutropenia after withdrawal from antibiotic therapy
- Suspected metastatic disease
- Abnormal hematopoietic disorder (leukemia, idiopathic thrombocytopenia, pancytopenia)
- Lymphoproliferative disorders, including lymphoma
- Immunodeficiency disorders, including HIV
- Fever of unknown etiology
- Suspected unusual presentation of an infectious disorder (fungal, tuberculosis)
- Chromosomal analysis
- Bone marrow transplantation

CONTRAINDICATIONS

- Severe osteoporosis
- Hemophilia
- Known radiation to bone site

▶ *Informed consent required*

PROCEDURE

Bone Marrow Aspiration and Biopsy

Equipment

Prepackaged disposable kits are available.

- Gloves—sterile
- Povidone-iodine (Betadine)
- Fenestrated drape—sterile
- 3-mL syringe
- Two needles—21 gauge and 25 gauge, 1½ inch
- 1% or 2% lidocaine without epinephrine
- 10-mL syringe prepared with ethylenediamine tetra-acetic acid (EDTA) solution rinse
- Complete blood count purple-top (EDTA) laboratory test tube
- No. 11 scalpel
- Bone marrow aspiration needle
- Jamshidi bone marrow biopsy needles (optional)
- Microscope glass slides
- Fixative specimen container
- 4 × 4 gauze—sterile
- Tape

Procedure

BONE MARROW ASPIRATION—ILIAC CREST

- Position the client comfortably on abdomen. A pillow under the area of the procedure may relax the individual.
- Identify the posterior-superior landmarks.
- Cleanse the area of the aspiration and 3 inches surrounding with povidone-iodine.
- Open the bone marrow kit.
- Put on sterile gloves.
- Draw up lidocaine in the 3-mL syringe with the 25-gauge needle.
- Insert the needle intradermally at the site, and inject a small amount of lidocaine until a wheal has formed.
- Replace the 25-gauge needle with the 21-gauge needle, and penetrate deeper into the tissue until the periosteum of the site is felt. Inject approximately 1 mL into the area; then slowly withdraw while infiltrating the needle tract with the remaining solution.
- While waiting for local anesthetic to work (5 to 10 minutes), confirm that the obdurator of the biopsy needle is locked in place and the cap is secured.
- When the skin is anesthetized, use the No. 11 scalpel and make a small (0.25 cm or less) stab wound.
- Insert the biopsy needle at a 90-degree angle into the incision with the capped end in the palm of the hand and the shaft between two fingers (usually index and middle fingers) until resistance of the periosteum is felt.
- Instruct the client that the next part of the procedure may cause a pressure sensation.
- Simultaneously begin to apply downward pressure and alternate clockwise and counterclockwise motions to penetrate the cortex of the bone.
- Continue this until penetration for approximately 1 cm until the "give" of the cortex is felt. Halt downward pressure, and advance approximately 1 to 2 mm farther to ensure placement in the marrow. The biopsy needle should be held in place by the skin and bone.
- Unlock the cap of the syringe, withdraw the obturator, and attach the EDTA-prepared 10-mL syringe.
- Counsel client that pain may be felt at this time and to remain as still as possible.
- Pull up on the plunger of syringe. This creates a vacuum, allowing bone marrow contents to be aspirated. If no material is withdrawn, advance the needle an additional 1 to 2 mm, and repeat aspiration.
- If still no response, withdraw the needle from that periosteum site, and try another site within the incision.
- Withdraw a minimum of 5 mL of marrow. A good specimen shows grossly visible bone **spicules**.
- Prepare the smears (may be performed by nonsterile assistant) in the following manner.
  - Thinly spread the bone marrow aspiration material over one glass specimen slide and cover with second slide.

- Gently squeeze the two slides together, and allow any excess blood to drain off the slides.
- After excess blood is removed, roll the slides apart lengthwise.
  - This allows thinning of any layering of the specimen.
- On successful aspiration, remove the needle, and apply pressure over the area using a quarter-folded 4 × 4 gauze and tape as a pressure dressing.
- Have the client remain supine for 1 hour with pressure dressing in place.
- After 1 hour, the client may get up and leave.

BONE MARROW BIOPSY—USUALLY PERFORMED ON THE ILIAC CREST

- Position the client comfortably on abdomen. A pillow under the area of the procedure may relax the individual.
- Identify the posterior-superior landmarks.
- Cleanse the area of the aspiration and 3 inches surrounding with povidone-iodine.
- Open the bone marrow kit.
- Put on sterile gloves.
- Draw up lidocaine in the 3-mL syringe with the 25-gauge needle.
- Insert the needle intradermally at the site and inject a small amount of lidocaine until a wheal has formed.
- Replace the 25-gauge needle with the 21-gauge needle, and penetrate deeper into the tissue until the periosteum of the site is felt. Inject approximately 1 mL into the area; then slowly withdraw while infiltrating the needle tract with the remaining solution.
- While waiting for local anesthesia to work (5 to 10 minutes), confirm that the obdurator of the biopsy needle is locked in place and cap is secured.
- When the skin is anesthetized, use the No. 11 scalpel and make a small (0.25 cm or less) stab wound.
- Insert the biopsy needle at a 90-degree angle into the incision with the capped end in the palm of the hand and the shaft between two fingers (usually index and middle fingers) until resistance of the periosteum is felt.
- Instruct patient that he or she may feel pain and pressure.
- Simultaneously begin to apply downward pressure and alternate clockwise and counterclockwise motions to penetrate the cortex of the bone.
- Continue this until penetration for approximately 1 cm until the "give" of the cortex is felt. Halt downward pressure, and advance approximately 1 to 2 mm farther to ensure placement in the marrow. The biopsy needle should be held in place by the skin and bone.
- When the biopsy syringe has been placed in the marrow, withdraw the needle 3 mm to have it placed in the cortex.
- Redirect the angle of the needle toward the anterior iliac spine, and advance it into the cortex until resistance decreases.
- Remove the obdurator and perform an alternate clockwise and counterclockwise motion for a distance of 2 cm.
- Proceed to rock the needle clockwise five times and then counterclockwise five times to ensure a good specimen.

- Change the angle approximately 15 degrees, and repeat previous step. This allows the specimen to be severed from the marrow.
- Cover the opening of bone marrow needle with your thumb and withdraw it.
- Insert the obturator and allow the specimen to be pushed out onto sterile 4 × 4 gauze.
- Prepare the smears (may be performed by nonsterile assistant) in the following manner.
  - Using a light touch, gently touch four glass slides to the specimen on the gauze.
- Place the specimen in a container with the fixative agent.
- On completion, remove needle, and apply pressure over the area using a quarter-folded sterile 4 × 4 gauze and tape as a pressure dressing.
- Have the client remain supine for 1 hour with pressure dressing in place.
- After 1 hour, client may get up and leave.

Client Instructions

- Infection rarely is associated with this procedure. Observe for signs and symptoms of infection, however, such as
  - Increased redness and warmth at the site
  - Red streaks
  - Swelling with drainage
  - Pus from site
- Contact your health-care provider if any of the following symptoms occur within 48 hours:
  - Fever
  - Abdominal pain
  - Unrelieved site pain
- Leave the pressure dressing on for 12 hours. After that time, the dressing may be removed and a standard dressing applied.
- Keep the site clean and dry for 24 hours.
- Avoid strenuous exercise for 48 hours.
- Pain is usually minimal and may be relieved with acetaminophen (Tylenol) or acetaminophen with codeine (Tylenol No. 3).
- Return to the office in 48 hours for recheck.

BIBLIOGRAPHY

Malempati S, Joshi S, Lai S, Braner AV, Tegtmeyer K. Bone marrow aspiration and biopsy. *N Engl J Med.* 2009;361:e28.

McCance K, Huether S. *Pathophysiology: The Biological Basis for Disease in Adults and Children.* 7th ed. St. Louis, MO: Mosby; 2014.

Paulman P. Marrow sampling. *Am Fam Physician.* 1989;40(6):85–87.

Pfenninger JL, Fowler GC. *Procedures for Primary Care Physicians.* St. Louis, MO: Mosby; 2019.

Trejo-Ayala RA, Luna-Perez M, Gutierrez-Romero M, Collazo-Jaloma M, Cedillo-Perez MC, Ramos-Penafiel CO. Bone marrow aspiration and biopsy, Technique and considerations. *Revista Médica Del Hospital General De México.* 2015;78(4):196–201.

29 Chapter

X-Ray Interpretation
Bones

Margaret R. Colyar

CPT Code
   Multiple listings based on area of body being x-rayed

X-rays of the musculoskeletal system are taken to determine the presence of disease, including arthritis, spondylitis, bone lesions, and fractures. The bone x-ray should be correlated with clinical history, physical examination, and additional diagnostic tool results.

OVERVIEW

- Densities
    - Air—DARK
    - Muscles—GRAY
    - Fat—Light GRAY
    - Muscle—Very light GRAY
    - Bones—WHITE
    - Foreign body—Varies based on density
        - Coin—DARK
        - Wood splinter—Difficult to see
- Inspect the posterior-anterior (PA) view to determine whether the x-ray is adequate using **RIPE.**
    - **R**otation—Do the clavicles and vertebrae form a cross?
    - **I**nspiration—Is there a minimum of eight ribs visible?
    - **P**enetration—Are the interspaces visible and the thoracic vertebral bodies well defined?
    - **E**xposure—Too much or too little?
- Approach must be systematic.
- Food and drinks are *not* restricted before musculoskeletal x-rays.
- Clothing, jewelry, hairpins, and dentures should be removed, depending on the area of the body being x-rayed.
- The genital area should be shielded unless the area to be x-rayed is the pelvis.
- In children or adolescents, the contralateral side always should be x-rayed for comparison purposes.

- Long bones should not be x-rayed without the joint.
- Always view a chest x-ray as if you are facing the client. The client's right will be on your left.

RATIONALE

- To determine the presence of
  - Fractures
  - Dislocations
  - Soft tissue injury
  - Disease processes

INDICATIONS

- Clinical suspicion of disease, injury, or deformity
- Pain of unknown origin

CONTRAINDICATIONS

- Pregnancy (unless shielded)

PROCEDURE

Interpretation of Musculoskeletal X-Rays

Equipment

- X-ray view box or digital viewing program

Procedure

Systematic approach to bone x-ray interpretation includes (Fig. 29.1)
- *Anatomical alignment and position*
- *Bone age*—Check epiphyseal growth plates. Epiphyses begin to appear at birth. Ossification usually is completed by age 20 in females and age 23 in males.
- *Bone density*—Density should be consistent over the entire bone. Changes in density indicate fractures, tumors, and sclerosis.
- *Continuity*—Check for fractures in bones and joint capsules (Fig. 29.2).
- *Cortex thickness*—As an adult ages, the cortex thins. If greater than 50% of the cortex is gone, REFER to an orthopedic surgeon.
- *Lucency*—Spotted lucency and dense sclerosis indicate
  - Bone metastases—spine and skull usually involved
  - Congenital diseases
  - Infectious diseases
  - Neoplastic diseases
  - Metabolical diseases—hyperparathyroidism or nutritional deficits—osteoporosis, malformation, and others
- *Periosteum*—Thickening indicates stress fractures or inflammation.
- *Size and shape of the bone*—Check for abnormalities in contour or excess calcification.
- *Soft tissue inflammation*—Inflammation indicates **osteomyelitis**.

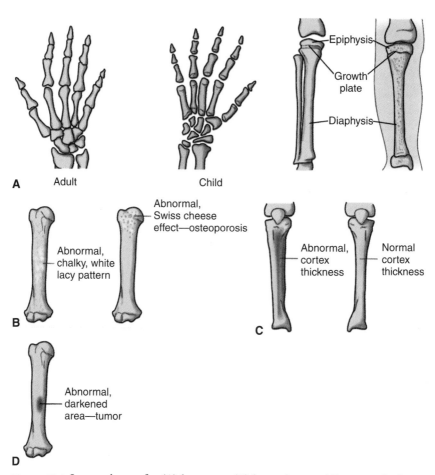

Figure 29.1 Inspect bones for (A) bone age, (B) bone density, (C) cortex thickness, and (D) lucency.

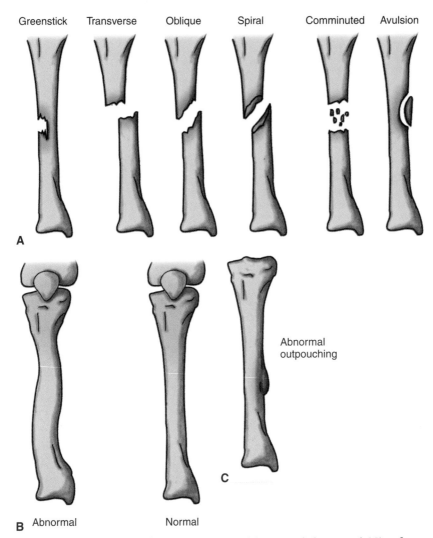

Greenstick   Transverse   Oblique   Spiral   Comminuted   Avulsion

A

Abnormal
outpouching

C

B Abnormal   Normal

Figure 29.2 Inspect bones for (A) continuity, (B) size and shape, and (C) soft tissue inflammation.

BIBLIOGRAPHY

Mayhew MS. *Procedures for the Primary Care Provider*. St. Louis, MO: Mosby; 2016.
Mercier LR. *Practical Orthopedics*. St. Louis, MO: Mosby; 2008.

30 Chapter

Arthrocentesis

Margaret R. Colyar

CPT Code
20600 Arthrocentesis, aspiration, or injection; small joint, bursa
20605 Arthrocentesis, intermediate joint or bursa
20610 Arthrocentesis, major joint or bursa

Arthrocentesis is the aspiration of fluid from a joint space. It is performed to decrease inflammation or differentiate the diagnosis between intra-articular and extra-articular origin. Knowledge of the injection site anatomy is crucial.

OPTIONS

- *Method 1*—Arthrocentesis only
  - Used to remove fluid for diagnostic purposes
- *Method 2*—Arthrocentesis with intra-articular corticosteroid injection
  - Used to remove fluid and inject corticosteroid to decrease inflammation and pain

RATIONALE

- To diminish inflammation of the joint
- To differentiate the diagnosis between intra-articular and extra-articular origin

INDICATIONS

- Remove joint fluid
- Decrease pain in a joint
- Diagnose the cause of joint inflammation

CONTRAINDICATIONS

- Anticoagulation therapy
- Presence of joint prosthesis
- Recent joint injury
▶ *Informed consent required*

PROCEDURE

- Sites for arthrocentesis (see Chapter 36)

Arthrocentesis
Equipment
- Methods 1 and 2
  - Alcohol prep pads
  - Povidone-iodine prep pads
  - Gloves—nonsterile
  - One or two syringes—10 to 20 mL
  - 18- to 20-gauge, 1½-inch needle
  - 4 × 4 gauze—sterile
  - Tape
  - Elastic bandage—3 or 4 inches
  - Culture tubes
  - **Hemostats**—sterile
- Method 2 only
  - 1% lidocaine (single-dose vial)
  - Corticosteroid of choice

Procedure
METHOD 1—ARTHROCENTESIS ONLY
- Position the client with the affected joint slightly flexed.
- Mark the injection site with your thumbnail.
- Cleanse the injection site with alcohol first, then with povidone-iodine.
- Let povidone-iodine air-dry.
- Put on gloves.
- Insert the syringe with the 18-gauge needle at a 90-degree angle, and aspirate the fluid.
- If blood is aspirated and a hematoma is not suspected, withdraw the needle.
- If more fluid needs to be removed (Fig. 30.1)
  - Stabilize the needle with the hemostats.
  - Remove the filled syringe and replace with an empty syringe.
  - Reaspirate.
- Withdraw the fluid, and inject into the culture tubes.
- Apply a pressure dressing with the 4 × 4 gauze and tape securely.
- Apply an elastic bandage.

METHOD 2—ARTHROCENTESIS WITH INTRA-ARTICULAR CORTICOSTEROID INJECTION
- Position the client with the affected joint slightly flexed.
- Mark the injection site with your thumbnail.
- Cleanse the injection site with alcohol first, then with povidone-iodine.
- Let povidone-iodine air-dry.
- Put on gloves.
- Insert the syringe with the 18-gauge needle at a 90-degree angle, and aspirate the fluid.
- If blood is aspirated and a hematoma is not suspected, withdraw the needle.

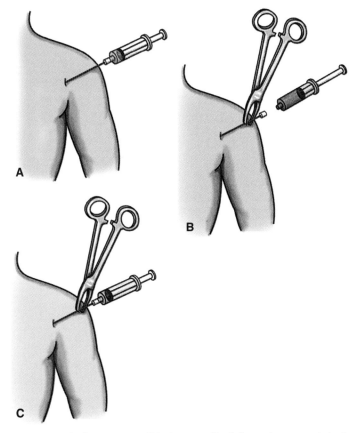

Figure 30.1 Arthrocentesis. (A) Aspirate fluid from the joint. (B) If more fluid needs to be removed, stabilize the needle with hemostats, remove the filled syringe, and (C) replace with an empty syringe.

- If more fluid needs to be removed
  - Stabilize the needle with the hemostats.
  - Remove the filled syringe and replace with an empty syringe.
  - Reaspirate.
- Withdraw the fluid, and inject into the culture tubes.
- If you are planning to inject the joint with a steroid and lidocaine mixture after the aspiration,
  - Stabilize the needle with the hemostat.
  - Remove the filled syringe and inject fluid into the culture tubes.
  - Replace the first syringe with the second syringe, holding the lidocaine and steroid mixture.
  - Inject the mixture steadily into the joint.
  - Remove the syringe from the joint.
  - Apply a pressure dressing with 4 × 4 gauze and tape securely.
  - Apply an elastic bandage.

Client Instructions

- Rest the joint for the next 24 hours.
- Remove the dressing and elastic bandage in 24 hours.
- Observe for signs of infection, such as
  - Increase in pain
  - Fever
  - Yellow or greenish discharge
  - Red streaks
- Sometimes fluid recollects in the joint. If this occurs, return to the office.
- Your culture should be back by _____. We will call you with the results.

BIBLIOGRAPHY

Pfenninger JL, Fowler GC. *Procedures for Primary Care Physicians*. St. Louis, MO: Mosby; 2019.

Thomsen TW, Shen S, Shaffer RW, Setnik GS. Arthrocentesis of the knee. *N Engl J Med*. 2006:354:e19.

Chapter **31**

Compartment Syndrome Assessment

Margaret R. Colyar

CPT Code
None

Compartment syndrome is more common in the lower leg (Fig. 31.1) and forearm (Fig. 31.2), but it can occur in the hand, foot, thigh, and upper arm. Thick layers of tissue (fascia) separate groups of muscles in the arms and legs from each other. Inside each layer of fascia is a confined space called a compartment that includes the muscle tissue, nerves, and blood vessels. Fascia surrounds these structures and does not expand. Any swelling of a compartment will lead to increased pressure, which will press on the muscles, blood vessels, and nerves.

If the pressure to the compartment is high enough, blood flow and oxygen will be blocked, leading to permanent injury to the muscle and nerves. As the

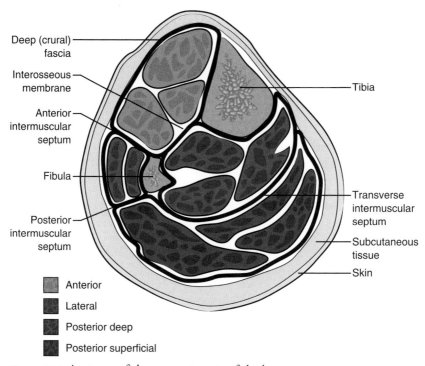

Deep (crural) fascia

Interosseous membrane

Anterior intermuscular septum

Fibula

Posterior intermuscular septum

Tibia

Transverse intermuscular septum

Subcutaneous tissue

Skin

Anterior

Lateral

Posterior deep

Posterior superficial

Figure 31.1 Anatomy of the compartments of the legs.

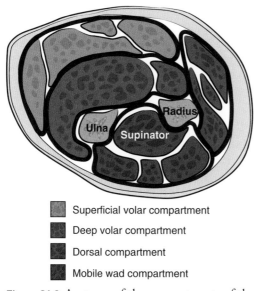

Radius

Ulna Supinator

Superficial volar compartment

Deep volar compartment

Dorsal compartment

Mobile wad compartment

Figure 31.2 Anatomy of the compartments of the forearm.

muscle cells lose their blood and oxygen supply, they use anaerobic metabolism and begin to die. If the pressure lasts long enough, the arm or leg will no longer function. When infection or necrosis develops, the limb may need to be amputated to prevent death.

OVERVIEW

Symptoms of compartment syndrome include
- Decreased sensation
- Numbness and tingling
- Paleness of skin
- Severe pain that gets worse
- Weakness
  On physical examination, suspect the compartment if
- Pain occurs when the area is squeezed
  - Pain that is dramatically out of proportion for the severity of the mechanism of injury
  - Usually described as dull, deep aching
  - Increases upon manipulation of the muscle and passive stretching
- Paresthesia, tingling (pins and needles), is the hallmark sign of compartment syndrome. Numbness not typically associated with limb injuries may indicate nerve damage.
- Paleness, a late sign, caused by vascular compromise—check distal to the injury
- Paralysis, a late sign, common in crush injuries—may imply significant muscle necrosis
- Pulselessness, a late sign—check distal to the extremity. However, a strong pulse and capillary refill do not rule out compartment syndrome, as the artery being palpated may bypass the affected compartment.
- Poikilothermia—the affected limb is cooler than the uninjured limb.
  Causes can be acute or chronic (Table 31.1).

RATIONALE

To prevent injury and death to the muscles and nerves

Tests

See Table 31.2.

Client Instructions

- Follow up with your provider if you experience
  - Pain that is not corrected with pain medication
  - Pain with stretching the affected limb
  - Numbness/tingling
  - Paleness of the skin over the area of pain
  - Paralysis—loss of motion of the affected limb
  - Affected limb cooler than unaffected limb

Table 31·1	Causes of Compartment Syndrome

Acute Causes

Traumatic injury
Crush injury
Fracture
Vein obstructions
Burns
Hemorrhage
Edema
Complication of surgery
Bandages—too tight
Casts—too tight
Snake envenomation
Anabolic steroid use
Venous obstruction
Extravasation of IV infusion
Aggressive fluid resuscitation

Chronic Causes

Repetitive activities such as running, bicycling, swimming
Immobility/compression can cause rhabdomyolysis (muscle breakdown).

Table 31·2	Tests to Determine Compartment Syndrome

Compartment pressure measurement (Fig. 31.3) is the gold standard. It measures pressure within the compartments of the affected limb. A difference of less than or equal to 20 mm Hg between diastolic BP minus compartment pressure is a strong indicator for a fasciotomy.

Lab

- Elevation of serum creatine kinase
- Elevation of urine myoglobin
- Basic metabolic panel (BMP)
- Comprehensive metabolic panel (CMP)—to evaluate organ functions
- Complete blood count (CBC)—to analyze the presence of various cells and substances found in the blood

Testing for Chronic Compartment Syndrome

- Near infrared spectroscopy (NIRS)—uses light wavelengths to measure tissue oxygen saturation in the blood to determine whether the muscle compartment has decreased blood flow
- MRI scan—can evaluate the structure of the muscles in the compartments and rule out other possible causes of the symptoms
- CT scan—combines a series of x-ray views taken from many different angles and computer processing to create cross-sectional images of the bones and soft tissues inside the body

Physical Testing

- Reflex testing
- Range-of-motion testing

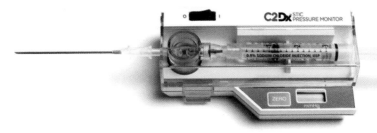

Figure 31.3 Compartment pressure testing device—slit catheter, tonometer.

BIBLIOGRAPHY

Curr Rev Musculoskelet Med. 2010 Oct; 3(1–4):32–37. Published online 2010 Sep 2. doi:
    10.1007/s12178-010-9065-4.
Mayo Clinic. Find Diseases & Conditions. http://www.mayoclinic.com/health/chronic
    -exertional-compartment-syndrome/DS00789/DSECTION=tests-and-diagnosis
https://www.ncbi.nlm.nih.gov/pmc/articles/PMC2941579/
Rakel RE. *Textbook of Family Medicine.* Philadelphia, PA: Saunders Elsevier; 2011.
Wedro B. MedicineNet. Compartment syndrome facts. Available at:
    https://www.orthobullets.com/knee-and-sports/3106/exertional-compartment-syndrome

Chapter **32**

Clavicle Immobilization Techniques
Clavicle Strap, Figure Eight, Sling and Swath

Margaret R. Colyar

CPT Code
23500   Closed treatment without manipulation
23505   Closed treatment with manipulation

Clavicle fractures usually result from a fall on the extended arm or a direct blow to
the shoulder. Fractures of the clavicle require immobilization for proper healing to
occur. Three types of immobilization are clavicle strap, figure eight, and sling and
swath. The clavicle strap technique holds the shoulder upward, outward, and away
from the thorax, as does the figure eight technique. The sling and swath technique
restricts the use of the arm on the side of the clavicle fracture.

OVERVIEW

- Clavicle fractures—80% occur in the middle or inner two-thirds of the clavicle.

OPTIONS

- *Method 1*—Clavicle strap technique
  - For fracture at the middle or inner two-thirds of the clavicle
  - Used to pull the shoulder back and hold the clavicle in **alignment**
- *Method 2*—Figure eight technique
  - For fracture at the middle or inner two-thirds of the clavicle
  - Used to pull the shoulder back and hold the clavicle in alignment
- *Method 3*—Sling and swath technique
  - For fracture at the distal third without displacement or ligament disruptions
  - Used to restrict use of the arm

RATIONALE

- To provide proper alignment
- To immobilize
- To promote proper healing

INDICATIONS

- Fracture of middle clavicle
- Fracture of inner two-thirds of the clavicle

CONTRAINDICATIONS

- Fracture of distal third of the clavicle with disruption and displacement—REFER

PROCEDURE

Clavicle Immobilization Techniques

Equipment

- Method 1
  - Clavicle strap
- Methods 2 and 3
  - Long (approximately 4 to 6 feet), 6-inch-wide bandage
  - 2 to 4 safety pins—nonsterile

Procedure

METHOD 1—CLAVICLE STRAP TECHNIQUE
See Figure 32.1.
- Place the straps over the client's shoulders, one strap over each shoulder.
- Pull straps gently toward the middle of the back and fasten.
- Palpate the fractured clavicle, checking that the displaced clavicle is pulled into alignment.
- Obtain an x-ray of the chest after placement of the clavicle strap to check for alignment. Tighten strap if needed.

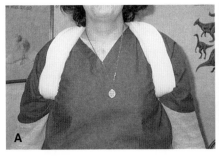 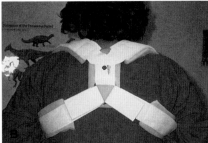

Figure 32.1 Clavicle strap. (A) Front. (B) Back.

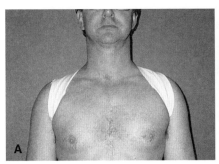 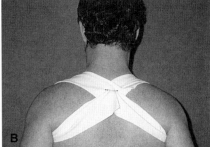

Figure 32.2 Figure eight clavicle strap. (A) Front. (B) Back.

METHOD 2—FIGURE EIGHT TECHNIQUE
See Figure 32.2.
- Starting at midback, go over, around, and under the right shoulder.
- Pull the end of the bandage across the back diagonally.
- Place the bandage over, around, and under the left shoulder.
- Pull across the back.
- Tie or pin in place.

METHOD 3—SLING AND SWATH TECHNIQUE
See Figure 32.3.
- Apply the sling.
- Wrap the 6-inch bandage around the torso and upper arm on the affected side.

Client Instructions
- Do *not* raise the arm above the shoulder for 6 weeks.
- Flex wrist, elbow, and fingers daily.
- Perform the following shoulder exercises after 6 weeks.
  - Pendulum—bend over and gently swing arm to and fro.
  - External rotation—lying down and using unaffected arm, push affected arm to lateral side.
  - Elevation—pull affected arm up in front of chest.

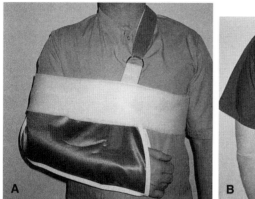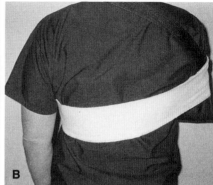

Figure 32.3 Sling and swath. (A) Front. (B) Back.

- Internal rotation—lying down and using unaffected arm, pull affected arm across chest.
- Wall climbing—walk fingers up a wall as far as possible.
- Heavy activity usually may be initiated after 3 months.

BIBLIOGRAPHY

Hinkle JL, Cheever KH. *Brunner and Suddarth's Textbook of Medical-Surgical Nursing.* Philadelphia, PA: Lippincott-Raven; 2017.
Pecci M, Kreher JB. Management of clavicle fractures. *Am Fam Physician.* 2008;55(1):121–128.

33
Chapter

Crutch Walking

Margaret R. Colyar

CPT Code
    None

Crutch walking is a method of support and balance for transferring or walking employed by a person who is lame, weak, or injured. Instruction in proper crutch-walking technique is essential in many orthopedic disorders.

OVERVIEW

* Incidence unknown

RATIONALE

* To ensure proper support and balance
* To prevent injury

INDICATIONS

* Fractured leg, knee, ankle, or foot
* Ankle sprain
* Postsurgical procedures of lower extremities

CONTRAINDICATIONS

* Client unable to balance well
* Elderly

PROCEDURE

Crutch Walking

Equipment

* Crutches—adjustable with rubber suction tips
* Measuring tape

Procedure

Measure the client for crutches using the following technique.

MEASUREMENTS—CRUTCH LENGTH

* Have client stand if possible.
* Measure from anterior axillary fold to sole of foot, then add 2 inches, or measure from 2 inches below the axilla to 6 inches in front of the client.
* Adjust crutches based on measurements.

MEASUREMENTS—HAND PIECE

* Have client position crutch under axilla and grasp hand piece. Armrest should be 1 to 2 inches below the axilla. Elbow should be flexed 20 to 30 degrees.
* Axilla should not rest on the crutch armrest because of the possibility of damage to the brachial plexus.
* Adjust crutches to fit the client's measurements.
* Demonstrate the following:
  * Tripod stance
    * Crutches 10 to 12 inches in front and to the side of the client. Weight is supported on hands, *not* axilla (Fig. 33.1).
  * Crutch gaits
    * Weight-bearing on both legs—use four-point gait (Fig. 33.2).
    * Advance in the following sequence: right crutch, left foot, left crutch, right foot.

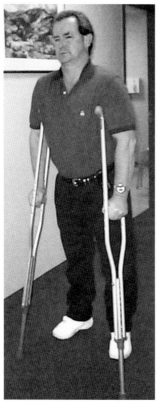

Figure 33.1 Tripod stance.

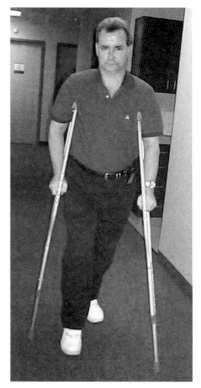

Figure 33.2 Four-point gait.

- Weight-bearing on one leg only—use three-point gait (Fig. 33.3).
  - Advance both crutches and swing the non–weight-bearing leg through while standing on the weight-bearing leg.
  - When the crutches are securely in place, put weight on the hand pieces and advance the weight-bearing leg.
- To sit down (Fig. 33.4)
  - Grasp both crutch hand pieces in one hand on the side of the weaker leg.
  - Grasp the hand rail of the chair.
  - Lower self into chair by bending the knee of the weight-bearing leg while lifting the weaker leg out in front.
- To stand up (Fig. 33.5)
  - Move forward to edge of the chair.
  - Grasp the hand pieces of both crutches in one hand on the side of the weaker leg.
  - Grasp the hand rail of the chair.
  - Use the weight-bearing leg to lift while pushing down on the hand pieces of crutches.

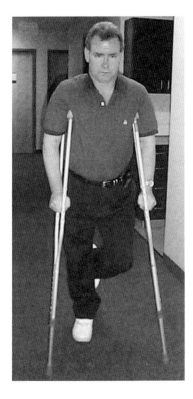

Figure 33.3 Three-point gait.

- To go down stairs (down with the weaker leg) (Fig. 33.6)
  - Stand on the weight-bearing leg.
  - Advance both crutches to the next step and advance the weaker leg.
  - Advance weight-bearing leg.
- To go up stairs (up with the weight-bearing leg) (Fig. 33.7)
  - While stabilizing self with hands on the hand pieces, advance the weight-bearing leg up to the next step.
  - Next, advance crutches and weaker leg up to the step.
- Have the client give a repeat demonstration.

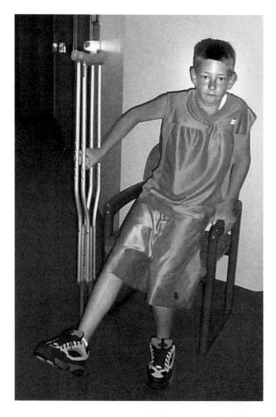

Figure 33.4 Sitting down with crutches.

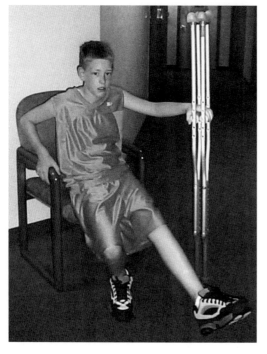

Figure 33.5 Standing up with crutches.

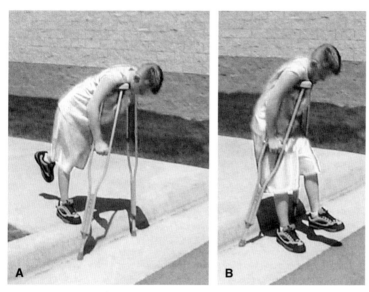

Figure 33.6 Going down stairs with crutches. (A) Stand on weight-bearing leg. (B) Advance both crutches to next step, then advance weaker leg, followed by weight-bearing leg.

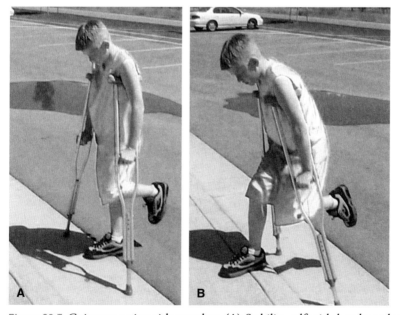

Figure 33.7 Going up stairs with crutches. (A) Stabilize self with hands on hand pieces. (B) Advance weight-bearing leg up to next step.

BIBLIOGRAPHY

Hinkle JL, Cheever KH. *Brunner and Suddarth's Textbook of Medical-Surgical Nursing.* Philadelphia, PA: Lippincott-Raven; 2017.

3 4 Chapter

Dislocation Reduction

Margaret R. Colyar

CPT Code

21480   Closed treatment of temporomandibular joint (TMJ) dislocation

23650–55 Closed treatment of shoulder dislocation, with manipulation

24600–05 Treatment of closed elbow dislocation

26700–05 Closed treatment of metacarpophalangeal (MCP) dislocation, single, with manipulation

26770–75 Closed treatment of interphalangeal joint dislocation, single, with manipulation

---

Dislocation indicates the partial or complete displacement of one bone from another bone. Displacement can occur spontaneously as a result of a structural defect, traumatic injury, or joint disease. A dislocated joint is reduced when it is restored to normal position. Reduction of a joint facilitates proper healing.

OVERVIEW

- Incidence
  - TMJ dislocations
    - 5% to 6% of the population. Dislocation is usually anterior but can be posterior, lateral, and superior.
  - Shoulder dislocation
    - 90% to 95% anterior
    - 5% posterior
    - 2% to 3% acromioclavicular (AC)
  - Recurrence of shoulder dislocations
    - Younger than 20 years of age—90% to 95%
    - Older than 40 years of age—10% to 15%
  - Elbow dislocations
    - Greater incidence than shoulder dislocations
  - Hand dislocations
    - Proximal interphalangeal (PIP) joint—most common dislocation in the body
    - MCP joint—index finger most common dislocation, then thumb and fifth digit
- Causes
  - TMJ dislocations
    - Spontaneous—eating, talking, yawning, or rinsing mouth
    - Traumatic—blow to mandible

- Shoulder dislocations
  - Anterior shoulder dislocation—trauma with arm abducted, extended, and externally rotated
  - Posterior shoulder dislocation—direct force to the shoulder while flexed, adducted, and internally rotated
  - AC shoulder dislocation—persistent upward displacement of lateral end of the clavicle
- Elbow dislocations
  - Posterior dislocations—direct trauma on outstretched forearm held in extension; also may have wrist injury
- Hand dislocations
  - MCP joint dislocations—hyperextension of finger at the MCP joint
  - PIP joint dislocations—hyperextension or "jamming" injury

OPTIONS

- TMJ dislocation reduction
  - *Method 1*—Passive reduction
    - Requires no anesthesia and can be done easily without force
  - *Method 2*—Manual reduction
    - Use if method 1 fails
- Shoulder dislocation reduction
  - Anterior shoulder dislocation
    - Method 1—Passive reduction
      - Requires no anesthesia and can be done easily without force
    - Method 2—Manual reduction
      - Use if method 1 fails
  - Posterior shoulder dislocation reduction
  - AC shoulder dislocation reduction
- Elbow dislocation reduction
- Hand dislocation reduction
  - MCP joint dislocation reduction
  - Dorsal PIP joint dislocation reduction
  - Volar PIP joint dislocation reduction
  - Thumb dislocation reduction

RATIONALE

- To diminish pain
- To prevent loss or decreased use of a joint
- To prevent structural defects

INDICATIONS

- Dislocation of mandible, shoulder, elbow, or finger

CONTRAINDICTIONS

- Dislocation with fracture of the mandible, shoulder, elbow, or finger
- Separation of the AC joint

- Fracture of the joint capsule
- Abnormal neurovascular status of the extremity
- Dislocation of the hip or knee

▶ *Informed consent required*

PROCEDURE

TMJ Dislocation Reduction

Equipment

- Methods 1 and 2
  - Gloves—nonsterile
  - Gauze—nonsterile
  - Tongue blade—nonsterile

Procedure

METHOD 1—PASSIVE REDUCTION—TMJ

- Examine the client. Your examination should show
  - Malocclusion
  - Mandibular fossa empty
  - Moderate pain
  - Mouth held open
- X-ray the TMJ if traumatic injury or if diagnosis of dislocation is in doubt.
  - Lateral view—check for fracture
  - Towne's view—shows medial or lateral offset (dislocation)
- Induce the gag reflex by probing the soft palate with tongue blade (Fig. 34.1).

METHOD 2—MANUAL REDUCTION—TMJ

- Position the client sitting on the floor with head stabilized by an assistant.
- Put on gloves.

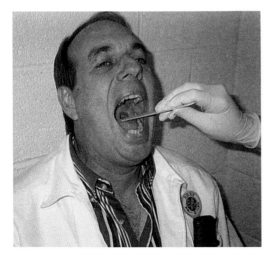

Figure 34.1 Passive reduction of TMJ. Probe the soft palate with a tongue blade to induce the gag reflex.

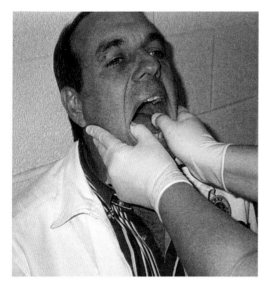

Figure 34.2 Manual reduction of TMJ. Place your thumbs on the bottom molars and fingers submentally. Ask the client to yawn.

- Stand above and in front of the client.
- Place your thumbs in the client's mouth on the bottom molars (Fig. 34.2). Place digits 3, 4, and 5 of each hand submentally.
- Place second digits of each hand at the mandibular angle.
- Ask the client to yawn.
- Apply your body weight downward on the mandible.
- Elevate the chin.
- Slide the mandible backward into position.
- Obtain an x-ray to determine whether the mandible is in the correct position.

Client Instructions

TMJ DISLOCATION REDUCTION

- Eat soft food for several days.
- Avoid opening the mouth wide for 3 to 4 weeks.
- Place your hand under your chin when yawning.
- Take acetaminophen every 4 hours as needed for pain.
- Perform jaw muscle–strengthening exercises.

Shoulder Dislocation Reduction

Equipment

- Method 1 only
  - Weights—5- to 10-lb free weights or sandbag
  - Towel—nonsterile
  - Roll of gauze
- Methods 1 and 2
  - 1% lidocaine, 20 mL, or muscle relaxer
  - Syringe—20 mL
  - 25-gauge, 1½-inch needle

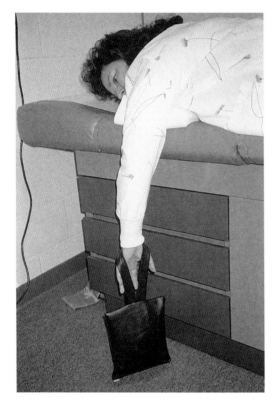

Figure 34.3 Passive reduction.

Procedure

ANTERIOR SHOULDER DISLOCATION REDUCTION

- Method 1—passive reduction (Fig. 34.3)
  - Examine the client. You should find
    - Fullness in the anterior capsule
    - Sulcus sign (space under the acromion)
    - Severe pain
    - Limited range of motion
    - Arm held slightly abducted and externally rotated
    - Shoulder contour flattened with protruding acromion
  - Examine the client's neurovascular status and document.
  - Give a muscle relaxer or inject 20 mL of 1% lidocaine inferiorly off the tip of the acromion (Fig. 34.4).
  - X-ray the shoulder (three views) to determine dislocation and whether a fracture is present. X-ray should show anterior and slight inferior displacement of the humerus out of the glenoid fossa. If a fracture is present, REFER.
    - Anteroposterior view—shows internal and external rotation of the shoulder, upper humerus, AC joint, and clavicle
    - Y view—needed to verify a dislocation

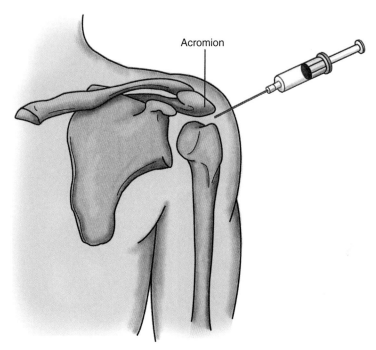

Figure 34.4 Passive reduction of anterior shoulder dislocation. Inject lidocaine inferiorly off the tip of the acromion.

- Load-bearing view—to differentiate an AC joint separation from a dislocation
- Position the client prone on an examination table with the affected arm hanging downward.
- Place a folded towel under the shoulder.
- Wrap gauze snugly around the wrist of the affected arm.
- Hook weights into the gauze.
  - If weights are not available, a sandbag may be used.
- Allow weights to pull on arm for 15 to 20 minutes.
- If no progress after 15 to 20 minutes, apply a sling and REFER to an orthopedic surgeon.
- If successful, immobilize the affected arm in a sling and swath to immobilize the shoulder.
- Method 2—Manual reduction (Fig. 34.5)
  - Position the client in a sitting position.
  - Grasp the wrist and elbow of the affected arm.
  - With the arm against the body
    - Flex the elbow 90 degrees.
    - Externally rotate the arm to approximately 70 to 85 degrees or until resistance is felt.
    - Lift the elbow in the sagittal plane as far as possible.

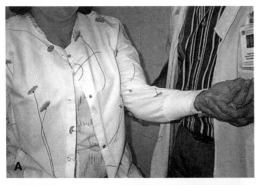

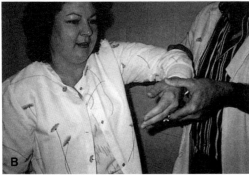

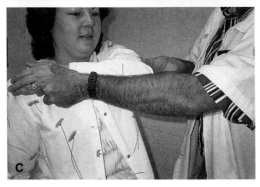

Figure 34.5 Manual reduction of anterior shoulder dislocation. (A) Flex the elbow 90 degrees, externally rotating the arm 70 to 85 degrees until resistance is felt; (B) lift the elbow in the sagittal plane while (C) internally rotating the arm.

- Internally rotate the arm. The head of the joint should slip into place; the pain immediately decreases.
- Obtain an x-ray of the shoulder to determine whether reduction was successful.
- Check neurovascular status and document.

POSTERIOR SHOULDER DISLOCATION REDUCTION
- Examine the client. You should find
  - Minimal posterior swelling
  - Severe pain with any motion
- Do not attempt to reduce; REFER to an orthopedic surgeon.

AC SHOULDER DISLOCATION REDUCTION
- Examine the client. You should find
  - Slight pain—worse on elevation of the arm
  - Lateral end of the clavicle prominent
  - Distinct step palpable between the clavicle and the acromion
- No active reduction is needed.
- Apply sling for 1 week or until the pain subsides.
- Instruct the client to avoid overhead work.

Client Instructions

SHOULDER DISLOCATION REDUCTION
- Apply an ice pack for the first 24 hours.
- Give acetaminophen every 4 hours as needed for pain.
- Start deltoid isometric exercises immediately.
- In 3 weeks, start the following exercises (Fig. 34.6)
  - Lean over with affected arm hanging, and make increasingly larger circles clockwise and counterclockwise.

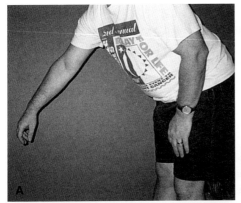
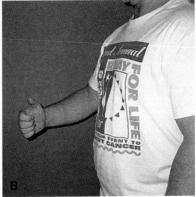
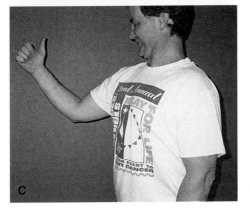

Figure 34.6 Shoulder exercises. (A) While leaning over, make hanging circles (clockwise/counterclockwise). (B) Flex the arm 90 degrees at the elbow, make a fist with the thumb up, and move the forearm and hand rotating at the elbow. (C) Flex the arm 90 degrees at the elbow, make a fist with the thumb up, and raise the arm at the shoulder in abduction.

- Standing upright with affected arm flexed 90 degrees at the elbow, make a fist with the thumb up. Move the forearm and hand rotating at the elbow to and away from the body.
- Standing upright with affected arm flexed 90 degrees at the elbow, make a fist with the thumb up; raise the arm at the shoulder in abduction.
- Return to the office in 1 week for recheck.

Elbow Dislocation Reduction

Equipment

- Metal splint with foam on one side
- Gauze—nonsterile
- Tape

Procedure

- Examine the client. You should find
  - Pain
  - Limited range of motion
- Assess and document neurovascular status.
  - Radial and brachial pulses
  - Capillary refill of the fingers
  - Nerve function of the median, ulnar, and radial nerves (Fig. 34.7)
  - Muscle function (Fig. 34.8)
- X-ray both arms for comparison—check for fat pad sign.
  - Anteroposterior, lateral, and oblique views
  - If fracture is present, REFER.
- Apply countertraction on the distal humeral shaft and continuous gentle downward traction to proximal portion of the forearm and bring the elbow into flexion (Fig. 34.9).
- X-ray the dislocated elbow to ensure that it is reduced.
- Repeat the neurovascular assessment and document.
- Apply a posterior splint (see Chapter 38) with the elbow at 100 to 110 degrees of flexion.

Client Instructions

ELBOW DISLOCATION REDUCTION

- Take acetaminophen every 4 hours as needed for pain.
- Return to the office in 1 week.
- Start range-of-motion exercises in 1 week if the elbow is stable. Gradually increase range-of-motion exercises (Fig. 34.10) after 10 to 14 days.
- Keep the splint in place until full extension is achieved.
- A follow-up x-ray must be taken in 2 to 3 weeks to determine stability of the elbow.

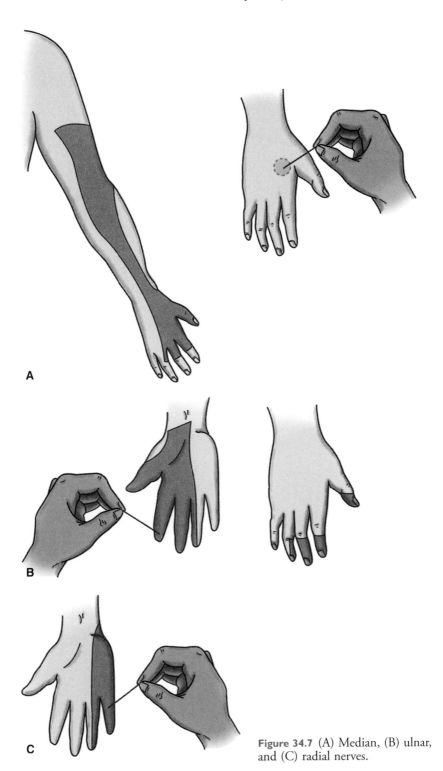

A

B

C

Figure 34.7 (A) Median, (B) ulnar, and (C) radial nerves.

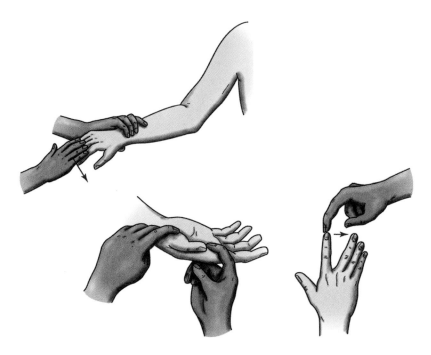

Figure 34.8 Muscle function.

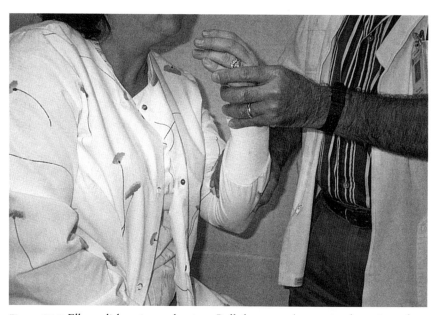

Figure 34.9 Elbow dislocation reduction. Pull down on the proximal portion of the forearm and bring the elbow into flexion.

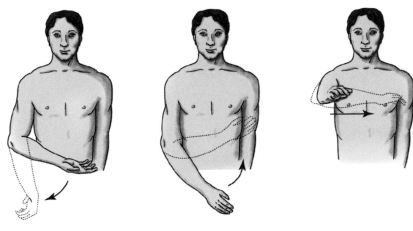

Figure 34.10 Elbow exercises.

Hand Dislocation Reduction

Equipment

- Splint
- Syringe—5 mL
- 25-gauge, 1½-inch needle
- 1% lidocaine—5 mL
- Gauze—nonsterile
- Tape

Procedure

MCP JOINT DISLOCATION REDUCTION

- Examine the client. You should find
  - Digit held in extension or hyperextension
  - Dimpling of the palmar skin over the protruding metacarpal head
- Assess neurovascular status and document.
- X-ray the affected hand.
  - Anteroposterior view shows obliteration of normal joint space.
  - Lateral view shows proximal phalanx is dorsal to the metacarpal head.
  - If a fracture is found, immobilize the joint and REFER to an orthopedic surgeon.
- Hyperextend the finger at the MCP joint.
- Apply traction by pulling the finger in an outward and upward direction.
- Apply pressure of the dorsal aspect of the base of the proximal phalanx (Fig. 34.11).
- Remove traction.
- Flex the finger.
- Obtain another x-ray of the hand to determine successful reduction.
- Assess neurovascular status and range of motion.

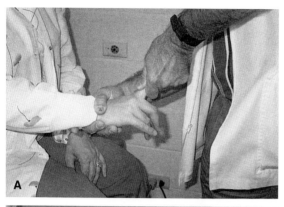

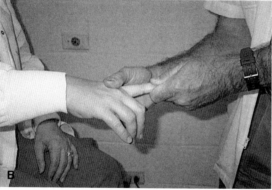

Figure 34.11 MCP joint dislocation reduction. (A) Hyperextend the MCP joint while pulling the finger outward and upward. (B) Apply pressure on the dorsal aspect of the proximal phalanx.

- Apply a posterior splint (see Chapter 38) with MCP flexed 70 degrees. Keep the posterior splint in place for 3 to 4 weeks.

DORSAL PIP JOINT DISLOCATION REDUCTION
- Examine the client. You should find
  - Finger swollen and malformed
  - Limited range of motion
- Assess neurovascular status and document.
- X-ray the hand.
  - Anteroposterior view shows obliteration of joint space.
  - Lateral view shows dorsal dislocation of middle phalanx.
  - If a fracture is present, immobilize, and REFER to an orthopedic surgeon.
- Perform a digital nerve block (see Chapter 8).
- Apply direct longitudinal traction.
- Obtain another x-ray of the hand to determine whether the PIP joint has been reduced.
- Reassess neurovascular status and document.

- Apply a dorsal extension block splint, blocking the last 15 degrees of extension. Keep splint in place for 3 to 4 weeks.

VOLAR PIP JOINT DISLOCATION REDUCTION

- Examine the client. You should find
  - Finger swollen and malformed
  - Limited range of motion
- Assess neurovascular status and document.
- X-ray the hand.
  - Lateral view shows base of middle phalanx is palmar to head of proximal phalanx.
  - If a fracture is present, immobilize, and REFER to an orthopedic surgeon.
- No active reduction is required.
- Splint in full extension of PIP joint on the volar side. Keep splint in place for 4 to 6 weeks.

THUMB DISLOCATION REDUCTION

- Usually a ligament tear is involved. REFER to an orthopedic surgeon.

Client Instructions

HAND DISLOCATION—MCP AND PIP—DORSAL

- Take acetaminophen every 4 hours as needed for pain.
- Return to the office in 1 week.
- Start flexion and extension exercises in 1 week.
- The splint can be removed in 3 to 4 weeks.

HAND DISLOCATION—PIP—VOLAR

- Take acetaminophen every 4 hours as needed for pain.
- Return to the office in 1 week.
- Keep the splint in place for 4 to 6 weeks.
- After 4 to 6 weeks, start flexion and extension exercises.

BIBLIOGRAPHY

Diamond S. The mechanism and management of shoulder pain. *Adv Nurs Pract.* 1996:16, 18, 20–21, 50.

Madden C, Putukian M, McCarty E, Young CMD. *Netter's Sports Medicine.* Philadelphia, PA: Saunders-Elsevier; 2017.

Pfenninger JL, Fowler GC. *Procedures for Primary Care Physicians.* St. Louis, MO: Mosby; 2019.

Thakur AJ, Narayan R. Painless reduction of shoulder dislocation by Kocher's method. *J Bone Joint Surg Am.* 1990;72(3):524.

35 Chapter

Ganglion Cyst Aspiration and Injection

Margaret R. Colyar

CPT Code

20600 Arthrocentesis, aspiration, or injection; small joint, bursa, or ganglion cyst (leg, fingers, toes)
20605 Arthrocentesis, aspiration, or injection; intermediate joint, bursa, or ganglion cyst (e.g., TMJ, acromioclavicular, wrist, elbow, ankle, olecranon bursa)
25111 Excision of ganglion, wrist; primary
25112 Excision of ganglion, wrist; recurrent
26160 Excision of lesion of tendon sheath or capsule (e.g., cyst, mucous cyst, or ganglion); hand or finger

A simple **ganglion** cyst is a cystic tumor that develops on or in a tendon sheath containing a thick, gel-like material. This gel-like material leaks from the joint into the weakened tendon sheath and forms a cyst sac (Fig. 35.1). The ganglion cyst usually is caused by frequent strains and contusions.

OVERVIEW

- Cause—joint inflammation
- Usual location—back of the wrist

RATIONALE

- To diminish pain
- To promote joint mobility

INDICATIONS

- Pain over a joint
- Limitation of joint movement

CONTRAINDICATIONS

- On anticoagulant therapy
- Problems with clotting
- Lack of response to previous injections
- Sepsis
- Recent joint fractures

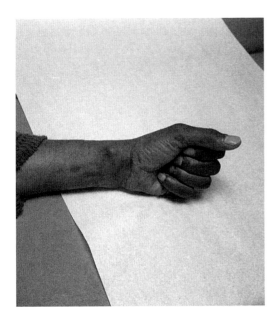

Figure 35.1 Ganglion cyst.

- Inform the client of the following
  - Chance of infection and recurrence
  - Chance of steroid flare 24 to 35 hours after injury
  - Chance of subcutaneous atrophy
- ▶ *Informed consent required*

PROCEDURE

Ganglion Cyst Aspiration and Injection

Equipment

- Antiseptic skin cleanser
- Gloves—sterile
- Drape—sterile
- 2 syringes—10 mL and 3 mL
- 18-gauge, 1½-inch needle
- 22- to 25-gauge, 1½-inch needle
- 1% lidocaine
  - Use single-dose vials because they do not contain preservatives that are likely to cause allergic reactions.
- Culture tubes
- Corticosteroid (Table 35.1)
- 4 × 4 gauze—sterile
- Tape

Procedure

- Position the client with the ganglion cyst easily accessible.

Table 35·1	Commonly Used Corticosteroids	
TYPE	**USE**	**DOSE**
Short-Acting		
Hydrocortisone	Quick relief in self-limiting disorders, such as bursitis	20 mg
Intermediate-Acting		
Methylprednisone		4 mg
Prednisolone (Depo-Medrol) 20 mg/mL		5–10 mg
Triamcinolone acetonide (Kenalog) 10 mg/mL		5–10 mg
Triamcinolone diacetate (Aristocort) 25 mg/mL		12.5–25 mg
Long-Acting		
Dexamethasone (Decadron) 4 mg/mL or 10 mg/mL	Chronic conditions such as tendinitis	0.6 mL
Betamethasone (Celestone) 6 mg/mL		0.6 mL

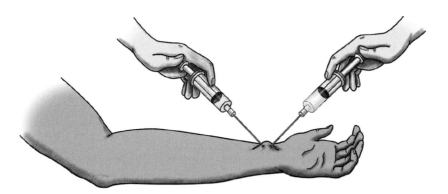

Figure 35.2 Aspirate the ganglion cyst with an 18-gauge needle, and inject the medication into the cyst with the second needle.

- Cleanse the skin in a 3-inch-diameter area around the ganglion cyst with antiseptic skin cleanser.
- Drape the ganglion cyst.
- Put on gloves.
- Using the 22- to 25-gauge needle on 3-mL syringe, draw up 2.5 mL of 1% lidocaine and 0.5 mL of corticosteroid. Mix well by gently rotating syringe back and forth.
- Insert the 10-mL syringe with the 18-gauge needle into the ganglion cyst (for aspiration) (Fig. 35.2).
- Insert the syringe with the medication into the ganglion cyst, and aspirate for blood.

- If no blood, aspirate the fluid from cyst. If the aspirate is cloudy, send it to the pathology laboratory for culture and sensitivity.
  - If blood is aspirated, remove the needle and dress the wound.
- Inject the medication.
- Remove both needles.
- Apply a pressure dressing.

Client Instructions

- Keep the wound covered for 8 to 12 hours.
- Some redness, swelling, and heat are normal. If you notice yellow or green drainage from wound or red streaks, return to the office.
- Take acetaminophen or ibuprofen every 4 to 6 hours as needed for pain.
- Rest the joint for 24 hours.
- Elevate the joint above the heart as much as possible for 24 hours.
- Return to the office in 1 week for recheck.
- If the cyst recurs, removal may be indicated.

BIBLIOGRAPHY

Hashimoto BE, Hayes AS, Ager JD. Sonographic diagnosis and treatment of ganglion cysts causing suprascapular nerve entrapment. *J Ultrasound Med.* 1994;13(9):671–674.
Pfenninger JL, Fowler GC. *Procedures for Primary Care Physicians.* St. Louis, MO: Mosby; 2019.

Chapter **36**

Intra-Articular and Bursa Corticosteroid Injection
Margaret R. Colyar

CPT Code
20550 Injection; tendon sheath, ligaments, trigger points
20600 Arthrocentesis, aspiration, or injection; small joint, bursa
20605 Arthrocentesis, aspiration, or injection; intermediate joint, bursa
20610 Arthrocentesis, aspiration, or injection; major joint or bursa

Injection of corticosteroids into a joint space or bursa is done to decrease pain in overuse injury and to improve function. Injection of corticosteroids may be done immediately after joint aspiration. Anesthetic agents are used in conjunction with corticosteroid injection to decrease injection pain. For overuse injuries, a general rule of thumb is that two injections can be done over 2 weeks and then in 3 to 4 months, if necessary. No more than three injections within a 12-month period are recommended.

OVERVIEW

- Familiarity with the anatomy of the injection site is crucial to effective intra-articular injection. Common conditions for which intra-articular injection is indicated are
  - Tendinitis
    - de Quervain's tendonitis
    - Tennis elbow
    - Plantar fasciitis
    - Trigger finger
  - Bursitis
  - Neuritis
    - Carpal or tarsal tunnel syndrome
    - Costochondritis
    - Tietze's syndrome
    - Postherpetic neuralgia
  - Myofascial pain syndrome
  - Arthritis
    - Osteoarthritis (degenerative)
    - Rheumatoid arthritis

Complications

- Tendon rupture
- Joint injection
- Postinjection flare (pain)
- Injection into a blood vessel
- Tissue atrophy

Commonly Used Corticosteroids

See Table 35·1.

Commonly Used Anesthetic Agents

- Lidocaine (Xylocaine) 1%—1 to 2 hours of relief
- Bupivacaine (Marcaine) 0.25%—6 to 8 hours of relief

RATIONALE

- To diminish pain
- To promote joint function

INDICATIONS

- Painful joint
- Inflamed joint

CONTRAINDICATIONS

- Infected joint
- Cellulitis over the joint
- More than three injections in a 12-month period
- Joint instability
- Joint surgery or prosthesis
- Fracture
- Sickle cell anemia
- Coagulation disorders
- Diabetes
- Children or adolescents
- ▶ *Informed consent required*

PROCEDURE

Intra-Articular and Bursa Corticosteroid Injection

Equipment

- Alcohol prep pads
- Povidone-iodine prep pads
- Gloves—nonsterile
- Syringe—3 to 10 mL
- 22-gauge, 1½-inch needle
- 1% lidocaine—single-dose vial (5 to 10 times the amount of steroid to be used—e.g., 2.5 mL of lidocaine to 0.5 mL of steroid)
- Corticosteroid of choice
- Adhesive bandage (Band-Aid)

Procedure

- Draw lidocaine and corticosteroid into the syringe.
- Mix by rolling or gently rocking the syringe back and forth.
- Mark the injection site with your thumbnail.
- Position the client with the joint slightly flexed to open the joint space (Fig. 36.1).
- Put on gloves.
- Cleanse the site with alcohol and then povidone-iodine.
  - Allow the povidone-iodine to air dry.
- Insert the needle at the thumbnail mark at 45- to 90-degree angle, depending on the site of injection.
- Aspirate.
  - If blood is obtained, remove the needle.
  - If using injection for a bursa, aspirate for cloudy bursal fluid. This indicates the appropriate site.
- Inject the corticosteroid mixture steadily and gently into the area.
- Remove the needle.
- Apply pressure for 1 minute.
- Cover with Band-Aid.

Text continued on page 173

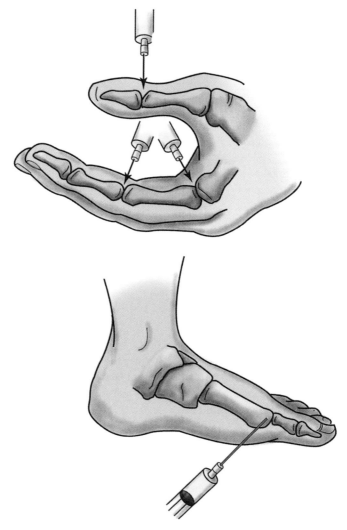

***Finger and toe joints* —**
• Flex the finger or toes to open the joint.
• Inject corticosteroid medial or lateral to the extensor tendon.

Figure 36.1 Injection sites.

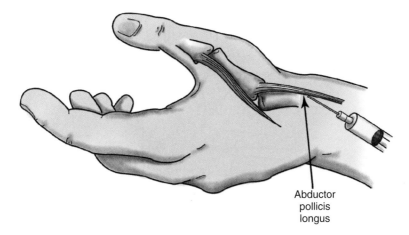

Abductor
pollicis
longus

***de Quervains Disease* —**
• Abduct the thumb.
• Inject parallel to the tendon at the point of tenderness.

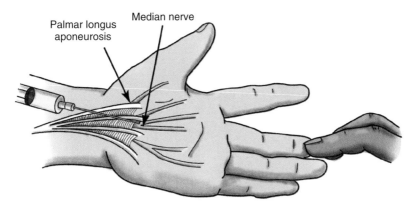

Palmar longus
aponeurosis

Median nerve

***Carpal Tunnel Syndrome* —**
• Dorsiflex the wrist.
• Insert the needle at the distal crease of the wrist lateral to the tendon toward the middle finger.
• 45-degree angle.
• 1–2 cm in depth.

Figure 36.1 cont'd   *Continued*

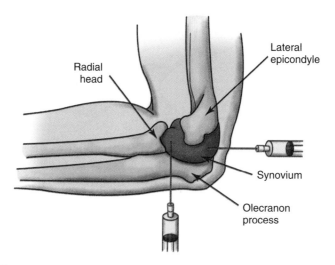

Tennis Elbow —
- Flex the elbow 45 degrees.
- Inject the corticosteroid in the joint
  space inferior to the lateral epicondoyle.
- Inject superior to the olecranon process.

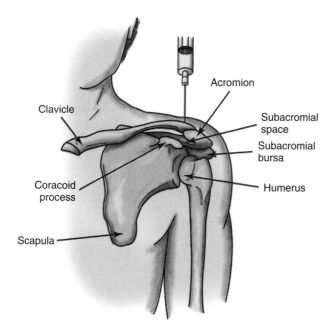

Shoulder (Acromioclavicular Joint) —
- Palpate distal clavicle until a moveable prominence is felt.
- Insert the needle anteriorally at a 90-degree angle.
- Inject the corticosteroid into the joint.

Figure 36.1 cont'd

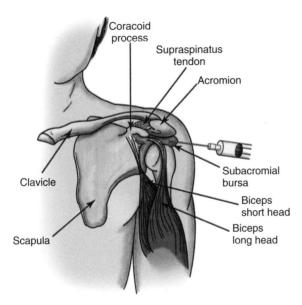

Shoulder (Subacromial Bursa) —
- Palpate the lateral edge of the acromion.
- The soft spot just below the acromion is the subacromial bursa.
- Insert the needle at a 90-degree angle into the bursa, which should feel soft.
- Be careful not to inject in the supraspinatus tendon or the deltoid.

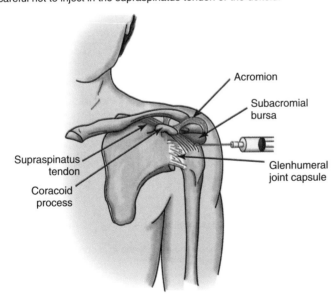

Shoulder (Rotator Cuff — supraspinatus tendonitis) —
- Use the same technique as for the subacromial bursa.
- Insert the needle farther into the area to the point of tenderness.
- Withdraw the needle slightly and inject the corticosteroid.

Figure 36.1 cont'd   *Continued*

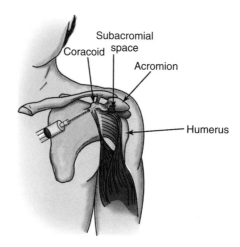

Shoulder (Short head of the biceps) —
• Identify the anterior coracoid bony process.
  • Inferior to the clavicle.
  • Medial to the humerus.
• Insert needle at the point of tenderness at a 90-degree angle until the bone is reached.
• Withdraw the needle 1–2 mm.
• Inject the corticosteroid.

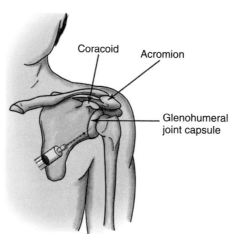

Shoulder (Glenohumeral or Scapulohumeral Joint) —
• *Anterior (Glenohumeral) —*
  • Rotate the shoulder joint toward the back and identify the joint space.
  • Insert the needle at a 90-degree angle into the glenohumeral joint.
  • No bone should be encountered.
  • Inject the corticosteroid.
• *Posterior (Scapulohumeral) —*
  • Rotate the shoulder anteriorly and identify the joint space.
  • Insert the needle at a 90-degree angle into the scapulohumeral joint.
  • No bone should be encountered.
  • Inject the corticosteroid.

Figure 36.1 cont'd

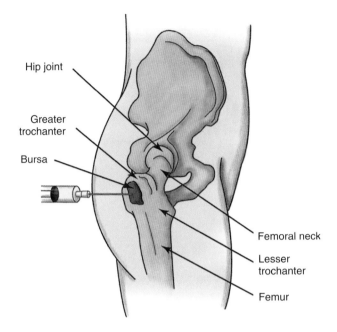

Hip Bursa —
- Identify the hip joint by having the client flex the joint.
- Insert the needle until you hit the bone.
- Withdraw 2–3 mm and inject the corticosteroid.

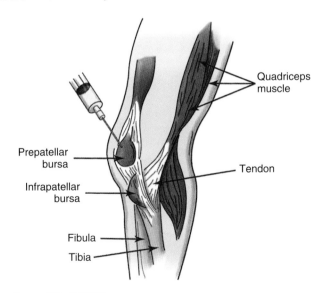

Knee Bursa (Prepatellar) —
- Inject above the patella.
- 90-degree angle.

Figure 36.1 cont'd   *Continued*

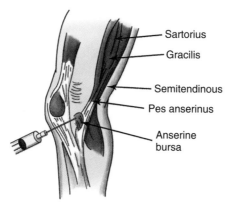

Knee-Anserine Bursa —
• Below patella find the lateral concavity.
• Inject the needle at 90-degree angle.
• Inject until you hit bone, then withdraw 2–3 mm.
• Inject the corticosteroid.
• Redirect the needle several times and inject in several areas.

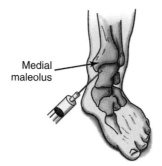

Ankle —
• Dorsiflex the ankle.
• Inject at the medial malleolous and tibia.

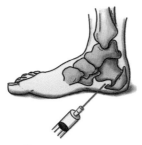

Heel Spur (Calcaneal) —
• Insert the needle on the lateral side of the foot at the heel at the point of maximal tenderness.
• Inject the corticosteroid.

Figure 36.1 cont'd

Client Instructions

- Rest the joint for the next 24 hours.
- You may remove the dressing and bandage in 24 hours.
- Observe for signs and symptoms of infection, such as
  - Increase in pain after 24 hours
  - Increase in temperature
  - Redness or swelling
  - Yellow or greenish drainage
  - Foul odor
- If any signs or symptoms of infection are found, return to the office.
- Steroid flare or postinjection pain lasting 36 hours may occur. If this does occur, do the following.
  - Apply an ice pack.
  - Take ibuprofen (Motrin) every 6 hours as needed.
  - Call the office if the pain does not subside within 36 hours.
- Sometimes fluid recollects in the joint. If this occurs, return to the office.
- Your culture should be back by _____. We will call you with the results.

BIBLIOGRAPHY ▰▰▰▰▰▰▰▰▰▰

Cardone DA. Diagnostic and therapeutic injection of the elbow region. *Am Fam Physician.* 2002;66(11):2097–2101.

Cardone DA. Diagnostic and therapeutic injection of the hip and knee. *Am Fam Physician.* 2003;67(10):2147–2152.

Tallia AF. Diagnostic and therapeutic injection of the shoulder region. *Am Fam Physician.* 2003;67(6):1271–1278.

Tallia AF. Diagnostic and therapeutic injection of the wrist and hand region. *Am Fam Physician.* 2003;67(4):745–750.

Chapter **37**

Sling Application

Margaret R. Colyar

CPT Code
None

Slings are devices used to immobilize, support, and elevate the shoulder, arm, and hand. A sling can be used by itself or in combination with other immobilization devices.

OVERVIEW

- Before sling application, always assess the extremity for and document
  - Pulse
  - Paresthesias
  - Paralysis
  - Pallor
  - Pain
  - Edema

OPTIONS

Sling Application

- Method 1—Manufactured sling application
- Method 2—Triangular sling application

RATIONALE

- To immobilize a joint
- To support and elevate the shoulder, arm, and hand

INDICATIONS

- Strain or sprain of the shoulder, elbow, or arm

CONTRAINDICATIONS

- Unstable fracture
- Loss of pulse
- Signs or symptoms of compartment syndrome

PROCEDURE

Sling Application

Equipment

- Method 1
  - Sling
- Method 2
  - Triangular piece of cloth 16 to 20 inches on each side
  - Two large safety pins—nonsterile

Procedure

METHOD 1—MANUFACTURED SLING APPLICATION

- Position the client sitting or supine with
  - Injured arm across the chest in 90-degree angle
  - Forearm slightly above the level of the elbow
  - Thumb pointed upward and toward the body
  - The sling outside the clothing
- Using manufactured sling
  - Secure the elbow snugly in the sling.

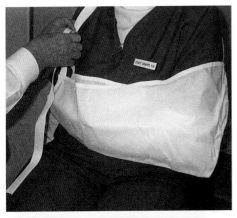

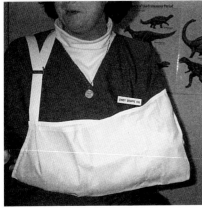

Figure 37.1 Manufactured sling application.

- Extend the sling to include the hand to the MCP joints.
  - This prevents ulnar deviation and supports the wrist.
- Cross the strap over the unaffected shoulder and around the back of the neck (Fig. 37.1).
- Buckle or tie the strap. Do not allow the buckle or knot to rest on a bony prominence or put pressure on the neck.
- Tighten the strap so that the arm is supported.

METHOD 2—TRIANGULAR SLING APPLICATION
- Fasten corner of cloth at elbow with safety pins (Fig. 37.2) with arm at a 45-degree angle across the chest.
- Tie ends around the neck.

METHODS 1 AND 2
- After application of the sling, assess the extremity for and document
  - Pulse
  - Grasp strength
  - Paresthesias
  - Warmth of hand

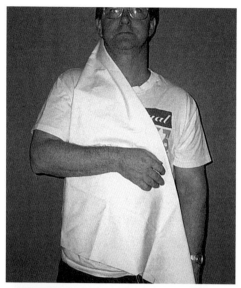

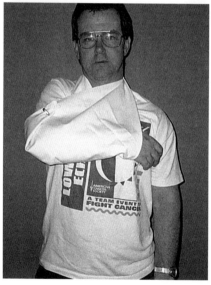

Figure 37.2 Triangular sling application.

- Color of hand
- Presence of edema

Client Instructions

- You must keep the sling in place for _____.
- If the hand becomes cold, pale in color, numb, or tingly, contact the nurse practitioner.
- Observe for signs of skin irritation around the neck. If skin irritation occurs, pad the strap with a soft cloth.

- Do the following exercises while the sling is in place
  - Isometrics of the deltoid—flex and relax.
  - Wiggle the fingers.
  - Return to the office for recheck on _____.

BIBLIOGRAPHY

Kenney DE, Klima RR. Modified arm sling for soft-tissue injuries of the shoulder and glenohumeral subluxation. *J Hand Ther.* 1993;6(3):215–216.

McConnell EA. Correctly positioning an arm sling. *Nursing.* 1991;21(7):70.

Potter PA, Perry AG. *Basic Nursing.* St. Louis, MO: Mosby; 2019.

Chapter **38**

Splinting and Taping
Cynthia R. Ehrhardt

CPT Code
29260–80 Strapping; elbow or wrist, hand or finger
29530–50 Strapping; ankle, knee, toes
99070 Splinting

Splinting and taping provide effective temporary methods of immobilizing a joint after a mild-to-moderate musculoskeletal joint inflammation or injury. Splinting frequently is used in place of casting.

OVERVIEW

- The most common musculoskeletal injuries involve the ankle joint following the mechanism of inversion and plantar flexion stretching of the lateral ligaments.
- The second most common musculoskeletal injury involves overuse syndrome of the wrist and thumb.
- General principles include the following.
  - During application, frequently reassess neurovascular status.
  - Apply material firmly but not tightly.
  - Avoid skin irritation wherever possible.
  - Instruct on precautions of skin irritation if stockinette is not used.
  - Remove splint at least four times a day for gentle range-of-motion exercises to reduce the incidence of "frozen joint syndrome."
  - Do not discharge client until 30 minutes after completion of the procedure, to ensure satisfactory application without compromise of neurovascular system.

- Determination of the appropriate appliance to use (taping versus splinting) depends on
  - Joint injured
  - Nature of joint injury and ligaments involved
  - Mechanism of joint injury
  - Time of injury
    - Immediate
    - Acute (within 24 hours without onset of swelling)
    - Intermediate acute (within 24 hours with onset of swelling)
    - Delayed acute (beyond 48 hours)
  - Previous history of injury to the joint
  - Severity of injury
    - Most grade II and grade III ligamental and musculoskeletal injuries respond well with splinting or immobilization.
  - Physical examination findings
  - Requirement to return to activity

HEALTH PROMOTION/PREVENTION

- Use of
  - Properly fitting athletic equipment
  - Appropriate footwear for participation in the sport
  - Proper stretching and warm-up exercises before sports participation
  - Proper conditioning to play the sport
  - Prophylactic use of taping of chronic joint injuries before sports participation

OPTIONS

See Table 38.1.

Splinting

- Ankle splinting
  - *Method 1*—Posterior splint
  - *Method 2*—Aircast technique
- Knee immobilization
  - Use with grade II and grade III knee strains
- Wrist splinting
  - *Method 1*—Premade wrist splint
  - *Method 2*—Volar splinting
- Thumb splinting
  - Use for adductor pollicis tendinitis
    - *Method 1*—Premade wrist splint with thumb support
    - *Method 2*—Aluminum thumb splint
    - *Method 3*—Thumb spica

Taping

- Ankle taping
  - *Method 1*—Louisiana ankle wrap technique

Table 38·1	Procedure Options

Splinting

Advantages
- Restricts movement 100%
- Allows stabilization of suspected joint fractures
- Prevents further trauma to the joint and skeletal structure
- Allows adjustment of the orthopedic device in the presence of soft tissue edema and its resolution
- Can replace bulky casting

Disadvantages
- Bulky prosthetic device
- Cannot be used as a prophylactic measure
- Can be overused and misused by client
- Can cause skin irritation
- More expensive than taping

Taping

Advantages
- Facilitates limiting movement
- Does not restrict movement 100%
- May immediately return to activity without an obtrusive prosthetic device
- Not as bulky as a prosthetic device
- Prophylactic use prevents further aggravation of a chronic injury

Disadvantages
- 50% of taping loosens within 10 minutes of application
- Requires some skill in application
- Can cause skin irritation
- Not as effective if joint immobilization is required

- *Method 2*—Open Gibney technique with heel lock
- *Method 3*—Open Gibney technique without heel lock
- *Method 4*—Basket-weave technique with heel lock
- Knee taping
- Wrist taping
- Elbow taping
  - Lateral epicondylar taping
- Foot taping
  - For plantar fasciitis, overuse, and blunt injury
    - *Method 1*—Figure eight technique
    - *Method 2*—Full plantar taping technique

RATIONALE

- To protect ligaments from abnormal stress

- To diminish muscle spasms
- To maintain range of motion

INDICATIONS

- Splinting and taping
  - Mild grade II or grade III ankle strains (Table 38.2)
  - Tenosynovitis from overuse syndrome, such as
    - Carpal tunnel syndrome
    - Abductor pollicis tendon inflammation (computer game syndrome)
    - Extensor retinaculum inflammation
  - Suspected peroneal tendon dislocation
  - Suspected fracture
  - Suspected unstable joint structure
- Taping only
  - Grade I and grade II strains (see Table 38.2)
  - Tenosynovitis from overuse syndromes, such as
    - Epicondylitis
    - Chondromalacia patellae
    - Iliotibial band tendinitis, also known as runner's knee
    - Osgood-Schlatter syndrome—occasionally beneficial
  - Plantar **fasciitis**

CONTRAINDICATIONS

- Sprains accompanied by soft tissue compression or open injury
- Neurovascular compromise
- Emergency department or orthopedic referral should be considered if
  - Injury is suspicious for fracture
  - Joint is unstable
  - Injury represents potential loss of limb or function
  - Internal derangement of ligamental structure is suspected
  - Pain persists
  - Injury is not resolved
  - Joint instability persists

PROCEDURE

Splinting

Equipment

- Tube stockinettes in various diameters
- Precast casting material or casting material of various widths (4 and 6 inches are used most often)
- Elastic wrap tape (2-, 4-, or 6-inch widths)
- Adhesive tape in various widths (1- or 2-inch widths)
- Bucket with water
- Soft padding material—optional
- Lubricated foam padding—optional

Table 38-2	**Grading of Injured Ligaments**

Grade I

- Injury history
- Short-lived or minimal experience of pain. Joint was forced beyond normal range of motion.
- Pain
- Momentary
- May proceed with activity but without significant interference of activity
- Physical examination
- Abnormal laxity of ligament present
- Localized tenderness at the insertion points of the ligament
- Minimal soft tissue edema

Grade II

- Injury history
- Sharp initial sensation with or without a "popping" or "snapping" sensation
- Joint is forced beyond normal range of motion
- Pain
- Generally progressive with continued stress to joint
- Eventually action must be halted
- Pathology
- Incomplete disruption of the musculotendinous unit
- Lengthening or partial tearing of the ligament
- Physical examination
- Laxity of the joint
- Soft tissue edema with obliteration of landmarks
- Possible ecchymosis

Grade III

- Injury history
- Sharp initial sensation with or without a "popping" or "snapping" sensation
- Joint was forced beyond normal range of motion
- Pain
- Short-lived and disappears within a few minutes
- Pathology
- Complete tearing of the ligament
- Complete disruption of the musculotendinous unit
- Physical examination
- Marked laxity
- Presence of drawer sign

- Scissors—nonsterile
- Sling—for upper extremity injuries
- Aluminum splits (1- or 2-inch widths)
- Wrist splints
- Knee immobilizer
- Arm sling

Procedure

ANKLE SPLINTING

- *Method 1*—Posterior splint (Fig. 38.1)
  - Position the client onto the abdomen with knee flexed at 90 degrees.
  - Have the ankle in a neutral position ensuring adequate stretching of the Achilles tendon.
  - Apply stockinette distal to proximal approximately 2 to 3 inches above and below the projected splint area.
  - Optional—Apply cotton web padding from distal to proximal until a 2-inch thickness is obtained.
    - Extra cushion and thickness may be necessary around the bony prominences of the ankle.
  - Select appropriate width of casting material (usually 6-inch width).
  - Cut casting material to the length needed.
    - If not precast with preset thickness, fold in 10 to 12 overlapping layers equaling the length plus 4 cm of the projected splint.
  - Moisten plaster (fiberglass, plaster, or precast) material by dipping in a bucket of cool water.

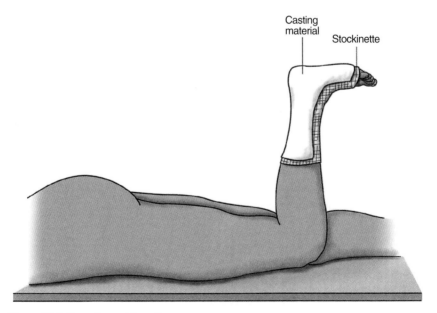

Figure 38.1 Posterior ankle splint.

- Apply casting material to the posterior portion of the leg and ankle.
- Mold the casting material to the shape and angle of the limb, ensuring a 90-degree flexion of the ankle.
- Wrap with elastic wrap proximally to distally. Sufficient elastic wrap should be used to hold the posterior splint snugly.
- Fold over the edge of stockinette and complete the elastic tape wrap. Secure end with tape.
- Allow casting material to dry.
- *Method 2*—Aircast technique
  - Position the ankle in neutral position, ensuring adequate stretching of the Achilles tendon (90-degree angle).
  - Apply stockinette or cotton sock.
  - Apply Aircast splint and secure straps.
  - Inflate as directed.

KNEE IMMOBILIZATION
See Figure 38.2.

- Position the client comfortably, and place a rolled towel underneath the knee sufficient to flex it 15 to 20 degrees.
- Optional—Apply stockinette extending to approximately 4 to 6 cm below the groin to midcalf (i.e., greater than the length of the immobilizer).

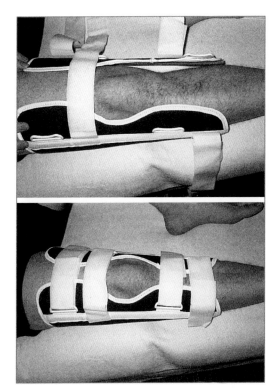

Figure 38.2 Knee immobilization.

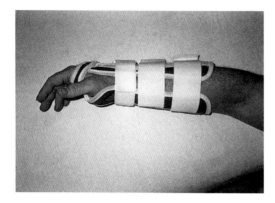

Figure 38.3 Premade wrist splint.

- Support pantyhose can be used in place of stockinette.
- Open the knee immobilizer and center the patellar notch of fabric.
- Close and secure the knee immobilizer with self-adhering straps.

WRIST SPLINTING
- *Method 1*—Premade wrist splint (Fig. 38.3)
  - Position the client comfortably with wrist in neutral position.
  - Optional—Apply stockinette and cut a small hole to slide the thumb through in a glovelike fashion. It should extend to a length approximately equal to the splint itself.
  - Position the splint to ensure adequate support of the joint structure.
  - Secure with self-adhering straps.
- *Method 2*—Volar splinting (Fig. 38.4)
  - Position the wrist slightly hyperextended (5 to 10 degrees).
  - Apply stockinette at least 6 to 8 cm longer than intended casting material, being sure to cut a hole to allow thumb through.
  - Optional—Apply cotton web padding to a thickness of at least 2 inches.
  - Select appropriate width of casting material (usually a 6-inch width).
  - Cut the casting material to the length needed.
    - If not precast with preset thickness, fold in 10 to 12 overlapping layers equaling the length plus 4 cm of the projected splint.
  - Moisten the plaster (fiberglass, plaster, or precast) material by dipping in a bucket of cool water.
  - Apply the casting material to the forearm, wrist, and palm of hand.
  - Apply casting material and mold it to the shape of the wrist.
  - If necessary, trim the distal edge of the casting material to the middle interphalangeal joint.
  - Fold excess stockinette over plaster.
  - Using elastic wrap, wrap from distal to proximal. Ensure secure fit with the use of two or three layers of elastic wrap.
  - Secure end with tape.
  - Apply sling until dry.

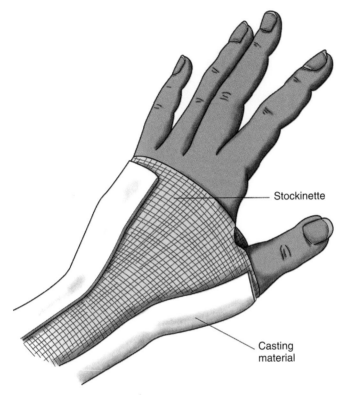

Stockinette

Casting
material

Figure 38.4 Volar wrist splint.

THUMB SPLINTING
- *Method 1*—Premade wrist splint
  - See method 1, premade wrist splint application.
- *Method 2*—Aluminum thumb splint (Fig. 38.5)
  - Position the wrist and hand comfortably, the thumb slightly flexed at the distal interphalangeal (DIP) joint. Have the client grasp an elastic wrap or 3-inch gauze roll in the web space of the hand.
    - Hyperflex the wrist approximately 5 to 10 degrees and in neutral radioulnar deviation position.
  - Measure the aluminum splint from the end of the thumb and 6 to 10 cm to the anatomical snuffbox of the forearm. Be sure to trim any sharp edges.
  - Optional—Apply stockinette to the thumb and forearm in the same length as the splint. Cut a hole in the stockinette to allow the thumb to slide through.
  - Optional—Apply cotton padding in 1- to 2-inch thickness.
  - Bend the aluminum splint to the position of the thumb and wrist.
  - Apply the splint to either the dorsal (most commonly performed) or the palmar side of the thumb.
  - Optional—Apply a single strip of tape to the aluminum splint at the DIP.

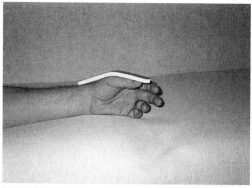

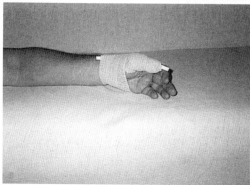

Figure 38.5 Aluminum thumb splint.

- Remove webbing used to maintain proper position.
- Wrap the aluminum splint distally to proximally with the elastic wrap, including the thumb. A modified figure eight pattern of thumb, wrist, and metacarpals can be used.
- Secure with tape.
- *Method 3*—Thumb spica (Fig. 38.6)
  - Position the wrist and hand comfortably, the thumb slightly flexed at the DIP joint. Have the client grasp an elastic wrap or 3-inch gauze roll in the web space of the hand.
    - Hyperflex the wrist approximately 5 to 10 degrees and in neutral radioulnar deviation position.
  - Measure the casting strips from just proximal to the distal palmar crease to midforearm. Use narrower width of casting material for the thumb, with the length being measured from the tip of the thumb to midforearm.
  - Apply stockinette to the thumb and forearm.
  - Optional—Apply cotton padding in 2-inch thickness, including the thumb.
  - Moisten all casting material by dipping in a bucket of cool water.
  - Apply wider casting material to the underside of the forearm.
  - Take narrower thumb strips and apply on lateral surface of thumb, molding them to the anatomical placement of the thumb.

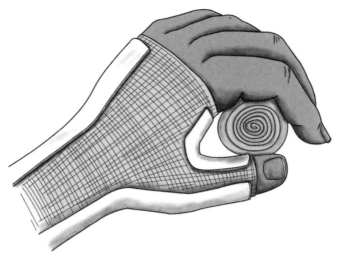

Figure 38.6 Thumb spica splint.

- Apply elastic wrap distally to proximally, including the thumb. A modified figure eight pattern of thumb, wrist, and metacarpals can be used.
- Apply a sling until dry.

Taping

Equipment
- Soft padding material
- Elastic wrap tape (2-, 4-, or 6-inch widths)
- Tape adherent spray (e.g., tincture of benzoin)
- Zinc white (cotton) tape in various widths (1-, 2-, 3-, or 4-inch widths)
- Scissors—nonsterile
- Arm sling
- Foam-cushion foot insert

Procedure

ANKLE TAPING
- *Method 1*—Louisiana ankle wrap technique (Fig. 38.7)
  - Position the ankle in a neutral position ensuring adequate stretching of the Achilles tendon (90-degree angle).
  - Optional—Apply stockinette to the ankle with it extending approximately 2 to 3 inches above and below the projected wrap area.
  - Spray tape adherent to the proposed taping site.
  - Begin wrap by anchoring across the top of the foot.
  - Continue wrap around instep, then proceed to around heel.
  - Continue wrapping in a layer format until satisfactory reduction of movement has been achieved.
  - Secure end of wrap with tape.

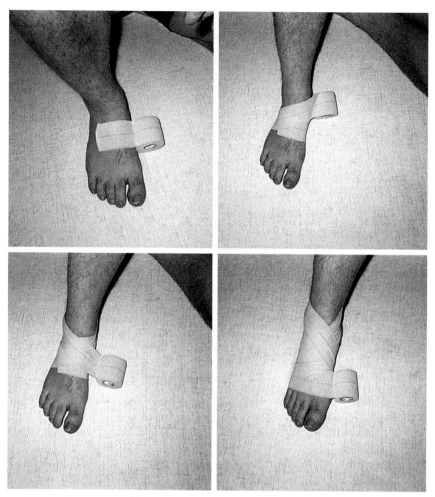

Figure 38.7 Louisiana ankle wrap technique.

- *Method 2*—Open Gibney technique with heel lock (Fig. 38.8)
  - Position the ankle in neutral position, ensuring adequate stretching of the Achilles tendon (90-degree angle).
  - Optional—Apply stockinette to ankle, with it extending approximately 2 to 3 inches above and below the projected wrap area.
  - Spray tape adherent to the proposed taping site.
  - Using zinc (cotton) tape 1 or 2 inches wide (depending on ankle size), apply a tape anchor approximately 10 to 12 cm above the lateral and medial malleolus encircling the leg.
  - Apply five to six overlapping circular tape layers over the stirrup strips.
  - Apply two to three diagonal overlapping circular tape layers to the arch region.
  - Apply two to three overlapping diagonal tape layers to the heel.

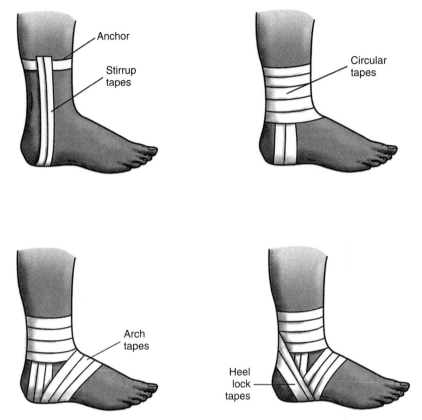

Figure 38.8 Open Gibney technique with heel lock.

- If using stockinette, fold the excess stockinette over the tape, anchor with tape, and trim.
- Apply two to three overlapping stirrup strips in a continuous fashion medially and laterally. These stirrup strips should extend from the anchor tape on the lateral side of the ankle under the bottom of the foot and back up to the anchor tape on the medial side of the ankle.
- *Method 3*—Open Gibney technique without heel lock (Fig. 38.9)
  - Position the ankle in neutral position, ensuring adequate stretching of the Achilles tendon (90-degree angle).
  - Optional—Apply stockinette to ankle with it extending approximately 2 to 3 inches above and below the projected wrap area.
  - Spray tape adherent to the proposed taping site.
  - Apply 6 to 10 overlapping semicircular tape strips to cover 50% of the posterior lower leg to approximately 1 to 2 cm above and 10 to 12 cm below the lateral and medial malleolus.
  - Apply four to six longer semicircular strips in an overlapping pattern to the long axis of the foot. Start at 2 cm proximal of the medial distal metatarsal

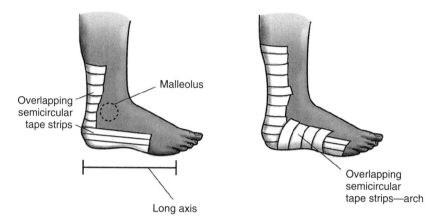

Figure 38.9 Open Gibney technique without heel lock.

head around the posterior heel extending to 2 cm proximal of the lateral distal metatarsal heads.
- Apply four to six semicircular strips in an overlapping pattern in the arch region of the foot extending from the distal calcaneus to midmetatarsal region.
- If using stockinette, fold over the excess stockinette, anchor with tape, and trim.
- *Method 4*—Basket-weave technique with heel lock (Fig. 38.10)
  - Position the ankle in neutral position ensuring adequate stretching of the Achilles tendon (90-degree angle).
  - Optional—Apply stockinette to ankle with it extending approximately 2 to 3 inches above and below the projected wrap area.
  - Spray tape adherent to the proposed taping site.
  - Apply two circular tape strips as follows.
    - One strip at the top of the projected area of taping approximately 10 to 12 cm above the lateral and medial malleolus
    - One strip at the bottom of the projected area of taping approximately 2 cm above the distal metatarsal head
  - Apply longitudinal and vertical tape strips in an overlapping pattern.
  - Apply a layer of circular tape strips covering the vertical tape strips.
  - Apply five to six circular strips across the arch region to approximately midmetatarsal.
  - If using stockinette, fold over the excess stockinette, anchor with tape, and trim.

KNEE TAPING
See Figure 38.11.
- Position the client comfortably, and place a rolled towel underneath the knee sufficient to flex it 15 to 20 degrees.
- Optional—Apply foam pad over the popliteal space to reduce chafing.

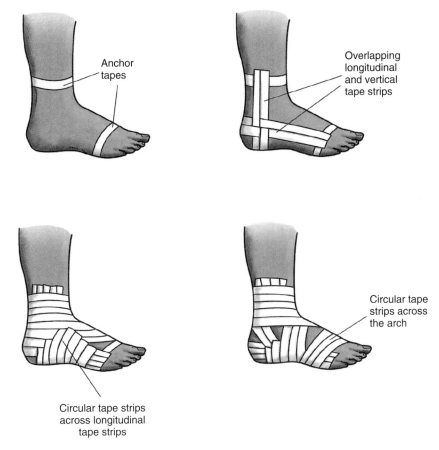

Figure 38.10 Basket-weave technique with heel lock.

- Optional—Apply stockinette extending to approximately 4 to 6 cm below the groin to midcalf.
- Spray tape adherent to the proposed taping site.
- Apply overlapping circular strips of tape (2- or 3-inch tape suggested) beginning either proximally or distally depending on personal preference in a basket-weave pattern.
- Apply 3- to 4-inch elastic tape (4-inch tape recommended) in a larger figure eight pattern, crossing over the medial and lateral collateral ligaments. This may be repeated in a layered fashion for three to four layers.
- If using stockinette, fold over the excess stockinette, anchor with tape, and trim.

WRIST TAPING
See Figure 38.12.
- Position the client comfortably with the thumb slightly flexed. Position of the thumb can be maintained with a roll of elastic tape or gauze in the web space.

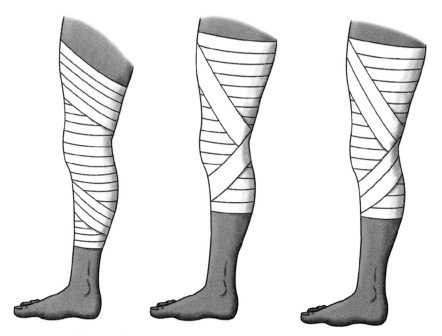

Figure 38.11 Knee taping.

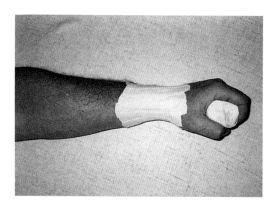

Figure 38.12 Wrist taping.

- Optional—Apply stockinette and cut a small hole to slide thumb through in a glovelike fashion. It should extend approximately 2 inches beyond the proposed taping area.
- Spray tape adherent to the skin.
- Cut approximately four to six 2-inch tape strips, and apply along the medial portion of the forearm covering the location of the distal insertion of the adductor pollicis across the distal radial head and the extensor carpi radialis longus and extensor carpi ulnaris brevis.
- If using stockinette, fold over the excess stockinette, anchor with tape, and trim.

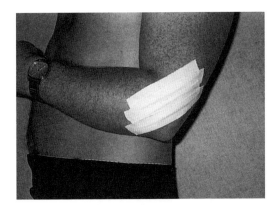

Figure 38.13 Lateral epicondylar elbow taping.

- Optional—Apply an elastic wrap in a figure eight pattern for further rigidity.

ELBOW TAPING—LATERAL EPICONDYLAR TAPING
See Figure 38.13.
- Position the client comfortably with the elbow flexed 90 degrees.
- Optional—Apply stockinette approximately 10 to 12 cm above and below the joint.
- Spray tape adherent to area to be taped.
- Apply 6-inch strips in an overlapping fashion over the lateral epicondylar process.
- If using stockinette, fold over the excess stockinette, anchor with tape, and trim.
- Apply an arm sling if only minimal relief was obtained from the taping.
  - Use the sling no longer than 72 hours.

FOOT TAPING
- *Method 1*—Figure eight technique (Fig. 38.14)
  - Position the client comfortably with foot in neutral position (90-degree angle).
  - Spray tape adherent to the area to be taped.
  - Apply a circular figure eight pattern with inclusion of the heel from the base of the first metatarsal to the base of the fifth metatarsal.
  - Continue in an overlapping pattern of at least three or four strips.
  - Apply three to four transverse strips in an overlapping pattern across the plantar surface at the metatarsal heads. They should not extend into the arch unless relief is not obtained.
  - Optional—Foam pad may be inserted in the shoe for added comfort.
- *Method 2*—Full plantar taping technique (Fig. 38.15)
  - Position the client comfortably with foot in neutral position (90-degree angle).
  - Spray tape adherent to the area to be taped.

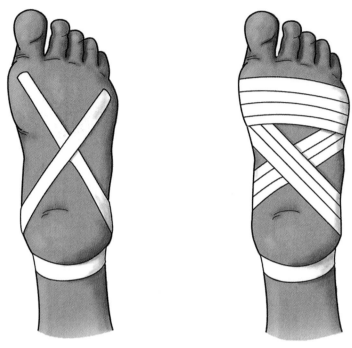

Figure 38.14 Foot taping—figure eight technique.

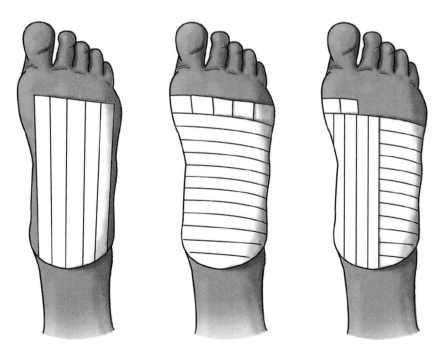

Figure 38.15 Foot taping—full plantar taping technique.

- Apply tape along the longitudinal axis of the plantar surface.
  - If necessary, reapply tape adherent spray if tape does not hold when using layering technique.
- Apply overlapping tape transversely.
- Apply overlapping tape longitudinally.
- If no improvement of the plantar fasciitis in 7 to 10 days, reevaluation of the diagnosis should be considered.

Client Instructions

SPLINTING AND TAPING

- RICE—Rest, Ice, Compression (splinting or taping as indicated by injury), and Elevate the injured joint for at least 48 hours to minimize further trauma.
- Avoid weight-bearing; use crutches for injuries of the knees or ankles.
- After 24 hours
  - Remove splint at least four times a day and begin gentle range of motion.
  - Remove taping once per day and begin gentle range of motion.
  - If pain occurs when range of motion is attempted, delay for an additional 24 hours.
  - If unable to resume gentle range of motion after 48 hours, return to the office for further evaluation of the injury.
- Observe for signs of neurovascular compromise, including
  - Pallor or decreased color of the fingers or toes
  - Decreased sensation or numbness in the fingers or toes
  - Increased pain
  - If any signs of neurovascular compromise occur, remove the tape and call health-care provider.
- To relieve pain and inflammation
  - Use acetaminophen every 4 to 6 hours.
  - NSAIDs, such as ibuprofen, may be initiated 12 to 24 hours after injury.
  - Elevate and rest the injured joint. This facilitates the effectiveness of medication.

BIBLIOGRAPHY

Birrer R, Poole B. Athletic taping part 3: The knee. *J Musculoskelet Med.* July 1995:43–45.
Mercier L. *Practical Orthopedics.* St. Louis, MO: Mosby; 2008.
Murtagh J. *Practice Tips.* New York, NY: McGraw-Hall; 2017.
Pfenniger JL, Fowler GC. *Procedures for Primary Care Physicians.* St. Louis, MO: Mosby; 2019.
Ryan J. Use of posterior night splints in the treatment of plantar fasciitis. *Am Fam Physician.* 1995;52(3):891–898.

39 Chapter

Trigger Point Injection

Margaret Colyar

CPT Code
20550 Injection; tendon sheath, ligament, trigger points, or ganglion cyst

Trigger points are areas of localized pain in various muscle groups, often near bony attachments. Focal tender areas are located by palpating the various muscle groups to determine the trigger point and the corresponding area of pain. Common points of maximum tenderness often are located at moving parts and sliding surfaces. Although exacerbations are not predictable, avoiding repetitive overuse of muscle groups might prevent occurrence.

OVERVIEW
- More common with myofascial pain syndromes and fibromyalgia

RATIONALE
- To interrupt the pain cycle and provide immediate relief

INDICATIONS
- Areas of localized tenderness without other pathology

CONTRAINDICATIONS
- Irritation or infection at injection site
- Anticoagulant therapy or increased bleeding tendency
- **Septicemia**
- Acute musculoskeletal trauma
- ❱ *Informed consent required*

PROCEDURE
Trigger Point Injection

Equipment
- Alcohol wipes
- Gloves—sterile
- 4 × 4 gauze pads
- Skin-marking pencil
- Topical skin cleanser
- 0.25% to 1% lidocaine *without* epinephrine (single-dose vials, if possible)

- Choice of steroid (0.5 to 1 mL of selected steroid, such as methylprednisolone acetate if used with lidocaine)
- 25- to 27-gauge needle of length appropriate for site injected
- 3-, 5-, or 10-mL syringe

Procedure

- Position patient in comfortable, safe position in the event of a syncopal reaction.
- Mark the point of maximal tenderness with a marking pencil.
- Cleanse the skin with topical antiseptic.
- Identify the trigger point (maximal area of tenderness) with sterile gloved finger using sterile technique.
- Using the 25- or 27-gauge needle, draw 3 to 5 mL of lidocaine (if using only lidocaine, begin with 5 mL of 0.25% to 1% lidocaine).
- If using the additional steroid, draw 3 to 4 mL of the lidocaine first; then draw 1 mL of the steroid into the same syringe.
  - *Note*—Change needles if drawing from both solutions to prevent dulling of the needle and contamination of multidose vials.
- Slowly advance the needle perpendicular to the skin until the point of tenderness is located.
- Aspirate for a blood return (relocate if identified).
- Inject 0.5 to 2 mL of the medication (the patient should have instant pain relief if properly located).
- Withdraw the needle slightly and inject the site two to four times at 30-degree angles from the first perpendicular injection (north, south, east, west).
- Remove the needle and wipe the skin with the disinfectant.
- Place an adhesive bandage over the injection site.
- Observe for immediate decrease in pain.
- Observe for light-headedness, tinnitus, peripheral numbness, slurring of speech, drowsiness, or seizures (may indicate reaction to the local anesthetic).

Client Instructions

- Observe for signs and symptoms of infection, such as
  - Increase in pain after 24 hours
  - Increase in temperature
  - Redness or swelling
  - Yellow or greenish drainage
  - Foul odor
- If any signs or symptoms of infection are found, return to the office.
- Observe for the following problems:
  - Hematoma formation
  - Reaction to local anesthetic
  - Rebound pain
  - Neuritis
- Trigger point injection may be repeated as needed if no steroids are used. If steroids are used, injections should be given at least 6 weeks apart.

BIBLIOGRAPHY

Alverez DJ, Rockwell DO. Trigger points: management and diagnosis. *Am Fam Physician.* 2002;65(4):653–661.

Bron C, Dommerholt JC. Etiology of myofascial trigger points. *Curr Pain Headache Rep.* 2012:16(5):439–444.

Pando JA, Klippel JH. Arthrocentesis and corticosteroid injections: An illustrated guide to technique. *Consultant.* 1996; 10:2137–2148.

Pfenninger JL, Fowler GC, eds. *Procedures for Primary Care Physicians.* St. Louis, MO: Mosby; 2019.

Genitourinary and Breast Procedures

Breast Biopsy
Fine Needle Aspiration
Margaret R. Colyar

CPT Code
10021   Fine needle aspiration without imaging guidance
19000   Puncture aspiration of cyst of breast
19001   Puncture aspiration, each additional cyst
19100   Biopsy of breast, needle core, without imaging guidance

Fine needle aspiration is a method of obtaining samples of a solid or cystic mass for laboratory evaluation. Tissues commonly obtained by this method are
• Breast
• Thyroid
• Lymph node
Thyroid masses and lymph node biopsies are not currently within the scope of practice for nurse practitioners and should be referred to a physician for aspiration.

OVERVIEW
• There are four common types of breast masses
  • Fibroadenomas—solid benign tumors usually found in younger women
  • Cysts—fluid-filled and usually seen during midlife
  • Benign masses—feel smooth, round, and freely moveable
  • Breast carcinomas—solid masses that increase in frequency with age and usually not seen in women younger than 30 years old
    • Usually feel solid and unmovable with poorly defined or irregular edges

RATIONALE

- To confirm etiology of a lesion for treatment
- To establish or confirm a diagnosis for treatment and/or intervention

INDICATIONS

- Palpable solitary breast mass
- Recurrent breast mass
- Anxiety concerning a mass

CONTRAINDICATIONS

- Coagulation disorder—REFER
- On anticoagulant therapy—REFER
- Bloody discharge from a nipple—REFER
- Definite cancerous breast—REFER
▶ *Informed consent required*

PROCEDURE

Biopsy—Fine Needle Aspiration

Equipment

- Antiseptic skin cleanser
- 1% lidocaine
- 3-mL syringe
- 21-, 22-, or 23-gauge, 1½-inch needle
- 12-mL syringe
- 4 × 4 gauze—sterile
- Gloves—sterile
- 27- to 30-gauge, ½-inch needle
- Optional—EURO-Med FNA 21 for fine needle aspiration
  - For solid core masses only
- Specimen jar with 10% formalin
  - For solid core cyst only
- Two sterile plain evacuated blood tubes
- Four microscope slides
- Fixative for slides
- Coverslips

Procedure

- Position the client with the mass easily accessible.
- Cleanse the mass and surrounding tissues with antiseptic skin cleanser.
- Inject 1% lidocaine around the mass, if desired (Fig. 40.1).
- If using a 12-mL syringe, aspirate one-fifth of syringe full of air.
  - Hold the mass immobile with nondominant hand.
  - Using dominant hand with syringe held like a pen, insert the 12-mL syringe with 21- to 23-gauge needle into the mass and aspirate.

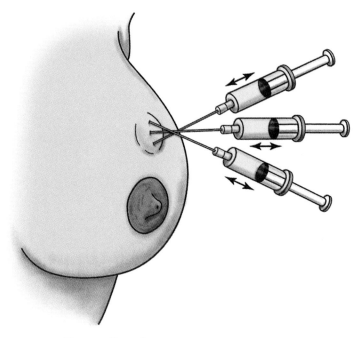

Figure 40.1 Fine needle aspiration.

- Move needle around into all areas of the mass. Aspirate in each area.
- Before withdrawing the syringe, return the plunger to the position before aspiration to prevent withdrawal of sample while leaving the mass. This prevents seeding the needle tract with malignant cells.
- Eject cell material onto slides (if fluid) or into specimen jar containing 10% formalin (if solid core).
- To decrease the chance of hematoma formation, either apply pressure with 4 × 4 gauze for 5 to 15 minutes or apply an ice pack for 15 to 20 minutes.

Client Instructions

- To prevent hematoma formation
  - Apply a pressure dressing and an ice pack for 24 hours.
- A moderate amount of pain, redness, and swelling is expected. Take acetaminophen (Tylenol) every 4 hours as needed.
- Observe for signs and symptoms of infection, such as
  - Increase in pain after 24 hours
  - Increase in temperature
  - Redness or swelling
  - Yellow or greenish drainage
  - Foul odor
- If any signs or symptoms of infection are found, return to the office.

BIBLIOGRAPHY

Casaubon JT, Regan J-P. Breast masses, fine needle aspiration. In *StatPearls [Internet]*. *StatPearls Publishing*; Treasure Island (FL): StatPearls Publishing; 2018. https://www.ncbi.nlm.nih.gov/books/NBK470268/. Accessed October 9, 2019.

Kline TS. Fine-needle aspiration biopsy of the breast. *Am Fam Physician*. 1995;52(7):2021–2025.

Layfield LJ, Chrischilles EA, Cohen MB, Bottles K. The palpable breast nodule: A cost-effectiveness analysis of alternate diagnostic approaches. *Cancer*. 1993;72(5):1640–1651.

Pfenninger JL, Fowler GC. *Procedures for Primary Care Physicians*. St. Louis, MO: Mosby; 2019.

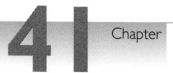

Chapter

Breast Examination

Margaret R. Colyar

CPT Code
None

Clinical breast examination is a screening examination done to differentiate normal physiological nodularity from a discrete breast mass. Using a systematic search pattern that ensures all breast tissue is examined increases the sensitivity of the clinical breast examination. Most breast cancers are found in the upper outer quadrant and under the areola and nipple.

OVERVIEW

- Breasts are least tender and least lumpy in the week following menses.
- Percentages of breast tissue are found
  - 50%—in the upper outer quadrant of the breast
  - 15%—in the upper medial quadrant
  - 11%—in the lower outer quadrant
  - 6%—lower medial quadrant
  - 18%—under the areola
- Malignancies usually originate in either the glandular tissues that secrete milk or in the ductal structures that transport the milk to the nipple.
- Major breast cancer risk factors are shown in Table 41.1.

Table 41·1	Major Breast Cancer Risk Factors

- Prior history of breast cancer
- Family history of first-degree relative with breast cancer
- Defective genetic mutations in the family—*BRCA1* and *BRCA2*
- Prolonged/uninterrupted exposure to estrogen
- Took diethylstilbestrol (DES) to prevent miscarriage
- Early age at onset of menstruation (before 12 y.o.)
- Never pregnant
- Increasing patient age
- Older age at first pregnancy
- Older age at menopause (after 55 y.o.)
- Obesity—more estrogen produced

- Use the acronym BREAST for an easy way to evaluate for physical signs associated with advanced breast cancer
  - B—Breast mass
  - R—Retraction
  - E—Edema
  - A—Axillary mass
  - S—Scaly nipple
  - T—Tender breast
- Use the 5 P's to guide breast tissue examination:
  - Position
    - Sitting—Evaluate axillary, supraclavicular, and infraclavicular lymph nodes
    - Lying—Breast palpation
  - Perimeter
    - Down the midaxillary line
    - Across the inframammary ridge at the fifth/sixth rib
    - Up the lateral edge of the sternum
    - Across the clavicle, back to the midaxilla
  - Pattern of search—circular, wedge, or vertical strip
  - Palpation—Use three middle fingers to palpate overlapping dime-sized circular motions.
  - Pressure—light, medium, and deep
- Type of nodularity is described in Table 41.2.
- Other examinations and tests are shown in Table 41.3.

RATIONALE

- To evaluate the breasts for masses

CONTRAINDICATIONS

- None
▶ *Informed consent required*

Table 41·2	**Types of Breast Nodularity**
TYPE	**HOW IT FEELS**
Physiological nodularity (fibrocystic breast) • Common in childbearing years	Dense with an irregular area of thicker tissue with a lumpy ridgelike surface OR Tiny beadlike masses scattered throughout the breast but most often found in the upper outer quadrant and under the areola
Mass—cyst • Increases before menses and decreases after menses	Fluid-filled Moveable; no dimpling/skin puckering Softer Round and smooth
Mass—malignant	Fixed, causes dimpling/skin puckering Hard Oddly shaped

Table 41·3	**Examinations and Tests**
TEST	**REASON**
Breast MRI	Better identify a breast lump An abnormal change on a mammogram
Breast ultrasound	Shows whether a lump is solid or fluid-filled
Breast biopsy	Aspirate nodule for testing
CT scan	To check if the cancer has spread
Mammography	To screen for breast cancer To help identify a breast lump
PET scan	To determine whether a breast cancer has spread
Sentinel lymph node biopsy	To check if the breast cancer has spread to the lymph nodes

PROCEDURE

Clinical Breast Examination

- Explain the procedure to the patient.
  - Discuss the monthly breast self-examination as you do the examination.
- Have the patient sit upright and open the gown.
- Instruct the patient to
  - Raise arms over the head
  - Press hands together just above the breasts
  - Press hands firmly on the hips—contracts pectoralis major muscles
- Observe for
  - Dimpling
  - Nipple asymmetry
  - Redness
  - Retraction
  - Skin changes/puckering

- Palpate the axillary, supraclavicular, and infraclavicular lymph nodes.
- Instruct the patient to lie down flat and place her right hand under the head.
- Uncover the right breast only.
- Examine the perimeter of the breast tissue from
  - The clavicle to the inferior portion of the breast
  - Medially to the midsternum
  - Laterally to the midaxillary line
  - The axillary tail of the breast tissue
  - The axilla for lymphadenopathy
- Use one of three techniques moving the three middle fingers in dime-sized circles, first with light pressure, then medium pressure, and then deep pressure (Fig. 41.1).
  - Circular
  - Wedge
  - Vertical strip
- Using the thumb and index finger, express the nipple.
- Then, using the same technique, examine the left breast.
- Describe any nodule in terms of
  - Location—more masses found in
    - Upper outer quadrant
    - Areola
  - Size—usually pea-sized before a mass can be detected
  - Mobility
    - Fixed—concerning for malignancy
    - Moveable—most likely benign
  - Texture
  - Color
    - Redness—infection or inflammation
    - "Peau d'orange"—aggressive inflammatory malignancy
  - Presence of nipple discharge
    - Blood—concerning for malignancy
    - Milk when not pregnant
      - Possible prolactin secretion from the pituitary
      - Possible side effect from some medications (Table 41.4)

Use the algorithms in Figures 41.2 and 41.3 as guides for further testing.

Client Instructions

Teach the following breast self-examination.
- Examine the breast one time each month, usually the week following menses as the breasts are least tender and least lumpy.
- In the shower, feel for lumps.
  - Fingers are flat.
  - Move gently over each breast.
  - Use the right hand to examine the left breast.
  - Use the left hand to examine the right breast.

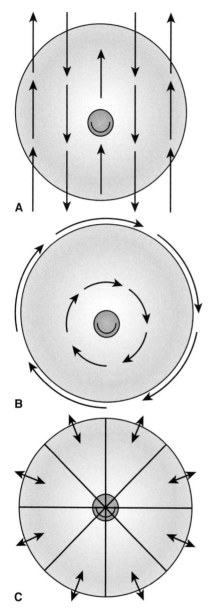

Figure 41.1 Three techniques for palpating breasts. (A) Vertical, (B) circular, (C) wedge.

Table 41·4	Medications That Increase Prolactin Levels
DRUG CLASS	**DRUG**
Antihypertensives	Beta blockers, methyldopa, verapamil
Tricyclic antipsychotics	Phenothiazines, Haloperidol
Atypical neuroleptics	Risperidone, olanzapine
Antidepressants, SSRIs	Paroxetine, escitalopram, sertraline, fluoxetine
H$_2$ antagonists	Cimetidine
Contraceptives	Combined oral contraceptive, Depo-Provera
Illicit drugs	Cannabis, opiates, amphetamines
Herbal remedies	Anise, blessed thistle, fennel, fenugreek seed, marshmallow, nettle, red clover, red raspberry
Others	Digoxin, spironolactone, danazol, sumatriptan, isoniazid, valproate, Buspar, alprazolam

- In front of a mirror, observe the breasts for swelling, dimpling, puckering, nipple changes
  - With hands at your sides
  - Raising hands overhead
  - Pressing your hands on your hips
- Lying down, feel for lumps.
  - With the right hand under your head, palpate the right breast with the left hand.
  - With the left hand under your head, palpate the left breast with the right hand.
  - Fingers flat, press in small circular motions around the breast. Then move in 1 inch and press around the breast. Follow this procedure until you complete the entire breast including the areola and nipple.
  - Squeeze the nipple of each breast between the thumb and index finger gently to check for discharge.

Lumps and discharge should be reported to your primary care provider immediately.

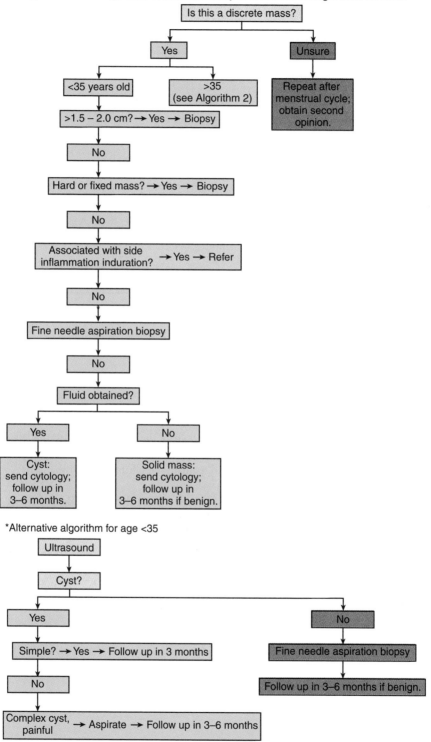

Figure 41.2 Algorithm for management of a breast lump in a woman younger than 35 years of age. *Image reprinted with permission from Medscape (http://www. medscape.com/), 2014, available at: http://www.medscape.com/viewarticle/408932.*

Algorithm 2: Management of a Breast Lump in a Woman 35 Years or Older

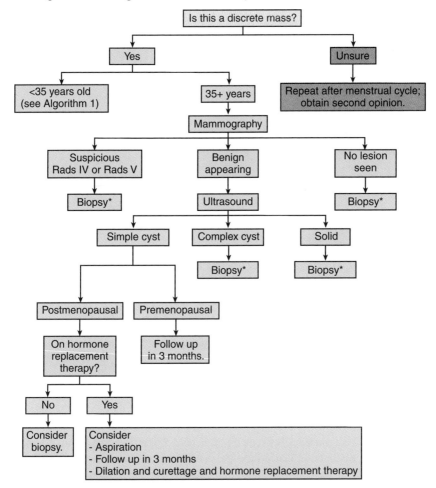

*Note that biopsy procedure may be excisional, core, or fine needle aspiration depending on the clinical situation.

Figure 41.3 Algorithm for management of a breast lump in a woman 35 years of age or older. *Image reprinted with permission from Medscape (http://www.medscape .com/), 2014, available at: http://www.medscape.com/viewarticle/408932.*

BIBLIOGRAPHY ▰▰▰▰▰▰▰▰▰▰▰▰▰

Breast Self-Exam. BREASTCANCER.ORG website. http://www.breastcancer.org/ symptoms/testing/types/self_exam/bse_steps?gclid=CKOjzJnm5b4CFXQiMgod LD8AQA. Last modified June 20, 2019. Accessed October 9, 2019.

Clinical Breast Exam. National Breast Cancer Foundation website. http:// www.nationalbreastcancer.org/clinical-breast-exam. Accessed October 9, 2019.

Fibrocystic Breast Changes: Lumps That Are Normal. Chiro.org website. http:// www.chiro.org/LINKS/FULL/Fibrocystic_Breast_Changes.shtml. Accessed October 9, 2019.

Freund KM. Rationale and technique of clinical breast examination. *Medscape Gen Med.*
2000;2(4):1–9.
Torre DL, Falorni A. Pharmacological causes of hyperprolactenemia. *Ther Clin Risk Manag.*
2007;3(5):929–951.

Chapter

42

Colposcopy
Endocervical Curettage and
Cervical Biopsy

Margaret R. Colyar

CPT Code
57452 Colposcopy
57454 Colposcopy with biopsy, single or multiple, of the cervix and/or
endocervical curettage
57500 Biopsy, single or multiple, or local excision of lesion, with or
without fulguration
57505 Endocervical curettage

A colposcopic examination is necessary after receiving an abnormal **Papanicolaou
(Pap) smear.** Endocervical **curettage** and cervical biopsy are done when abnormalities are found on the colposcopic examination.

OVERVIEW

- The use of a colposcopic examination form is helpful in documenting findings
  (Fig. 42.1).
- Questions to ask each client include
  - Menstrual history
  - Medications—especially hormones and anticoagulants
  - History of abnormal Pap smears
  - History of previous treatment for abnormal Pap smears
  - Signs of pelvic or vaginal infection
  - History of human papillomavirus (HPV) infection
  - History of diethylstilbestrol (DES) exposure
  - History of sexually transmitted diseases, sexual abuse, or partner with genital
    condyloma acuminatum
  - History of cervical, vaginal, or vulvar cancer

COLPOSCOPY

Date _____

Name _____ Age _____ DOB _____

Reason for colposcopy _____

LMP _____ Pap smear date _____ Result _____

# of pregnancies ___ # of children ___ Type of contraception _____

History of STDs _____ Vaginal warts _____ Vaginal infections _____

Do you smoke? _____ How much? _____

Conclusions of the colposcopy

Vaginal vault_____ Urethra _____

Labia _____ Perineum _____ Rectum_____

Signs of vaginal infection_____

Complete transformation zone seen?_____

Biopsy site _____

Impressions _____

_____

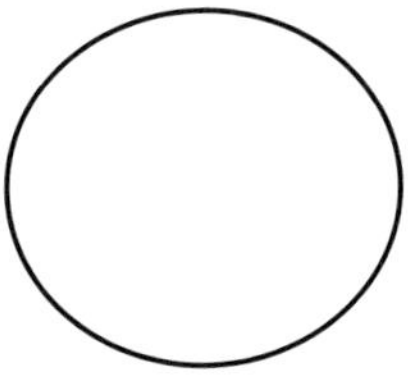

Recommendations: (Circle one)

Cryotherapy   Loop

Referral to _____

Signature _____

Key: WE - White epithelium

L - Leukoplakia

P - Punctation

M - Mosaicism

ATZ - Abnormal TZ

AV - Abnormal vessels

X - Biopsy sites

Figure 42.1 Sample colposcopic examination form.

RATIONALE

- To evaluate cervical abnormalities

INDICATIONS

- Abnormal Pap smear
- Observed cervical lesion
- HPV infection
- Unexplained vaginal bleeding
- History of DES exposure in utero

CONTRAINDICATIONS

- Pregnancy—REFER to gynecologist for testing.
- Current heavy menses
- ▶ *Informed consent required*

Ask client to take 600 mg of ibuprofen 1 hour before the testing time to decrease uterine discomfort.

PROCEDURE

Colposcopy, Endocervical Curettage, Cervical Biopsy

Equipment

- Drape—sterile
- Gloves—nonsterile
- Syringe—3 mL
- Vaginal **speculum**—large
- Colposcope with
  - 3× to 20× power
  - Green light filter
- Ring **forceps**—sterile
- Cotton balls—sterile
- 0.9% sodium chloride—sterile
- Cotton-tipped applicators—small and large—sterile
- White vinegar—5% acetic acid solution
- Containers with 10% **formalin**
- Cervical biopsy punch forceps—sterile
- Cervical brush or broom
- Monsel's solution or other topical hemostatic agent

Procedure

COLPOSCOPY

- Have the client void immediately before the procedure.
- Position the client in the lithotomy position.
- Drape the perineum.
- Put on gloves.
- Insert the warmed speculum into the vagina and bring the cervix into view.
- Inspect the cervix with the naked eye.
- Wash the cervix and vagina gently with large cotton-tipped swab or cotton balls soaked in sterile saline.
- Remove mucus with ring forceps and cotton balls.
- Position the colposcope. Visualize the cervix and vaginal walls using the 5× setting.
- Switch to green filter light (enhances visibility of blood vessels) and visualize.
- Using cotton balls soaked in vinegar for 3 to 5 minutes, wash the cervix with warm vinegar.
  - *Note*—Vinegar dissolves mucus, constricts blood vessels, and allows better visualization of the cervix.

- Reapply vinegar every 5 minutes to maintain acetowhiteness during the procedure.
- Systematically examine the cervix for the squamocolumnar junction, **transformation zone**, and abnormalities using
  - Low power and white light
  - Higher power and white light
  - Lower power and green filter light
  - Higher power and green filter light
- Document findings.

CERVICAL BIOPSY
- Biopsy areas that show (Fig. 42.2)
  - Acetowhite after application of vinegar
    - Shiny white indicates a low-grade lesion.
    - Dull grayish white indicates a high-grade lesion.

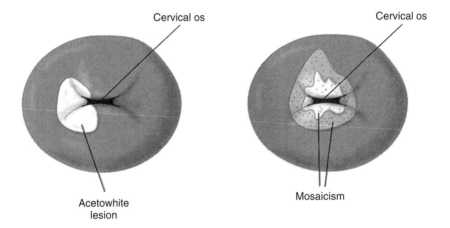

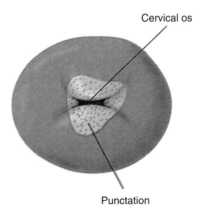

Figure 42.2 Abnormalities found on cervical biopsy that must be biopsied.

- **Mosaicism**—abnormal chicken wire, cobblestone, or tile-floor pattern
- **Punctation**—abnormal stippled appearance
- To biopsy
  - Using the cervical biopsy punch forceps, start at the bottom of the cervix and work upward, taking 3-mm specimens (Fig. 42.3).
- Apply topical hemostatic agent to areas of bleeding.
- Put each specimen in a different specimen jar and label with location.

ENDOCERVICAL CURETTAGE

- After the cervical biopsies are completed, take a specimen from the endocervical canal.
- Insert the cervical brush or broom into the cervical os, and make a complete 360-degree turn.
- Remove and place scrapings into a container with 10% formalin and label.
- Remove the speculum.
- After examination of the cervix, apply vinegar to the vagina and external genitalia. Take biopsy specimens as necessary, when acetowhiteness appears.

Client Instructions

- You may have dark or black vaginal discharge for 2 days after the procedure.
- Observe for and report the following
  - Heavy vaginal bleeding (greater than one sanitary pad change per hour)
  - Low abdominal pain
  - Fever, chills, or foul-smelling vaginal odor
- Do *not* use tampons for at least 1 week.
- Do *not* have sexual intercourse for 1 week.
- Do *not* douche for 3 weeks.

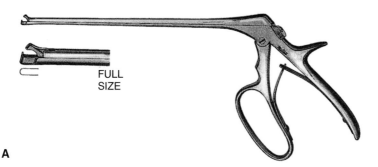

A

Figure 42.3 (A) Cervical biopsy forceps. *(Reproduced with permission from Miltex Instrument Company, Inc.)*

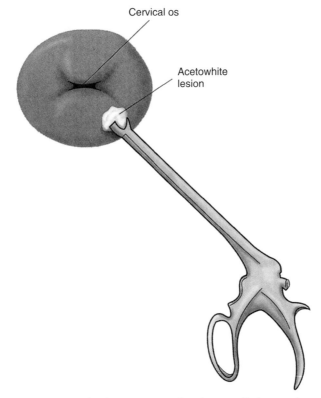

Cervical os

Acetowhite
lesion

B

Figure 42.3 cont'd (B) The forceps are used to biopsy all abnormal cervical lesions.

BIBLIOGRAPHY

Barbara SA, Kaufman AJ, Bettcher C, Parker-Featherstone E. Gynecologic procedures: Colposcopy treatment, cervical intraepithelial neoplasia, and endometrial assessment. *Am Fam Physician.* 2013;87(12):836–843.

Colodny CS. Procedures for your practice: Colposcopy and cervical biopsy. *Patient Care.* June 1995:66–71.

Frisch LE, Milner F, Ferris D. Naked-eye inspection of the cervix after acetic acid application may improve the predictive value of negative cytologic screening. *J Fam Pract.* 1994;39(5):457–460.

Johnson BA. The colposcopic examination. *Am Fam Physician.* 1996;53(8):2473–2482.

43 Chapter

Endometrial Biopsy

Margaret R. Colyar

CPT Code
58100 Endometrial sampling

Endometrial biopsy is a procedure used to obtain cells directly from the lining of the uterus to evaluate dysfunctional uterine bleeding. If endometrial cancer is suspected, refer for diagnostic curettage.

OVERVIEW

Factors that may interfere with an endometrial biopsy are
- Acute vaginal or cervical infections
- Acute pelvic inflammatory disease
- Cervical cancer

RATIONALE

- To diagnose
  - Cancer
    - Take the specimen any time.
  - Infertility (to determine corpus luteum function)
    - Take the specimen during the last half of the menstrual cycle (days 21 or 22).
  - Menstrual disturbances (especially anovulatory bleeding)
    - Take the specimen immediately before menstruation. Get index of progesterone influence and ovulation.

INDICATIONS

- Suspicion of endometrial cancer
- Infertility
- Amenorrhea

CONTRAINDICATIONS

- Pregnancy

PROCEDURE

Endometrial Biopsy

Equipment
- Antiseptic skin cleanser
- Drape—sterile

- Light source
- Endometrial suction **curette**
- Vaginal **speculum**
- Water-soluble lubricant—K-Y jelly
- Gloves—sterile
- Ring **forceps** or **tenaculum**
- 4 × 4 gauze—sterile
- Container with 10% **formalin**

Procedure

- Have the client void immediately before the examination.
- In women of childbearing age, perform a urine pregnancy test.
- Place the client in the lithotomy position.
- Cleanse the perineum.
- Drape the perineum.
- Lubricate the vaginal speculum.
- Put on gloves.
- Insert the speculum into the vagina, and lock in place with the cervix and os in view.
- Using ring forceps or the tenaculum, cleanse the vagina and cervix with sterile gauze.
- Insert the endometrial suction curette into the cervical os 3 to 4 inches (7 to 10 cm) (Fig. 43.1).
- If entry is difficult, use the tenaculum to pull the bottom of the os gently down to increase the opening size (Fig. 43.2). The cervix has little nervous innervation up to the transformation zone. The client should feel no pain if you are careful not to grasp the os into the transformation zone.
- Pull back on the inner cannula of the suction curette to aspirate cells from the uterine lining.
- Withdraw the entire curette.
- Expel the specimen from the curette into the container with formalin.
- Label and send the specimen to the laboratory.

Client Instructions

- You may experience some cramping and bleeding after the procedure. If this occurs, take 400 to 600 mg of ibuprofen every 6 hours as needed.
- Observe for signs and symptoms of infection, such as
  - Increase in pain after 24 hours
  - Increase in temperature
  - Foul odor
- If any signs or symptoms of infection are found, return to the office.

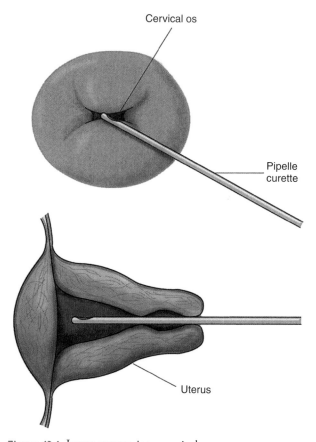

Cervical os

Pipelle
curette

Uterus

Figure 43.1 Insert curette into cervical os.

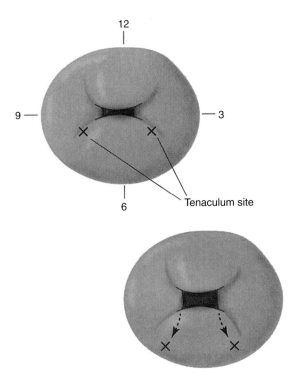

12

9 —   — 3

6   Tenaculum site

Figure 43.2 Pull the os down to increase the opening.

BIBLIOGRAPHY

Guido RS, Kanbor A, Ruhlin M, Christopherson WA. Pipelle endometrial sampling: Sensitivity in the detection of endometrial cancer. *J Reprod Med.* 1995;40(8):553–555.

Ignatavicius DD, Workman ML. *Medical-Surgical Nursing: Patient-Centered Collaborative Care.* 8th ed. Philadelphia, PA: Saunders; 2016.

Youssif SN, McMellan DL. Outpatient endometrial biopsy: The pipelle. *Br J Hosp Med.* 1995;54(23):198–201.

44 Chapter

Specimen Collection
Gram Stain, Wet Mount (Saline and KOH)
Margaret R. Colyar

CPT Code
87205 Gram stain
87210 Wet smear
87220 KOH prep

Gram stain technique is a procedure used to differentiate gram-positive and gram-negative organisms. The technique was named after Christian Gram, who developed it in 1884. Knowing if an organism is gram-positive or gram-negative helps the practitioner determine the etiology of the infection and determine appropriate treatment.

The wet mount (wet prep, wet smear) is a tool used to evaluate the etiology of abnormal vaginal secretions. Saline and 10% potassium hydroxide (KOH) preparations are used. With the saline preparation, white blood cells, bacteria, trichomonads, and clue cells can be detected. With the 10% KOH preparation, hyphae and buds can be detected.

OVERVIEW

- Potentially reportable vaginal infections include gonorrhea, syphilis, *Chlamydia trachomatis,* herpes genitalis, **condyloma acuminatum,** pelvic inflammatory disease, and nonspecific urethritis (male). Check the regulations for reporting sexually transmitted diseases in the state in which you practice.

HEALTH PROMOTION/PREVENTION

- To prevent vaginal, uterine, tubal, and ovarian infections, the use of condoms during intercourse is suggested.

RATIONALE

- To aid in assessment of all suspected vaginal infections
- To assist in determination of disease etiology

INDICATIONS

- Unusual foul-smelling vaginal discharge
- Lower abdominal pain

- Vaginal itching
- Dysuria

CONTRAINDICATIONS

- Recent douching
- Menses
- Intravaginal medications

PROCEDURE

Wet Smear (Saline and KOH)

Equipment

- Vaginal **speculum**—small, medium, or large
- Drape—nonsterile
- Two pairs of gloves—nonsterile
- Test tube with 1 mL 0.9% sodium chloride
- Cotton-tipped applicators—sterile
- 0.9% sodium chloride
- 10% KOH solution—two drops
- Two microscope slides
- Two coverslips
- Microscope

Procedure

- Place the client in the lithotomy position and drape.
- Insert the vaginal speculum and observe the vaginal wall and cervix for inflammation and/or infections, cysts, lesions, and bleeding.
- Using cotton-tipped applicators, collect specimen of vaginal secretions.
- Place one cotton-tipped applicator in the test tube with 1 mL 0.9% sodium chloride and mix well.
- Remove the speculum.
- With the cotton-tipped applicator, place a smear on each slide.
  - On one slide, add one or two drops of saline and cover with the coverslip.
  - On the second slide, add one or two drops of 10% KOH and cover with the coverslip.
    - Gently heat the KOH slide for 2 to 3 seconds.
    - Allow the KOH slide to sit for 15 to 20 minutes at room temperature.
- Place the saline slide (Fig. 44.1) on the microscope at 10× (low power) and focus. Change to 40× (high power) and focus. Look for the following in five different fields
  - White blood cells
  - Trichomonads
  - Clue cells (large epithelial cells with indistinct borders with multiple cocci clinging to them)
    - Clue cells often are described as appearing like "pepper on a fried egg"; they indicate bacterial vaginosis.

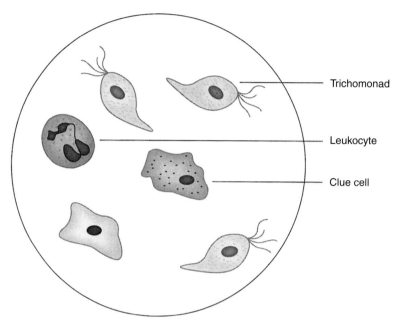

Figure 44.1 Saline preparation.

- Place the KOH slide (Fig. 44.2) on the microscope at 10× and 40×. Look for the following in five different fields
  - Hyphae
  - Spores (buds, candidiasis)

Client Instructions

- Based on the results of your vaginal smears, you have _____.
- You will need to take _____ for _____ days.
- Return to the office 1 week after you finish your medications for recheck or sooner if your symptoms worsen.

Gram Stain

Equipment

- Vaginal speculum
- Drape—nonsterile
- Cotton-tipped applicators—sterile
- One microscope slide
- Gram stain kit
- Microscope
- Gloves—nonsterile

Procedure

- Place client in lithotomy position and drape.

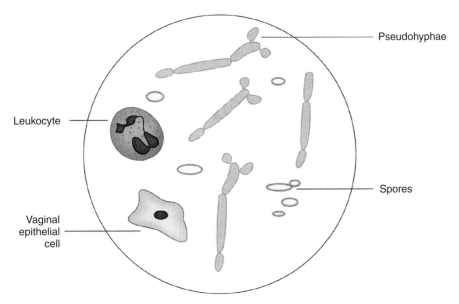

Figure 44.2 KOH preparation.

- Insert vaginal speculum, and observe vaginal wall and cervix (see Chapter 45).
- Using cotton-tipped applicators, collect specimen of vaginal secretions.
- Remove speculum.
- With cotton-tipped applicator, place drop of secretions on the slide and follow the directions in the Gram stain kit.
  - Let specimen air-dry.
  - Apply solutions from the Gram stain kit in the following manner
    - Stain with crystal violet and Gram iodine solution.
      - All bacteria become blue-purple.
    - Rinse with a decolorizer (usually a 95% alcohol or alcohol-acetone mixture).
      - Gram-negative bacteria become transparent and lose their color.
      - Gram-positive bacteria retain the blue-purple color.
    - Apply safranin (a red dye) to the slide.
      - Gram-negative bacteria become red. Gonorrhea bacteria are gram-negative.
      - Gram-positive bacteria remain blue-purple.

Client Instructions

- Based on the results of your vaginal smears, you have _____.
- You will need to take _____ for _____ days.
- Return to the office 1 week after you finish your medications for recheck, or sooner if your symptoms worsen.

BIBLIOGRAPHY

Dino-lite: https://www.microscope.com/education-center/how-to-guides/mount-slides. Accessed October 9, 2019.

Ferris DG, Hendrich J, Payne PM, et al. Office laboratory diagnosis of vaginitis. *J Fam Pract.* 1995;46 (6):575–581.

Heimbrook ME, Wang WL, Campbell G. Staining bacterial flagella easily. *J Clin Micro.* 1989;27(11):2612–2615.

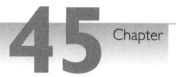

Chapter

Specimen Collection
Papanicolaou (Pap) Smear
Margaret R. Colyar

CPT Code
18811 Sure Path with reflex
88150 Pap smear interpretation
Not used by the clinician; used by the pathologist who interprets the specimen.

The **Pap smear** is a tool for screening of cervical cancer. Appropriate smear collection is paramount to detection of cancer cells. In addition, if a lesion is seen or palpated, other tests, such as ultrasound examination of the pelvis or **colposcopy**, should be performed in conjunction with the Pap smear.

OVERVIEW

- Adequacy of the specimen is shown by the presence of
  - Endocervical cells
  - Squamous metaplasia (found in the **transformation zone**) (Fig. 45.1)
    - The transformation zone is found inside the cervical os; this is an area of replacement of endocervical columnar cells by squamous cells and varies with age. In perimenopausal women, the transformation zone is found high in the endocervical canal (Fig. 45.2).
- The practitioner should be familiar with the classification of cervical smears (Table 45.1).

RATIONALE

- To detect cervical carcinoma
- To detect early cervical dysplasia related to infection with HPV

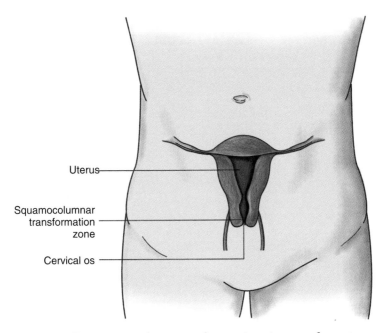

Figure 45.1 Premenopausal squamocolumnar junction transformation zone.

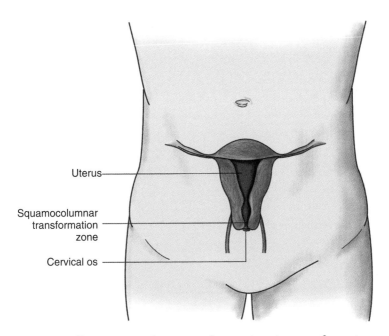

Figure 45.2 Perimenopausal squamocolumnar junction transformation zone.

Table 45·1	**Cervical Smear Classifications**		
CLASS	**DESCRIPTIVE**	**BETHESDA**	**CIN**
Class I	Negative	WNL	Negative
Class II	Inflammatory, squamous, koilocytotic atypia	Reactive, reparative changes, ASCUs, LSIL (HPV)	
Class III	Mild dysplasia	LSIL (HPV)	CIN I
	Moderate dysplasia	HSIL	CIN2
	Severe dysplasia	HSIL	CIN3
Class IV	Ca in situ	HSIL	CIN3
Class V	Invasive	Invasive	Invasive

ASCU = Atypical squamous cell undetermined; CIN = cervical intraepithelial neoplasia; HPV = Human papilloma virus; HSIL = high-grade intraepithelial lesion; LSIL = low-grade intraepithelial lesion; WNL = within normal limits.

INDICATIONS

- Abnormal vaginal bleeding or discharge
- Lower abdominal pain
- Yearly screening
- Visible or palpable cervical lesions
- Report of cervical dysplasia or malignancy on previous Pap smear
- DES-exposed female—REFER to gynecologist for treatment.
- History of sexually transmitted disease
- History of multiple sexual partners

CONTRAINDICTIONS

- Pelvic inflammatory disease
- Active vaginitis
- Active cervicitis

PROCEDURE

Pap Smear

Equipment

- Vaginal speculum—small, medium, or large
- Drape—nonsterile
- Gloves—nonsterile
- Light source
- Pap smear kit or liquid-based kit (usually provided by the reference laboratory)
  - Wooden paddle and cotton-tipped applicator
  - Optional—cytobrush (decreases the chance of a false-negative result)
  - Cervical broom (Fig. 45.3)
  - Microscope slides
  - Fixative

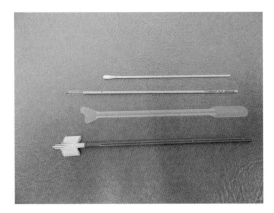

Figure 45.3 Four types of specimen collection tools. From top to bottom: cotton-tipped applicator, cytobrush, plastic paddle, and cervical broom.

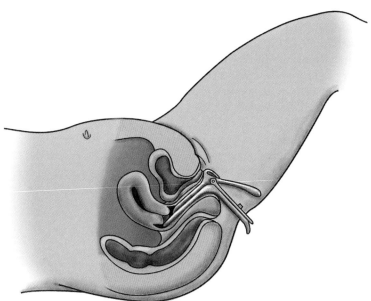

Figure 45.4 Direct the vaginal speculum in a downward posterior direction.

- Water-soluble lubricant—K-Y jelly
- Large cotton-tipped swabs

Procedure

- Place the client in the lithotomy position and drape.
- Put on gloves.
- Examine the vulva and Bartholin's and Skene's glands.
- Warm the speculum with water or lubricate with water-soluble lubricant.
- Ask the client to relax and breathe deeply (this may help the client to relax).
- Insert the speculum at a slight diagonal angle and rotate to a horizontal angle as inserting. Direct the speculum in a downward posterior direction, applying gentle pressure (Fig. 45.4).

- Open the speculum and adjust the position until the cervix is easily visible.
- Observe the cervix and vaginal wall for inflammation and/or infection, cysts, lesions, or bleeding.
- If necessary, absorb discharge or blood with large cotton-tipped swab.
- **Pap smear kit**:
  - Insert the wooden paddle into the cervix and rotate 360 degrees.
  - Place the smear on the slide indicated in the Pap smear kit.
  - Insert other end of the wooden paddle and brush the ectocervix and vaginal wall.
  - Apply this specimen to the slide indicated in the Pap smear kit.
  - Next, insert the cytobrush, broom, or cotton-tipped applicator in the cervical os and rotate 360 degrees.
  - Apply this specimen to the slide indicated in the Pap smear kit.
  - Apply fixative provided to the slides.
  - Label and send to reference laboratory.
- **Liquid based kit**:
  - Insert the cytobrush in the cervix and rotate 360 degrees.
  - Insert the paddle into the cervix and rotate 360 degrees.
  - Put both specimens in the specimen bottle.
  - Snap off the handles and apply the lid.
  - Label and send to reference laboratory.
- *Hint*—With postmenopausal and obese clients, the vaginal walls may prolapse into the open speculum, occluding your view of the cervix. To prevent this complication, a special splint (Fig. 45.5) using a glove and the speculum can be used. You can make this splint by
  - Inserting the speculum into the finger of a nonsterile glove
  - Removing the excess glove
  - Cutting off the fingertip
- The glove provides a splintlike effect when the speculum is opened in the vagina.

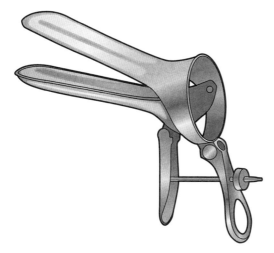

Figure 45.5 Speculum splint.

Client Instructions

- There may be minor bleeding after the examination. This is normal.
- If your Pap smear is class II through V, further testing is necessary.
- The nurse from the office will call you in 5 to 10 days with the results of your Pap smear.

BIBLIOGRAPHY

Boskey E. Overview of the Pap smear procedure. verywellhealth website. Dec 2018. https://www.verywellhealth.com/what-is-it-like-to-get-a-pap-smear-3132772. Updated July 1, 2019. Accessed October 9, 2019.

Helderman G, Graham L, Cannon D, Waters K, Feller D. Comparing two sampling techniques of endocervical cell recovery on Papanicolaou smears. *Nurse Pract.* 1990;15(11):30–32.

Lieu D. The Papanicolaou smear: Its value and limitations. *J Fam Pract.* 1996;45(4):391–399.

Chapter **46**

Administration of Vaginal Medications and Condoms

Margaret R. Colyar

CPT Code
None

Vaginal medications come in the form of creams, suppositories, and inserts. Creams and suppositories are inserted with a plastic applicator that accompanies the medication. Inserts are applied manually.

There are two types of condoms: male and female. Either may be made of latex, lamb intestines, or polyurethane. As a method of contraception, male condoms are inexpensive, easy to use, and have few side effects. Latex/polyurethane condoms offer protection against sexually transmitted diseases. Lamb intestine condoms do not protect against sexually transmitted diseases.

OVERVIEW

- Effectiveness
  - Male condom users experience a 2% per year pregnancy rate.
  - Female condom users experience a 5% per year pregnancy rate.

- Use only water-based lubricants such as K-Y jelly or AstroGlide with latex condoms.
- Oil-based lubricants (petroleum jelly, butter, cold cream, mineral or vegetable oils) can damage latex.

RATIONALE

- To prevent pregnancy
- To prevent sexually transmitted diseases

CONTRAINDICATIONS

- Latex allergy

PROCEDURE

Vaginal Creams and Suppositories

Equipment

- Vaginal cream
- Vaginal suppository
- Applicator
- Gloves—nonsterile

Procedure

- Fill the applicator
  - For cream dosage forms
    - Screw the applicator onto the tube.
    - Squeeze the medicine into the applicator slowly until it is measured properly.
    - Remove the applicator from the tube. Replace the cap on the tube.
  - For suppository dosage form
    - Place the suppository into the applicator.
- Position the patient on her back with knees bent.
- Put on gloves.
- Slide the applicator slowly into the vagina until resistance is met.
- Slowly press the plunger until it stops.
- Withdraw the applicator.
- Clean the applicator after use by pulling the plunger out of the applicator and washing both parts completely in warm, soapy water.
- Rinse well.
- After drying the applicator, replace the plunger.

PROCEDURE

Vaginal Inserts

Equipment

- Vaginal insert
- Gloves—nonsterile

Procedure

- Insertion of the vaginal insert
  - Position the patient on her back with knees bent.
  - Pinch or press the sides of the vaginal insert between your forefinger and middle finger.
  - With one hand, part the folds of skin around the vagina.
  - Slide the vaginal insert slowly into the upper third of the vagina.
- Removal of the vaginal insert
  - Position the patient on her back with knees bent.
  - Slide one finger into the vagina and hook it around the closest part of the vaginal insert.
  - Slowly pull the vaginal insert out.
  - Wrap the vaginal insert and dispose in the trash.

PROCEDURE

Applying Male Condoms

- Put a drop or two of spermicide or lubricant inside the condom.
- Have the patient pull back the foreskin, unless circumcised, then roll the condom over the tip of the hard penis.
- Have the patient pinch the air out of the tip while placing it on the penis.
- Leave a half an inch of space at the tip to collect semen.
- Teach the patient to unroll the condom over the penis all the way down to the base of the penis and smooth out any air bubbles gently.
- Lastly, instruct the patient to lubricate the outside of the condom.
- To remove the condom, prevent any sperm transfer into the vagina by holding the condom around the base of the penis.
- Dispose in the trash.

PROCEDURE

Applying Female Condoms

- Put spermicide or lubricant on the outside of the closed end of the condom.
- Have the patient stand with one foot on a chair, sit on the edge of a chair, lie down, or squat.
- Have the patient squeeze together the sides of the inner ring at the closed end of the condom like a pencil and insert it into the vagina like a tampon.
- After the inner ring is inserted, the patient should place two fingers inside the condom and push the inner ring into the vagina until it reaches the cervix. She will feel the inner ring open up.
- Have her pull out her fingers and let the outer ring hang about an inch outside the vagina.
- To remove the female condom, twist it around a finger and pull it out.
- Dispose in the trash.

Client Instructions

- Use a condom only one time.

- Check expiration date.
- Be careful while unwrapping a condom. If it is torn, brittle, stiff, or sticky, throw it away and use another.

BIBLIOGRAPHY

Condom. Planned Parenthood Web site. Video. http://www.plannedparenthood.org/
health-topics/birth-control/condom-10187.htm.
Internal Condom. Planned Parenthood Web site. Video. http://www.plannedparenthood
.org/health-topics/birth-control/female-condom. Accessed October 9, 2019.

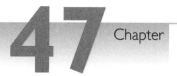

Chapter

Bartholin Cyst Abscess Incision and Drainage

Margaret R. Colyar

CPT Code
56420 Incision and drainage of Bartholin's gland abscess
56740 Excision of Bartholin's gland or cyst

Bartholinitis is inflammation of one or both of the Bartholin's glands at the opening of the vagina (Fig. 47.1). Obstruction of the main duct of these glands causes retention of secretions and dilation of the gland. Incision and drainage of abscessed Bartholin's glands are needed if the gland is swollen and painful. A culture of the abscess material should be taken to determine the etiology of the abscess and to provide treatment guidance.

OVERVIEW

- Approximately 2% of adult women develop an abscess of the Bartholin's glands.
- Recurrence rate is high.
- Most common causes are
  - **Inspissated** mucus
  - Congenital narrowing of the gland
  - *Neisseria gonorrhoeae*
  - *Staphylococcus*
  - *Streptococcus*
  - *Escherichia coli*

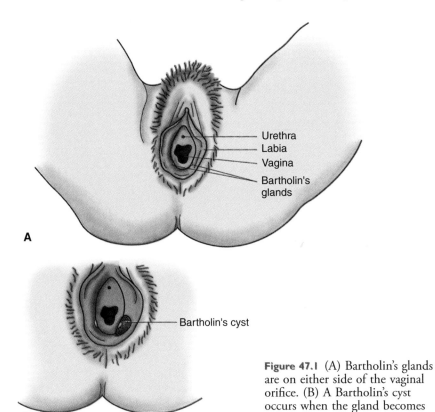

Figure 47.1 (A) Bartholin's glands are on either side of the vaginal orifice. (B) A Bartholin's cyst occurs when the gland becomes inflamed or infected.

- *Trichomonas*
- *Bacteroides*
- Symptoms of bartholinitis include
  - Swelling of the labia
  - Tenderness/pain in the labia when walking and/or sitting
  - Enlarged inguinal nodes
  - **Dyspareunia**
  - Palpable mass
- Prevention includes
  - Protected sexual intercourse
  - Meticulous cleansing of the perineum

RATIONALE
- To relieve pain
- To determine the etiology and provide treatment guidance

INDICATIONS
- Infected Bartholin's glands

CONTRAINDICATIONS

- Pregnancy—REFER to a gynecologist.

▶ *Informed consent required*

PROCEDURE

Bartholin's Cyst Abscess—Incision and Drainage

Equipment

- Antiseptic skin cleanser
- Drape—sterile
- Gloves—sterile
- 1% lidocaine—5 to 10 mL
- Two syringes—10 and 20 mL
- Two needles—18- and 25-gauge, ½-inch needle
- 0.9% sodium chloride—250 mL
- No. 11 scalpel
- 4 × 4 gauze—sterile
- Iodoform gauze—¼- or ½-inch wide
- Scissors—sterile
- Curved **hemostats**—sterile
- Pickups—sterile
- Vaginal culture swab
- Peri pads—nonsterile

Procedure

- Instruct the client to empty her bladder.
- Position the client in the lithotomy position.
- Cleanse perineum with antiseptic skin cleanser.
- Open gauze, scalpel, needle, and syringes onto a sterile field.
- Put on gloves.
- Inject 5 to 10 mL of 1% lidocaine along the top of the abscessed Bartholin's gland using the 10-mL syringe with the 25-gauge needle.
- Incise the cyst along the top. Make the incision deep enough and long enough to allow drainage.
  - A longer incision is considered better than a smaller incision.
- Culture the drainage.
- Insert a gloved finger into the vaginal orifice, and apply gentle pressure toward the abscess to express the exudate.
- After all exudate is expressed, inspect the wound with curved hemostats and break up any **loculations** (small cavities).
- Irrigate with 0.9% sodium chloride using the 20-mL syringe with the 18-gauge needle.
- Insert iodoform gauze into the wound, leaving approximately ½ inch protruding from the wound.
- Cover with 4 × 4 gauze sponges and apply a peri pad.

Client Instructions

- To prevent further infection, the following antibiotic has been ordered: (doxycycline, erythromycin, or a cephalosporin) _____.
- Remove half of the gauze in 24 hours. Remove the remaining gauze in 48 hours.
- Change the 4 × 4 sponges and peri pad every 4 to 6 hours.
- Soak in a basin or tub of warm water four times per day for 1 week.
- Return to the office in 1 week for recheck, or sooner if your symptoms worsen.

BIBLIOGRAPHY

Kellerman RD, Bope ET. *Conn's Current Therapy*. Philadelphia, PA: Saunders; 2018.
Pfenninger JL, Fowler GC. *Procedures for Primary Care Physicians*. St. Louis, MO: Mosby; 2019.
Youngkin EQ, Davis MS. *Women's Health: A Primary Care Clinical Guide*. Norwalk, CT: Appleton & Lange; 2012.

Chapter **48**

Cervical Cap Fitting, Insertion, and Removal

Margaret R. Colyar

CPT Code
57170 Diaphragm/cervical cap fitting with instructions

A cervical cap is a helmet-shaped, rubber device that fits over the cervix. It is much smaller than a diaphragm. When used with spermicide, the cervical cap acts as a physical and chemical barrier to sperm. Cervical caps come in several sizes and must be fitted by a professional. It is a nonsystemic, nonhormonal, and reversible method of contraception.

OVERVIEW

- Prevention of pregnancy—sources differ
  - Among nulliparous women, cervical caps are 80% to 91% effective; 9% to 20% become pregnant within the first year.
  - Among parous women, cervical caps are 60% to 74% effective; 26% to 40% become pregnant within the first year.

Potential Complications

- Pregnancy
- Conversion from normal to abnormal cervical cytology
- Urinary tract infections
- Cervical or vaginal lesions with prolonged use
- Toxic shock syndrome
- Allergy to latex rubber or spermicide
- Sexually transmitted disease transmission

Assess

- Comfort with and ability (woman/partner) to insert, check placement, and remove cap
- Ability to understand instructions for proper use
- Length of cervix—a long or short cervix can compromise fit of cap
- Willingness to return after pregnancy or weight change of more than 10 lb

RATIONALE

- To provide a reliable, nonhormonal, nonsystemic, and reversible form of contraception

INDICATIONS

- Contraception
- Patient choice
- Contraindications to other methods of contraception

CONTRAINDICATIONS

- History of toxic shock syndrome
- Allergy to latex, rubber, or spermicide
- Suspected or known cervical or uterine malignancy
- Unusually long or short cervix
- Extensive cervical scarring or lacerations
- Unresolved abnormal Pap smear
- Inability to learn proper use

▶ *Informed consent required*

PROCEDURE

Cervical Cap Fitting, Insertion, and Removal

Equipment

- Cervical cap
  - The clinician must order a set of cervical caps to use in the office for fitting the client. The caps are available in various internal rim diameter sizes.
- Speculum
- Water-soluble lubricant—K-Y jelly
- Gloves—nonsterile

Procedure

CERVICAL CAP FITTING AND INSERTION

- Have client empty her bladder before fitting and insertion.
- Position the client in the lithotomy position.
- With a gloved hand, perform a bimanual examination to evaluate the size and position of the uterus and cervix.
- Apply K-Y jelly to a speculum.
- Insert the speculum to visualize the cervix to estimate the cap size, and note any scarring, lacerations, and length of the cervix. The cervix must be symmetrical, be long enough to apply the cap, and have a proper seal.
- Fold the rim of the cap and compress the cap dome to insert it into the vagina, and place it over the cervix. Unfolding the dome creates suction between the rim of the cap and the cervix.
- After applying the cap to the cervix, run a finger around the entire rim to check for gaps. Note the stability of the cap by determining how easily it is displaced with your finger. There should not be any gaps, and the cap must cover the cervix completely and fit snugly, but not tightly.
- After 1 to 2 minutes, check again for fit and suction. Try to rotate the cap; it should rotate with slight resistance and not come off the cervix.
- Try at least one other cap size, either smaller or larger, to determine which one fits best.
- Have the client feel the cap in place and give her instructions for use.
- Provide a written prescription for the patient to fill at a pharmacy that carries cervical caps.

CERVICAL CAP REMOVAL

- To remove the cap, insert one finger between the rim of the cap and the cervix to break the suction, then gently pull the cap down and out. Have the client practice putting the cap on and off in the office.

Client Instructions

- Check cap for holes, tears, and cracks by holding the cervical cap up to a light.
- Apply a teaspoon of spermicidal cream to the dome of the cap before inserting.
- Empty bladder before insertion.
- Insert the cap in a squatting position.
- Do not remove the cap for at least 8 hours after last coitus.
- To reduce risk of toxic shock syndrome, the cap must be removed within 48 hours after use.
- To remove, push the rim away from the cervix to break the suction and pull the cap out.
- Use of additional spermicide with repeated intercourse is optional. Do not remove cap. Use a plastic introducer to insert fresh spermicide.
- Do not use during vaginal bleeding.
- After removal, clean the cervical cap with soapy water, rinse thoroughly in plain water, and air dry. Do not use powders, oils, or petroleum jelly (Vaseline) with the cap.

- Check fit yearly with annual examination and refit if client has had a pregnancy or gained or lost more than 10 lb.

BIBLIOGRAPHY

Hatcher R. *Contraceptive Technology.* 21st ed. New York, NY: Ardent Media; 2018.
Planned Parenthood Web site. http://www.plannedparenthood.org.
The Fem Cap. https://www.plannedparenthood.org/learn/birth-control/cervical-cap.

49 Chapter

Cervical Lesions
Cryotherapy
Margaret R. Colyar

CPT Code
57511   Cryocautery of cervix, initial or repeat

Cryotherapy is a technique in which the outermost layer of cervical cells is frozen. The transformation zone is destroyed. If the lesion is confined to the exocervix, cryotherapy is appropriate.

OVERVIEW
- Depth of tissue destruction is 3 to 4 mm.
- Cryosurgery is not recommended if
  - It is 5 to 7 days before menses. Edema of cervical tissue may occur.
  - The lesion cannot be entirely visualized.
  - There is greater than grade II cervical dysplasia. Appropriate depth of tissue will not be able to be removed.
  - The patient is immunocompromised or on high-dose steroids. Patient may develop secondary infection.

OPTIONS
- *Method 1*—Freeze, thaw, freeze
- *Method 2*—Freeze, thaw

RATIONALE
- To diminish pain
- To prevent further tissue destruction
- To prevent spread of lesion

INDICATIONS

- Cervical dysplasia—grade I or II—if lesion can be covered by the cryoprobe
- Precancerous cervical lesions
- Carcinoma in situ

CONTRAINDICATIONS

- Pregnancy
- Cervical cancer
- Cervical dysplasia—greater than grade II
- Positive endocervical curettage
- Entire lesion cannot be seen
- Positive for sexually transmitted disease
- 5 to 7 days before menses
- Immunocompromised
- On high-dose steroids

◗ *Informed consent required*

PROCEDURE

Cervical Lesions—Cryotherapy

Equipment

- Methods 1 and 2
  - Nitrous oxide cryoprobe unit
  - Cryoprobes—flat or cone
  - Water-soluble lubricant (K-Y jelly, Cryogel, lidocaine jelly)
  - Drape—nonsterile
  - Cotton-tipped applicators
  - Vaginal speculum with retraction device (see Chapter 45)
  - Light source
  - Gloves—nonsterile
  - NSAIDs

Procedure

METHOD 1—FREEZE, THAW, FREEZE

- Have the client take a dose of an NSAID 0.5 to 1 hour prior to the procedure.
- Position the client in the lithotomy position.
- Drape the client.
- Put on gloves.
- Select the appropriate cryoprobe (Fig. 49.1).
  - Must cover the entire lesion
  - Must be flat or slightly conical
- Apply a water-soluble lubricant to the cryoprobe tip.
- Activate the nitrous oxide unit according to the manufacturer's directions.
- Insert the vaginal speculum in the vaginal vault.

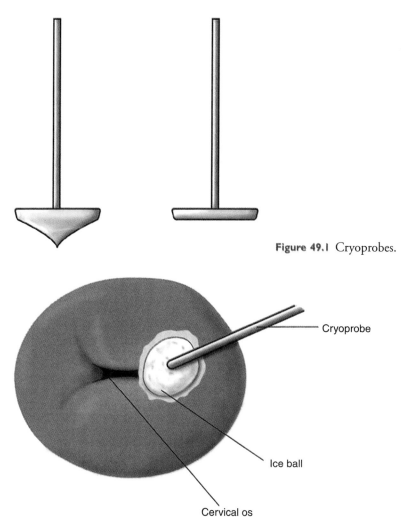

Figure 49.1 Cryoprobes.

Figure 49.2 Cervical lesions. Freeze for 3 minutes or until a 5-mm ice ball surrounds the lesion. Thaw for 5 minutes; then refreeze.

- Position the probe over the area to be treated and start the freeze (Fig. 49.2).
  - Be sure the probe does not touch the vaginal wall (very sensitive).
  - Freeze for 3 minutes or until a 5-mm ice ball is beyond the lesion.
- Thaw. Wait 5 minutes.
- Refreeze for 3 minutes or until a 5-mm ice ball is beyond the lesion.

METHOD 2—FREEZE, THAW
- Have the client take a dose of an NSAID 0.5 to 1 hour before the procedure.
- Position the client in the lithotomy position.
- Drape the client.
- Put on gloves.

- Select the appropriate cryoprobe (Fig. 49.1).
  - Must cover the entire lesion
  - Must be flat or slightly conical
- Apply a water-soluble lubricant to the cryoprobe tip.
- Activate the nitrous oxide unit according to the manufacturer's directions.
- Insert the vaginal speculum in the vaginal vault.
  - Position the probe over the area to be treated and start the freeze (Fig. 49.2).
  - Be sure the probe does not touch the vaginal wall (very sensitive).
- Freeze for 3 minutes or until a 5-mm ice ball is beyond the lesion.
- Thaw.

Client Instructions

- Expect some mild cramping and watery, foul-smelling discharge for 3 weeks.
- Take acetaminophen or ibuprofen as directed for abdominal cramping.
- Do not put anything inside the vagina for 3 weeks, such as
  - Tampons
  - Douching solutions
- Do not engage in vaginal intercourse for 3 weeks.
- A follow-up Pap smear in 6 months will be needed. Your next appointment is
  _____.

BIBLIOGRAPHY

Beckman CRB, Ling F. *Obstetrics and Gynecology.* 7th ed. Philadelphia, PA: Lippincott Williams Wilkins; 2018.

Pfenniger JL, Fowler GC. *Procedures for Primary Care Physicians.* St. Louis, MO: Mosby; 2019.

Youngkin EQ, Davis MS. *Women's Health: A Primary Care Clinical Guide.* Norwalk, CT: Appleton & Lange; 2012.

Chapter **50**

Condyloma Acuminata Removal

Cynthia Ehrhardt

CPT Code

54050	Destruction of lesion(s), penis; simple, chemical
54054	Destruction of lesion(s), penis; simple, cryosurgery
54065	Destruction of lesion(s), penis; extensive, any method
56501	Destruction of lesion(s), vulva; simple, any method
56515	Destruction of lesion(s), vulva; extensive, any method

Condyloma acuminatum (or HPV genital infection) is a viral infection responsible for causing genital warts. These warts usually are located in the dermal layers

of the body. Currently, 60 types of HPV have been identified. These viruses can be classified in three categories:
- Viruses causing benign and low-risk lesions
- Viruses causing lesions with a moderate oncogenic risk
- Viruses causing lesions with a high oncogenic risk

Genital warts typically have a hypertrophic or cauliflower-type appearance.

In the male, most of the lesions are located on the prepuce, glans, urethra, penile shaft, and scrotum. In the female, most lesions are found on the vulva, perianal area, vagina, and cervix.

OVERVIEW

- Incidence
  - It is estimated that 1 million individuals are newly diagnosed with condyloma acuminatum in the United States each year.
  - Incidence of success of treatment modalities is broken down into several categories (Table 50.1).
- Complications of condyloma acuminatum include
  - Increased risk for skin, cervical, and urethral cancers
  - Bladder, testicular, and prostate cancers in men

Table 50-1 Incidence of Success of Treatment Modalities for Condyloma Acuminatum		
CATEGORY OF TREATMENT MODALITY	**TREATMENT MODALITY**	**PERCENTAGE OF SUCCESS (WHERE KNOWN)**
Destruction of lesion	Cryosurgical techniques	83
Surgical techniques	Electrocautery	93
	CO_2 laser ablation	89
	Excision	93
	Cutterage by loop electrosurgical excision procedure (LEEP)	90
Immunotherapy with local intralesional injection	Interferon	52
Antiviral agents	Cimetidine (Tagamet) Acyclovir (Zovirax) Famciclovir (Famvir) Zidovudine (Retrovir)	
Chemotherapy techniques	Acid treatment (trichloroacetic and dichloroacetic)	81
	Podophyllin	65
	Podofilox (Condylox)	61
	5-Fluorouracil	71
	Silver nitrate	60

- General principles
  - Universal precautions should be followed.
  - If uncertain about the malignancy of the lesion, perform a biopsy before attempting a treatment modality.

HEALTH PROMOTION/PREVENTION

- Regular self-examination of the genital and perianal region
- Regular **Pap smear** examinations by all sexually active women and women with a history of HPV
- Prevention of the contraction of the infection by
  - Avoidance of multiple sexual partners
  - Use of condoms with new sexual partners to reduce the likelihood of disease transmission
  - Regular use of condoms during intercourse

OPTIONS

- *Method 1*—Intralesional injection (Table 50.2)
- *Method 2*—Topical agent administration
- *Method 3*—Cryosurgery

RATIONALE

- To reduce the risk of the occurrence of oncogenic changes in tissue
- To promote cosmetic improvement

Table 50·2 **Treatment Options**

METHOD OF TREATMENT	ADVANTAGES	DISADVANTAGES
Intralesional injection	None	Painful, expensive, limited effectiveness
Topical agents Fluorouracil	Can be done at home Relatively inexpensive	Not FDA approved High risk of skin irritation and ulceration
Podophyllin and podofilox	Inexpensive Low systemic absorption rate	Skin irritation Must abstain from sexual activity during treatment Cannot use during pregnancy
Trichloroacetic and dichloroacetic acid	Relatively inexpensive Shorter treatment period	Difficult to control skin penetration rate Skin irritation Requires special kit for treatment* Requires special membership from pharmacy to purchase†

*Available from Professional Compounding Pharmacies of America, Houston; 800-331-2498. www.pccarx.com.
†Available from Glenwood, Inc., 83 N. Summit St., Tenafly, NJ 07670; 800-542-0772. www.glenwood-llc.com.

INDICATIONS

- All visible condyloma acuminatum
- Symptomatic condyloma acuminatum
- Documented abnormal Pap smear with or without suggestion of HPV infection

CONTRAINDICATIONS

- Lesions treated by ablation, which require biopsy to determine malignancy
- Prior history of adverse reaction to treatment regimen
- Pregnancy
- ▶ *Informed consent required*

PROCEDURE

Condyloma Acuminatum Removal

Equipment

- Methods 1 and 2
  - Povidone antiseptic or antiseptic skin cleanser
  - Gloves—sterile
  - Cotton-tipped applicators—sterile
  - 4 × 4 gauze—sterile
- Method 1 only
  - Tuberculin syringes
  - Interferon
- Method 2 only
  - Silver nitrate sticks
- Method 3 only (see Chapter 14)

Procedure

METHOD 1—INTRALESIONAL INJECTION

- Position the client in a comfortable position with lesions easily accessible.
- Cleanse the lesions with povidone antiseptic or other antiseptic skin cleanser.
- Put on gloves.
- Draw up 0.05 mL of interferon in a tuberculin syringe for each lesion.
- Insert the needle into the wart, and inject the solution. A wheal should be noted in the lesion.
- Repeat the procedure for each lesion treated.
- Repeat intralesional injection twice a week for 8 weeks.

METHOD 2—TOPICAL AGENT ADMINISTRATION

- Position the client in a comfortable position with lesions easily accessible.
- Cleanse the lesions with povidone antiseptic or other antiseptic skin cleanser.
- Put on gloves.
- Apply the fenestrated drape.
- Using two digits, apply tension to the skin surrounding the lesion.

- Apply the chemically impregnated silver nitrate stick to the desired site for approximately 15 seconds.
- Remove the silver nitrate stick, and release the skin.
- Repeat this procedure to each wart.

METHOD 3—CRYOSURGERY
See Chapter 14.

Client Instructions

- Use "safe sex" behaviors to reduce the risk of disease transmission.
- Observe for signs and symptoms of infection. If any of the following signs and symptoms of infection are found, return to the office.
  - Increase in pain after 24 hours
  - Increase in temperature
  - Redness or swelling
  - Yellow or greenish drainage
  - Foul odor
- Keep follow-up treatment appointments.
- Closely follow instructions on self-administered medication.
  - Fluorouracil (topical 5-FU, Efudex, Fluoroplex)
    - Apply a thin coat of 5% cream to the lesion at bedtime once or twice a week for up to 10 weeks.
      - Leave on overnight.
    - For penile lesions, apply thin film over the lesion and wrap penis in gauze or condom three times a week for 3 to 4 weeks.
      - Rinse off in 3 hours.
  - Podophyllum and podofilox agent
    - Apply petroleum jelly approximately 3 to 5 mm away from the lesion to reduce irritation of normal tissue and prevent running of the liquid.
      - Do not get any petroleum jelly on the lesion because it reduces the effectiveness of treatment.
    - Apply the liquid drop in sufficient quantity to cover the entire lesion.
    - Leave the chemical on for 4 to 6 hours.
    - Rinse off agent gently with soapy water.
    - Repeat the procedure twice a week until full resolution has occurred (usually 4 to 8 weeks).
    - Treat promptly if warts recur.
  - Trichloroacetic acid (Tri-Chlor) and dichloroacetic acid (bichloroacetic acid) agents
    - Apply petroleum jelly approximately 3 to 5 mm away from the lesion to reduce irritation of normal tissue and prevent running of the liquid.
    - Apply to the affected lesion three times per week with maximum treatment of 4 weeks.
    - Optional—Apply once or twice daily for 3 consecutive days per week for a maximum of 4 weeks.

BIBLIOGRAPHY

Carson S. Human papillomatous virus infection update: Impact on women's health. *Nurse Practitioner.* 1997;22(4):24–27.

Habif T. *Clinical Dermatology: A Color Guide to Diagnosis and Therapy.* St. Louis, MO: Mosby; 2015

Miller D, Brodell R. Human papillomavirus infection treatment options for warts. *Am Fam Physician.* 1996;53(1):68–74.

Pfenninger JL, Fowler GC. *Procedures for Primary Care Physicians.* St. Louis, MO: Mosby; 2019.

Chapter

51

Diaphragm Fitting, Insertion, and Removal

Margaret R. Colyar

CPT Code
57170 Diaphragm/cervical cap fitting with instructions

A **diaphragm** is a soft latex rubber dome contraceptive barrier device that is supported by a round metal spring on the outside. Diaphragms come in various sizes and must be fitted to each individual. A diaphragm is a nonsystemic and reversible method of contraception and is not a 100% effective method of contraception. It does not protect against sexually transmitted diseases.

OVERVIEW

- Prevention of pregnancy
  - Among first-year users: 2.2 pregnancies per 100 women
  - Among established users: 1.9 to 2.4 pregnancies per 100 women per year
  - Among women older than age 35: fewer than 1.9 pregnancies per 100 women per year
- Potential complications include
  - Pregnancy
  - Increased risk of urinary tract infections
  - Increased risk of cervicitis and vaginal infections
  - Increased incidence of toxic shock syndrome
  - Associated with a slightly increased risk of abnormal **Pap smears**

- Types of diaphragm kits
  - Arching spring (most common)
  - Coil spring
  - Flat spring
  - Wide spring

RATIONALE

- To provide a reversible form of contraception

INDICATIONS

- Contraception protection during sexual intercourse
- Other methods of contraception ruled out

CONTRAINDICATIONS

- Allergy to latex rubber products
- Allergy to spermicide gel
- Prior history of toxic shock syndrome
- **Cystocele**
- Rectocele
- Uterine retroversion
- Uterine prolapse
- History of frequent lower urinary tract infections

PROCEDURE

Diaphragm Fitting, Insertion, and Removal

Equipment

- Diaphragm kit with sizes ranging from 50 to 105 mm
- Lubricant (diaphragm gel or K-Y jelly)
- Gloves—nonsterile
- Light source
- Mirror for patient to watch—optional

Procedure

DIAPHRAGM FITTING

- Have the client empty her bladder before fitting.
- Place the client in the lithotomy position with feet in stirrups.
- Put on gloves and lubricate finger with gel.
- Insert a finger (usually middle) into the vaginal vault until it is deep in the posterior fornix.
- Using the thumb tip of the inserted hand, mark where the pubic bone touches the middle finger.
- Remove and match the width of the diaphragm to the distance measured on the middle finger.
  - This is the approximate width of the diaphragm.

DIAPHRAGM INSERTION

- After lubricating the chosen diaphragm, hold it between the thumb and finger and gently squeeze the rim together.
- Separate the labia with the opposite hand, and use the free hand to insert a finger at the base of the vaginal os and apply pressure downward to open the os wider.
- Gently insert the diaphragm into the vagina with the diaphragm dome facing downward until it reaches the posterior fornix behind the cervix.
  - A finger may need to be used to guide the diaphragm in place.
- As the diaphragm expands, feel that it fits snugly against the vaginal walls. The finger may be used as a guide.
- When fully in place, use the inserted finger to follow the edges of the diaphragm ring, feeling for gaps; if none are felt, remove finger.
- Several insertions and removals of different ring sizes may be required until the proper size is found.
- Have the client try the size larger and smaller before making a final selection.
- The diaphragm should be posterior to the symphysis pubis if inserted properly.
- Use the largest size that is comfortable for the client because the vaginal vault enlarges during sexual arousal.
  - Too small a diaphragm may not cover the cervix properly and may increase the risk of trauma to the cervix and vaginal vault.
  - Too large a diaphragm may cause vaginal pressure, abdominal pain and/or cramping, ulceration of the vaginal wall, and increased risk of urinary tract infections.
- With the diaphragm inserted, have the client squat and move around to ensure a proper fit.
- The client should not be able to feel the diaphragm.

DIAPHRAGM REMOVAL

- Place a finger behind the front rim of the diaphragm near the symphysis pubis, and pull it down and out.
  - Have the client demonstrate the correct insertion, placement, and removal of the diaphragm at least three times in the office.

Client Instructions

- Preinsertion checklist includes
  - Check diaphragm for holes, tears, and cracks by holding it up against a light.
  - Apply a teaspoon of spermicidal gel or cream to the dome of the diaphragm.
  - Apply additional spermicidal gel or cream to the ring of the diaphragm.
  - If the diaphragm has been in place for 2 hours or more before intercourse, add spermicidal gel or cream into the vaginal vault.
  - Check for proper placement before coitus.
- During coitus
  - Use of condom increases contraceptive protection.
  - Without removing the diaphragm, apply additional spermicidal gel or cream into the vaginal vault after each episode.

- Postcoitus care
  - Do not remove for at least 6 hours after last coitus.
  - Do not douche with diaphragm in place because it will wash away the spermicidal gel or cream barrier. Recheck for proper placement between acts of coitus.
  - After removal, clean the diaphragm with soapy water, rinse thoroughly in plain water, and air dry. Avoid oil-based products because they can weaken the latex and accelerate deterioration.
  - Avoid douching after removal of the diaphragm.
  - Avoid wearing the diaphragm for 2 to 3 days before Pap smear testing.
  - Refit
    - At annual visit
    - If increase or decrease in weight of 5 lb or more
    - After full-term pregnancy and delivery
    - After an abortion
    - If complaining of dyspareunia, cramping, bladder pain, or rectal pain or partner complains of penile pain
    - After pelvic surgery

BIBLIOGRAPHY

DeCherney A, Bathan L, Laufer N, Roman AS. *Current Obstetric & Gynecologic Diagnosis & Treatment.* Los Altos, CA: Lange Medical Publications; 2013.

Hatcher R, Trussell J, Nelson A, Cates W. *Contraceptive Technology.* 21st ed. New York, NY: Ardent Media; 2018.

Pfenninger JL, Fowler GC. *Procedures for Primary Care Physicians.* St. Louis, MO: Mosby; 2019.

Chapter **52**

IUD Fitting, Insertion, and Removal

Margaret R. Colyar

CPT Code
58300 Insertion of intrauterine device (IUD)
58301 Removal of intrauterine device (IUD)

An IUD is a small plastic device that is inserted through the cervix and is retained in the uterus to prevent pregnancy. A string or strings hang from the IUD through

Table 52·1   Medical Eligibility Checklist for IUDs

- Ask the client the following questions, before inserting an IUD:
  - Do you think you are pregnant, or have you had a recent pregnancy?
  - When was your last menstrual period, and was it normal?
  - Are your periods unusually heavy, or do you experience severe cramping?
  - Do you have any abnormalities of the uterus?
  - What contraception have you been using?
  - Are you having any unusual bleeding between periods?
  - Do you have multiple sexual partners, or does your partner have multiple partners?
  - Have you ever had a sexually transmitted disease? If yes, which ones?
  - Do you think you have HIV?
  - Have you ever had pelvic inflammatory disease?
  - Have you ever had cancer of the reproductive organs?
  - Do you have any other medical conditions (i.e., bleeding disorders, anemia, steroid therapy, heart disease or murmur, hepatitis, leukemia)?

the cervix and into the vagina to ensure the presence of the IUD and for removal. The IUD is a reversible form of contraception that does not offer protection against and may increase the risk of sexually transmitted diseases.

Types of IUDs include ParaGard Copper T (wrapped with copper wire and hormone-free) and Mirena. The Mirena IUD has a levonorgestrel-releasing system that thickens cervical mucus and alters the endometrial lining and decreases the ability of sperm to enter the uterus and implant.

Use a medical checklist to determine eligibility for IUD placement (Table 52.1).

OVERVIEW

- Perform the following laboratory tests before insertion
  - Urine pregnancy test
  - Chlamydia and gonorrhea culture
  - Offer HIV screening
  - Pap smear

POTENTIAL COMPLICATIONS

- Increased risk of pelvic inflammatory disease
- Increased risk of infertility
- Increased risk of menorrhagia and dysmenorrhea with Copper-T-380/ParaGard

RATIONALE

- To provide a reliable and reversible form of contraception
- To treat menorrhagia (Mirena) due to progesterone effect

INDICATIONS

- Contraception
- Patient choice
- Menorrhagia (Mirena)
- Contraindications to other forms of contraception
- Emergency contraception (ParaGard Copper T insertion within 5 days of unprotected intercourse)

CONTRAINDICATIONS

- Pelvic inflammatory disease within the past 12 months or recurrent pelvic inflammatory disease (more than one episode in the past 2 years)
- Postabortal or postpartum endometritis or septic abortion in the past 3 months
- Known or suspected untreated endocervical gonorrhea, chlamydia, or mucopurulent cervicitis
- Undiagnosed abnormal vaginal bleeding
- Pregnancy or suspicion of established pregnancy
- Small uterine cavity with sounding less than 6.5 cm
  - A *sound* is a long, narrow plastic disposable or metal calibrated rod that measures the internal length of the uterine cavity, including the length of the cervix.
- Suspected or known uterine perforation occurring with the placement of a uterine sound during the current insertion procedure
- History of ectopic pregnancy
- HIV/AIDS
- History of symptomatic pelvic actinomycosis confirmed by a culture (not asymptomatic colonization)
- Known or suspected allergy to copper or history of Wilson's disease (for copper IUD only)
- Acute liver disease or tumor—benign or malignant (levonorgestrel IUD only)
- Known or suspected breast cancer (levonorgestrel IUD only)
- Known or suspected cervical and uterine cancer

▶ *Informed consent required*

PROCEDURE

IUD Insertion

Equipment

- IUD
- Stabilizing rod (Mirena only)
- Insertion tube
- Gloves—nonsterile
- Gloves—sterile
- Speculum—sterile
- Uterine sound
- Light source

- K-Y jelly
- Povidone-iodine swabs
- Large cotton-tipped applicator
- Tenaculum
- 1% lidocaine—optional
- Silver nitrate—optional

Procedure—Both ParaGard Copper T and Mirena

See Figure 52.1.
- Screen client for copper sensitivity, if using the ParaGard Copper T IUD.
- Determine if the client is menstruating or in the follicular phase of the cycle.
- Advise client to take 400 to 800 mg of ibuprofen 1 to 2 hours before appointment.
- Have client read the medical checklist and sign consent form.
- Put on nonsterile gloves.
- Apply K-Y jelly to second and third digits.
- Place client in the lithotomy position with feet in stirrups, and perform a bimanual examination to determine the size and position of the cervix and uterus.
- Change into sterile gloves.
- Using a sterile speculum, visualize the cervix.
- Wash the cervix three times with povidone-iodine swabs.
- Consider using a **paracervical block** (see Chapter 55) if the patient has never had a full-term pregnancy, has cervical stenosis, or has a history of vasovagal reactions.

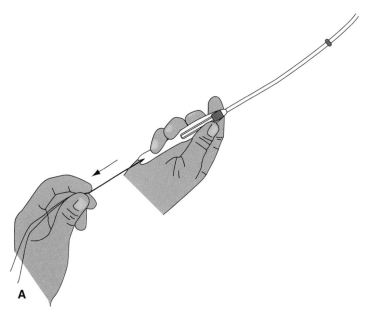

A

Figure 52.1 IUD insertion. (A) System being drawn in insertion tube.

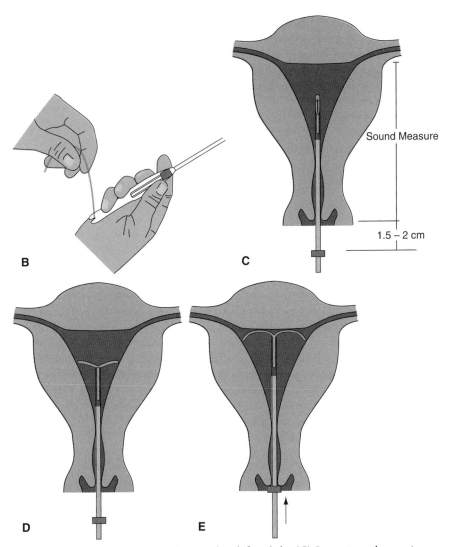

B

C

Sound Measure

1.5 – 2 cm

D

E

Figure 52.1 cont'd (B) Pull threads into the cleft tightly. (C) Insert into the cervix. (D) Release the arms of the IUD. (E) Release and withdraw the inserter.

- **Sound** the uterus prior to insertion of the IUD.
  - Insert a speculum into the vagina.
  - Cleanse the cervix and vagina with an antiseptic (povidone-iodine or chlorhexidine).
  - Place a tenaculum at the 2:00 and 10:00 positions.
    - If you have not used a paracervical block, alert the patient that she will feel a sharp cramp with the placement of the tenaculum. The cramping subsides within 1 minute.

- With gentle traction on the tenaculum, pull the uterus to align the uterus, cervical opening, and vaginal canal.
- Insert the sound into the vagina and through the cervical opening.
- Advance the sound into the uterine cavity until a slight resistance is felt.
  - Alert the client she will feel another cramp when the sound reaches the uterine fundus.
- Remove the sound and assess the level of mucus/blood to determine the depth of the uterus.
  - Most uteri sound between 7 and 9 cm. Do not insert the IUD if the uterus sounds only to 6.5 cm or less, owing to increased expulsion rates.

Procedure

ParaGard Copper T

- Using sterile technique, load the IUD into insertion tube by bending the T arms of the device **downward**. The positioning rod is pushed back into the insertion tube when the IUD is loaded. The device has an approximate 5-minute memory to spring back into the T shape.
- Adjust the flange on the insertion tube to depth measured by the sound. The flange is oval shaped, and the flattest part of the flange should be lined up with the T arms of the IUD to ensure proper positioning inside the uterus.
- With gentle traction on the tenaculum, alert the client she will feel another uterine cramp as the IUD is being placed. Insert the IUD and insertion device into the cervix to the level of the flange, making sure the flange is in a horizontal orientation to the cervix.
- Holding the stabilizing rod in one hand and the insertion tube in the other, withdraw the insertion tube toward you.
  - Never push the stabilizing rod deeper into the uterus; this would increase the possibility of uterine perforation.
- Withdraw the stabilizing rod with the insertion tube.
- Cut the string of the IUD to approximately 3 cm from the cervical os.
- Remove the tenaculum, and observe for bleeding at the tenaculum site on the cervix.
- Apply pressure to the site with a large cotton swab. If bleeding does not cease within 1 to 2 minutes, dab the site gently with silver nitrate or Monsel's solution.
- Give a piece of the IUD string to the client for her to feel and have her check her own cervix to feel the protruding IUD string.

Client Instructions—ParaGard Copper T

- Give client the card to have ParaGard Copper T removed after 10 years.
- Take 400 to 800 mg of ibuprofen for several days if needed for cramping.
- Your menstrual periods may be heavier, or you may experience severe cramping.
- Return to the clinic in 6 weeks for a follow-up visit to check string length and side effects.

- Check strings after each menstrual period and call immediately if unable to locate the strings.
- If you miss a menstrual period, perform a pregnancy test and come into the clinic immediately for removal of the IUD if you are pregnant.

Procedure

LEVONORGESTREL-RELEASING IUD (MIRENA)
- Carefully release the threads from behind the slider so that they hang freely.
- The slider should be in the farthest position away from you (positioned at the top of the handle nearest the IUD).
- The arms of the system must be horizontal, before loading the system.
- Without touching the IUD arms, load the IUD by pulling on both strings. This draws the IUD into the insertion tube, with the arms in an upward extended position.
- When the IUD is fully loaded, the end of the rounded knobs of the arms protrude from the end of the insertion tube.
- Fix the strings tightly in the cleft at the end of the handle.
- Set the flange to the depth measured by the sound.
- Advise the client she will feel a cramping sensation with the insertion of the IUD.
- Insert the IUD by using gentle traction on the tenaculum. **Stop advancing the IUD insertion tube when the flange is within 1.5 to 2 cm of the cervix.**
- While holding the inserter steady, release the arms of the IUD by pulling the slider back until it reaches the horizontal line on the handle. You will feel a popping sensation as the IUD is released.
- Push the inserter gently into the uterine cavity until the flange touches the cervix. The IUD now should be in the fundal position of the uterus.
- Holding the inserter firmly in position, release the IUD by pulling the slider down all the way. The strings release automatically.
- Remove the inserter from the uterus.
- Remove the tenaculum from the cervix.
  - Observe for bleeding and apply pressure at the tenaculum site with a large cotton swab.
  - If the bleeding does not cease within 1 to 2 minutes, dab the site with silver nitrate.
- Cut the string to approximately 3 cm from the cervical os.
- Give a piece of the IUD string to the client for her to feel, and have her check her own cervix to feel the protruding IUD string.

Client Instructions—Levonorgestrel-Releasing IUD (Mirena)

- Give client the card to have Mirena IUD removed after 5 years.
- Return to the clinic in 6 weeks for a follow-up visit to check string length and side effects.
- Check strings after each menstrual period and call immediately if you are unable to locate the strings.

- You may have some irregular menstrual bleeding for the first 3 to 6 months after insertion.
  - These symptoms decrease over time; 90% of women have lighter periods in the future, and 20% will stop menstruating altogether.
- If you do become pregnant on the IUD, you need to have it removed as soon as possible.

Removal of an IUD

Equipment

- Gloves—nonsterile
- Speculum
- Light source
- K-Y jelly
- Pelvic ultrasound—optional

Procedure

- Put on gloves.
- With the patient in the lithotomy position, insert a speculum into the vagina.
- Grasp the IUD strings with a ring forceps, and with gentle traction withdraw the IUD from the uterus.
- If the strings are not present, obtain a pelvic ultrasound to determine the location of the IUD.

Client Instructions

- Client will feel slight cramping when the IUD is pulled. This should quickly abate.
  - Only minimal bleeding should be experienced.
  - If bleeding does not stop, contact health-care provider immediately.
- Fertility status returns immediately on removal of the IUD.

BIBLIOGRAPHY

Hatcher R, Trussell J, Nelson A, Cates W. *Contraceptive Technology.* 21st ed. New York, NY: Ardent Media; 2018.

Johnson BA. Insertion and removal of IUD. *Am Fam Physician.* 2005;71(1):95–102.

Zieman M, Hatcher R. *Managing Contraception.* Tiger, GA: Bridging the Gap Foundation; 2012.

Chapter **53**

Nexplanon Insertion
Margaret R. Colyar

CPT Code
11975   Insertion, implantable contraceptive capsules

Nexplanon, a radiopaque implant, is a mode of contraception that is reversible. Nexplanon is implanted under the skin of the upper arm, using daily release of etonogestrol to prevent pregnancy by stopping the release of the egg from the ovary and thickening cervical mucus to prevent sperm from reaching the egg.

OVERVIEW
- It is necessary to ensure that a woman who is to receive a Nexplanon implant is not pregnant at the time of implantation. The Nexplanon should be implanted in the first few days after the menstrual cycle begins or right after an abortion.

RATIONALE
- To initiate the contraception process
- To prevent pregnancy

CONTRAINDICATIONS
- Active or history of thrombophlebitis
- Thromboembolic disorder
- Undiagnosed genital bleeding
- Known or suspected pregnancy
- Acute liver disease and/or benign or malignant liver tumors
- Known or suspected breast carcinoma
- Allergy to progesterone or etonogestrol
- Nursing mother—4 weeks after birth
- History of coronary artery disease
Client teaching includes advising of potential side effects such as
- Acne
- Bleeding irregularities
- Breast carcinoma
- Ovarian cysts
- Dizziness
- Ectopic pregnancy
- Foreign-body carcinogenesis
- Gallbladder problems
- Headache

- Hirsutism
- Hypertension
- Increase in thromboembolic disorder and other vascular problems if the client smokes
- Liver tumors
- Mood swings
- Nervousness, depression, and anxiety
- Nausea and vomiting
- Pain in breasts
- Rash
- Vaginitis
- Weight gain
- Scalp hair loss

Decreased efficacy of Nexplanon occurs with

- Phenobarbital
- Carbamazepine
- Rifampicin
- Griseofulvin
- Oxcarbazepine
- Phenytoin
- St. John's wort
- Topiramate

▶ *Informed consent required*

PROCEDURE

Nexplanon Insertion

Equipment

The following equipment comes in the package with Nexplanon

- Trochar for Nexplanon system
- Scalpel
- **Forceps**
- Syringe
- Two syringe needles
- **Steri-Strips**
- Gauze sponges
- Stretch bandage
- One surgical drape (fenestrated)
- Two surgical drapes
- Antiseptic skin cleanser
- Gloves—sterile
- Drape—sterile
- 1% lidocaine—2 mL

Procedure

- Position the client on her back with the nondominant arm flexed at elbow and externally rotated parallel to the ear.

- Identify the insertion site.
- Cleanse the insertion site with antiseptic skin cleanser.
- Drape the arm above and below the insertion site.
- Fill a syringe with 2 mL 1% lidocaine.
  - Inject lidocaine into insertion site.
- Remove the sterile preloaded disposable Nexplanon applicator carrying the implant from its blister pack. The applicator should not be used if sterility is in question.
- Hold the applicator just above the needle at the textured surface area.
- Remove the transparent protection cap by sliding it horizontally in the direction of the arrow away from the needle. If the cap does not come off easily, the applicator should not be used.
- Stretch the skin around the insertion site with thumb and index finger.
- Puncture the skin with the tip of the needle angled about 30 degrees.
- Lower the applicator to a horizontal position. While lifting the skin with the tip of the needle, slide the needle to its full length. You may feel slight resistance, but do not exert excessive force.
- Keeping the applicator in the same position, unlock the purple slider by pushing it slightly down. Move the slider fully back until it stops.
- Remove the applicator.
- Verify the presence of the implant in the upper arm by palpation.
- Place a small adhesive bandage over the insertion site.
- Apply a pressure bandage with sterile gauze to minimize bruising and secure with a stretch bandage.

Client Instructions

- Remove the pressure bandage in 24 hours.
- You can expect some pain at the incision site.
  - Take acetaminophen or ibuprofen every 4 to 6 hours as needed.
- To limit bruising
  - Avoid heavy lifting for 2 to 3 days.
  - Keep the incision covered with a small bandage over the insertion site for 3 to 5 days.
- Observe for signs and symptoms of infection, such as
  - Increase in pain after 24 hours
  - Increase in temperature
  - Redness or swelling
  - Yellow or greenish drainage
  - Foul odor
- If any of the signs and symptoms of infection are found, return to the office.

BIBLIOGRAPHY ▮▮▮▮▮▮▮▮▮▮▮▮▮▮▮▮▮▮▮▮▮▮

Nexplanon. Drugs.com Web site. http://www.drugs.com/pro/nexplanon.html. October 1, 2018. Accessed October 9, 2019.
Palomba S, Fallbo A, Cello AD, et al. Nexplanon: the new implant for long-term contraception. *Gynecol Endo.* 2012;28(9):710–721.

54 Chapter

Nexplanon Removal

Margaret R. Colyar

CPT Code
11976 Removal, implantable contraceptive capsules
11977 Removal with reinsertion, implantable contraceptive capsules

---

Nexplanon removal consists of removing an implanted contraceptive capsule that is used to prevent pregnancy. After removal of the implanted contraceptive capsule, fertility is returned immediately.

RATIONALE

- To reverse the contraception process
- To diminish unwanted side effects

INDICATIONS

- Request of the client
- Five years elapsed since insertion
- Prolonged vaginal bleeding
- Pain at the implant site

CONTRAINDICATIONS

- None

▶ *Informed consent required*

PROCEDURE

Nexplanon Removal

Equipment

- Antiseptic skin cleanser
- Two drapes—sterile
- Gloves—sterile
- 1% lidocaine
- 2-mL syringe
- 25- to 27-gauge, 1½-inch needle
- No. 11 scalpel
- **Hemostats**—sterile
- Topical antibiotic ointment (Bactroban or Polysporin)
- **Steri-Strips**—⅛ to ¼ inch

- Tape adhesive **(benzoin)**
- Cotton-tipped applicators—nonsterile
- 4 × 4 gauze—sterile
- Kerlix or stretch bandage

Procedure

REMOVAL OF NEXPLANON

- Verify the location of the implant.
- Cleanse the site where the incision will be made with antiseptic skin cleanser.
- Mark the site.
- Drape above and below the Nexplanon implant.
- Anesthetize the arm with 2 mL 1% lidocaine at the marked site where the incision will be made under the implant.
- Push down the proximal end of the implant and a bulge may appear indicating the distal end of the implant. Make a 2-mm incision at the distal end of the implant.
- Gently push the implant toward the incision until the tip is visible.
- Grasp the implant with forceps and gently remove the implant.
- If you have difficulty withdrawing the capsule, gently break away the tissue around the capsule; then pull it out.
- Apply topical antibiotic.
- Close the incision with a Steri-Strip (see Chapter 20) and apply an adhesive bandage.
- Apply a pressure dressing and secure with Kerlix or a stretch bandage.

Client Instructions

- Bruising may occur.
  - To avoid bruising, avoid heavy lifting for 2 to 3 days.
  - Keep the dressing in place for 24 hours.
- Watch for signs and symptoms of infection.
  - Keep incision clean and dry.
  - Return to the clinic if any yellow or greenish drainage occurs.
- You can expect some pain at the incision site.
  - Take acetaminophen every 4 hours or NSAID drug as needed.

BIBLIOGRAPHY

Nexplanon. Drugs.com Web site. http://www.drugs.com/pro/nexplanon.html. October 1, 2018.

Palomba S, Fallbo A, Cello AD, et al. Nexplanon: The new implant for long-term contraception. *Gynecol Endo.* 2012;28(9):710–721.

Paracervical Nerve Block

Margaret R. Colyar

CPT Code
64435   Injection, anesthetic agent; paracervical (uterine) nerve

---

The **paracervical** nerve block is a technique used to anesthetize the uterus, cervix, and upper vagina during cervical conization. The cervical block is of short duration (30 to 60 minutes). This procedure previously was used in the first stage of labor, but it no longer is considered safe during labor.

RATIONALE

*   To anesthetize the uterus, cervix, and upper vagina
*   To diminish pain

INDICATIONS

*   Cervical conization
*   Cervical biopsy

CONTRAINDICATIONS

*   Presence of infection or inflammation
*   Pregnancy
▶ *Informed consent required*

PROCEDURE

Paracervical Block

Equipment

*   Topical antiseptic cleanser
*   Syringe with ring plunger—10 mL
*   Iowa trumpet
*   22-gauge, 1½-inch needle
*   1% lidocaine—10 mL
*   Gloves—sterile
*   4 × 4 gauge—sterile
*   K-Y jelly

Procedure

*   Position the client in the lithotomy position.

- Cleanse the perineum with antiseptic skin cleanser.
- Put on gloves.
- Lubricate fingers and insert into the vagina.
- Locate the cervicovaginal junction.
- Insert the Iowa trumpet into the vagina at the cervicovaginal junction (Fig. 55.1).
- Insert the needle and syringe in the end of the trumpet outside the vagina.
- Insert the needle 0.5 cm into the tissue.
- Aspirate for the presence of blood.

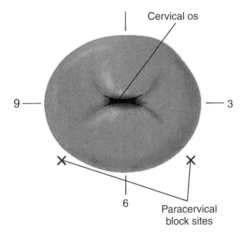

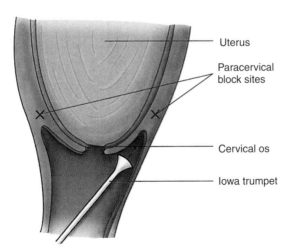

Figure 55.1 Insert the Iowa trumpet into the vagina at the cervicovaginal junction, and inject 1% lidocaine at the paracervical block sites.

- Inject 5 to 10 mL of 1% lidocaine.
- Repeat the procedure on the opposite side of the cervix.

BIBLIOGRAPHY ▮▮▮▮▮▮▮▮▮▮▮▮▮▮▮▮▮▮▮▮▮▮▮▮▮▮▮

Beckmann CRB, Ling F. *Obstetrics and Gynecology*. Philadelphia, PA: Lippincott, Williams & Wilkins; 2018.

Chapter 56

Pessary Insertion
Margaret R. Colyar

CPT Code
57160 Pessary insertion

A pessary is a hard rubber or plastic prosthetic device that serves to elevate the uterus in the vaginal vault. Pessaries are indicated for women who have uterine **prolapse** or **cystocele**. Elderly women most commonly use pessary devices, especially if surgery is contraindicated or undesirable.

OVERVIEW
- Used to maintain
  - Uterine position
    - Prevention of uterine prolapse
    - Alleviation of **menorrhagia, dysmenorrhea**, or **dyspareunia**
  - Bladder and rectum position
    - Prevention of incontinence
  - Support of the pelvic floor in genital hernias because pessaries increase the tension of the pelvic floor
- Frequent complications
  - Vaginal infection
  - Urinary tract infections
- Symptoms associated with pessary use
  - Vaginal burning
  - Vaginal itching
  - Urinary retention
  - Urinary frequency

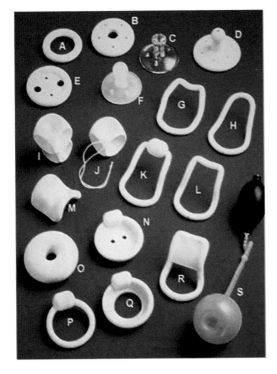

Figure 56.1 Types of pessaries.
(A) Ring; (B) Shaatz;
(C) Gellhorn; (D) Gellhorn;
(E) ring with support;
(F) Gellhorn; (G) Risser;
(H) Smith; (I) tandem cube;
(J) cube; (K) Hodge with
knob; (L) Hodge;
(M) Gehrung;
(N) incontinence dish
with support; (O) donut;
(P) incontinence ring;
(Q) incontinence dish;
(R) Hodge with support;
(S) Inflatoball (latex).

- Urinary urgency
- Dysuria

OPTIONS

There are several types of pessaries to choose from (Fig. 56.1).
- For cystocele only
  - Gehrung
- For cystocele and/or rectocele
  - Ring
  - Doughnut
  - Ball
  - Bee cell
  - Inflatable
- For uterine prolapse
  - Gellhorn
  - Hodge
  - Napier

RATIONALE

- To elevate the uterus in the vaginal vault
- To provide relief with cystocele, rectocele, and uterine prolapse
- To assist in fertility

INDICATIONS

- For women who have one of the following problems but are unable or do not wish to have surgery
  - Uterine prolapse
  - Menorrhagia, dysmenorrhea, or dyspareunia caused by retroposition of the uterus or adnexa prolapse
  - Cystocele
  - Rectocele
  - Bladder or rectal incontinence
  - Hernia of the pelvic floor
  - Obstetric reasons
    - To tilt the cervix into the midline if indicated in infertility

CONTRAINDICATIONS

- Acute genital tract infection
- Adherent retroposition of the uterus

PROCEDURE

Pessary Insertion

Equipment

- Pessary—sterile
- Drape—nonsterile
- Gloves—nonsterile
- Povidone-iodine solution
- Basin—sterile
- Ring **forceps** or claw forceps—sterile
- Light source
- K-Y jelly

Procedure

- Position the client in the lithotomy position.
- Drape the lower half of the client's torso.
- Put on gloves.
- Measure the client for a pessary by
  - Length—measure from the introitus to the top of the posterior vaginal vault and subtract 1 cm.
  - Width—insert ring forceps into the vagina to the level of the cervix, and open until the blades touch the walls of the vagina.
    - Note the distance between the handles of the forceps.
    - Remove the forceps and open again the same distance.
    - Measure between the tips of the blades.
  - Average the two measurements. This is the diameter of the pessary.
- Soak the pessary in a sterile basin filled with povidone-iodine before insertion.
- Lubricate the pessary with K-Y jelly.
- Depress the perineum with the opposite hand to widen the introitus.

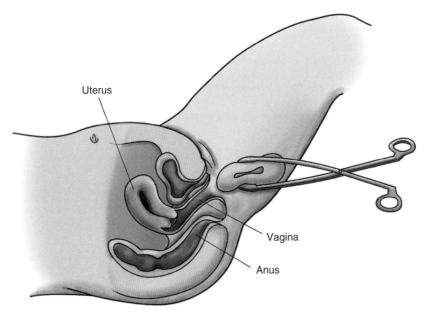

Figure 56.2 Squeeze the pessary with forceps, and insert toward the posterior vagina.

- Grasp the pessary with the forceps and squeeze together (Fig. 56.2).
- Insert the pessary toward the posterior of the vagina.
- When resistance is met, remove forceps.
- Using gloved finger, push the pessary into place behind the suprapubic bone.
- Have the client urinate to determine adequacy of placement.
- Have the client ambulate and squat to evaluate if the client has pain or discomfort or if the pessary gets displaced with position changes.

Client Instructions

- You have a _____ type of pessary inserted to maintain the position of the uterus. Bladder. Rectum. Pelvic floor. Your pessary should be removed _____ daily _____ weekly _____ monthly and cleaned with soap and water.
- Vaginal douching with half water and half vinegar is suggested to decrease the chance of infection and vaginal odor.
- Report the following symptoms as soon as possible
  - Urinary retention
  - Urinary frequency
  - Urinary urgency
  - Difficulty urinating
  - Foul vaginal odor
  - Vaginal discharge
- Your next appointment to check your pessary placement is _____.

BIBLIOGRAPHY

Beckmann CRB, Ling F. *Obstetrics and Gynecology*. Philadelphia, PA: Lippincott, Williams & Wilkins; 2018.

Davila GW. Vaginal prolapse: Management with nonsurgical techniques. *Postgrad Med.* 1996;99(4):171–176, 181, 184–185.

Youngkin EQ, Davis MS. *Women's Health: A Primary Care Clinical Guide*. Norwalk, CT: Appleton & Lange; 2012.

Zeitlin MP, Lobherz TB. Pessaries in the geriatric patient. *J Am Geriatr Soc.* 1992;40(6), 635–639.

57 Chapter

Vaginal Examination

Margaret R. Colyar

CPT Code
None

The routine vaginal examination consists of a visual external inspection and bimanual examination of the lower and upper soft tissue of the genital tract. Insertion of a speculum is done to perform a Pap smear (see Chapter 45). Vaginal examinations may sometimes be done during pregnancy. Table 57.1 reviews the physical signs that should be observed. See Figure 57.1.

OVERVIEW

- During examination, always inform the patient of what will be done beforehand. Bimanual examinations are performed for a number of clinical reasons.
  - Problems relating to menstruation
  - Irregular bleeding
  - Dyspareunia
  - Abnormal vaginal discharge
  - Pelvic pain
  - Check for infection
  - Making decisions about induction methods

RATIONALE

- To assess gynecological health
- To diagnose a medical condition

Table 57·1	Physical Signs During Pregnancy Seen on Vaginal Examination	
SIGN	**WHEN DURING PREGNANCY**	**CHANGE**
Jacquemier's	By the 8th week	Color of cervix is more purplish/blue.
Hegar's	Between 6 and 12 weeks	Uterus is usually enlarged and softer, pear shaped.
Oslander's	By the 8th week	Feeling of blood pulsing through the uterus.
Softening of the cervix	By the 10th week	Cervix feels softer, more like touching the lips rather than the tip of the nose

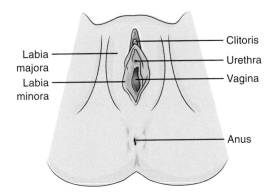

Figure 57.1 Female anatomy.

CONTRAINDICATIONS

None
▶ *Informed consent required*

PROCEDURE

Bimanual Vaginal Examination

Equipment

* Gloves—nonsterile
* K-Y jelly
* Hemoccult card (optional)

Procedure

* Explain the procedure to the patient.
* Position the patient supine with knees bent, ankles together, and legs apart.
* Put on gloves.
* Observe the external genitalia (Table 57.2).
* Apply K-Y jelly to index and middle fingers of the dominant hand.
* Palpate the external genitalia for any lumps or bumps.

Table 57·2	**Basic Evaluation of the External Genitalia Area**

Evaluate the external genitalia for
- Developmental assessment
- Symmetry
- Hair quality
- Hair growth distribution
- Skin abnormalities
  - Labial fusion of the majora and minora
- Swelling
- Varicosities
- Ulcerations
- Cystocele
- Rectocele
- Growths
  - Genital warts
  - Nevi
  - Tumors
- Rashes
- Lacerations
- Piercings
- Bruising
- Discharge

- Separate the labia with your nondominant hand.
- Instruct the patient to cough so that the vaginal orifice opens.
- Insert the lubricated fingers into the vaginal orifice.
  - Palpate the Bartholin's glands at 5:00 and 7:00.
  - Palpate the Skene's glands anterior to the vagina.
  - Palpate the vaginal walls.
  - Palpate the cervix, feeling for size, shape, mobility, and tenderness.
- Place your nondominant hand on the patient's abdomen just above the symphysis pubis and push downward while pushing upward on the cervix with your dominant hand (Fig. 57.2).
  - Palpate the top of the uterus.
  - Direct your fingers inside the vagina to the left fornix and place your nondominant hand outside on the left iliac fossa. Ask the patient to exhale as you compress to facilitate muscle relaxation while palpating the ovaries.
- Repeat for the right ovary.
- Remove your fingers.
- Inform the patient of the rectal/vaginal examination.
  - Insert the gloved index finger into the vagina and the middle finger into the rectum and palpate for lumps and bumps.

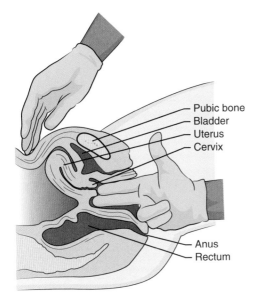

Figure 57.2 Bimanual examination of the uterus.

- Remove your fingers and check for any blood or discharge.
- If there is stool on the middle finger, do a hemoccult test (see Chapter 105).
- Cover the patient.
- Hand the patient a tissue.

Client Instructions

- A small amount of vaginal bleeding is expected.

BIBLIOGRAPHY

Pelvic Examination Technique. Medscape Web site. http://emedicine.medscape.com/article/1947956-technique#showall. Updated September 25, 2018.
https://www.medistudents.com/en/learning/osce-skills/obstetrics-and-gynaecology/bimanual-vaginal-examination/
https://www.jove.com/science-education/10163/pelvic-exam-iii-bimanual-and-rectovaginal-exam

Obstetrical Procedures

Chapter 58

At-Risk Fetal Assessment
Third Trimester Testing

Margaret R. Colyar

CPT Code
76818   Fetal biophysical profile with non-stress testing
76819   Fetal biophysical profile without non-stress testing

Non-stress testing (NST), biophysical profile (amniotic fluid index [AFI], fetal breathing movements, fetal movement, and fetal tone), and Doppler evaluation of fetal circulation are all assessment tools used when a pregnancy is considered to be at risk.

Non-stress testing is usually done during the third trimester to check for fetal well-being. It is performed using an external fetal heart rate monitor to assess the fetal heart rate response to fetal movements. NST is conducted when the baby is overdue, the baby appears to be small or growing slowly, the baby is more or less active than usual, there is a small or a large amount of fluid around the baby, or the mother has a condition such as high blood pressure or diabetes or has abdominal pain.

Amniotic fluid is the clear or slightly yellowish liquid surrounding the fetus in the uterus and contains water, fetal wastes (mainly urine), and fetal skin cells. The AFI is an ultrasound procedure used to assess the amount of amniotic fluid by dividing the uterus into four imaginary quadrants using the linea nigra to divide the uterus into right and left halves and the umbilicus as the dividing point for the upper and lower halves.

OVERVIEW

- Other fetal assessment is done by
  - Assessing fundal height (see Chapter 60)

- Assessing fetal lie (see Chapter 59, Leopold's Maneuver)
  - Longitudinal (normal)
  - Transverse
  - Oblique
- Assessing fetal presentation
  - Breech presentation
  - Cephalic presentation
  - Vertex presentation (normal attitude: full flexion)
  - Face presentation (abnormal attitude: head extends)

RATIONALE

- To evaluate fetal circulation.

INDICATIONS

- Protocols for maternal complications (Table 58.1)
- Protocols for fetal complications (Table 58.2)

CONTRAINDICATIONS

None

PROCEDURE

Obstetric Ultrasound (See Chapter 61)

Non-Stress Test

- Place the mother in a supine position.
- Using elastic bands, place the sensors over the abdomen—one above and one below the umbilicus.
- Attach the sensors to the monitor.
- Turn on the monitor to record the fetal heart rate and movement.
  - One sensor records the baby's movements or any contractions the mother is having.
  - The other sensor measures how fast the baby's heart is beating.
- Interpretation of results
  - Reactive (normal)—presence of two or more fetal heart rate accelerations within a 20-minute period, with or without fetal movement
    - Accelerations: 15 beats per minute (bpm) above baselines for at least 15 seconds if beyond 32 weeks' gestation, or 10 bpm for at least 10 seconds if at or below 32 weeks
  - Nonreactive: less than two fetal heart rate accelerations within a 20-minute period over a 40-minute testing period

Amniotic Fluid Index

- Apply gel over the umbilicus.
- Place the ultrasound transducer parallel over the umbilicus.
  - The linea nigra divides the uterus into right and left halves.
  - The umbilicus divides the uterus into upper and lower halves.

Table 58-1	Protocols for Various Maternal Complications		
MATERNAL COMPLICATION	**NON-STRESS TESTING**	**AMNIOTIC FLUID INDEX**	**ULTRASOUND**
Gestational Diabetes			
Diet controlled, no complications	Biweekly starting at 40 weeks	Biweekly starting at 40 weeks	
Insulin controlled, no complications	Biweekly starting at 32 weeks	Biweekly starting at 32 weeks	Monthly starting at 36 weeks
Diet or insulin controlled, poor control	Biweekly starting at 32 weeks	Biweekly starting at 32 weeks	Monthly starting at 32 weeks
Hypertension			
Chronic, low risk	Weekly starting at 34 weeks	Weekly starting at 34 weeks	Monthly starting at 32 weeks
Chronic, high risk	Weekly starting at 32 weeks	Weekly starting at 32 weeks	Monthly starting at 28 weeks
Pregnancy induced hypertension	Biweekly starting at time of diagnosis	Biweekly starting at time of diagnosis	
Other Problems			
Anemia, sickle cell disease (hematocrit <28%)	Weekly starting at 34 weeks	Weekly starting at 34 weeks	
Seizure disorder	Weekly starting at 34 weeks	Weekly starting at 34 weeks	
Hyperthyroidism	Weekly starting at 34 weeks	Weekly starting at 34 weeks	
Heart disease	Weekly starting at 34 weeks	Weekly starting at 34 weeks	Monthly starting at 28 weeks
Renal disease	Weekly starting at 28 to 30 weeks	Weekly starting at 28 to 30 weeks	Monthly starting at 28 weeks
Collagen vascular disease	Weekly starting at 28 to 30 weeks	Weekly starting at 28 to 30 weeks	Monthly starting at 28 weeks
Advanced maternal age >34 y.o.	Weekly starting at 36 weeks	Weekly starting at 36 weeks	
Asthma (symptomatic)	Weekly starting at 34 weeks	Weekly starting at 34 weeks	
Third trimester abdominal surgery (e.g., appendectomy)	Weekly starting at date of surgery	Weekly starting at date of surgery	
Postterm (>41 weeks)	Biweekly starting at 41 weeks	Biweekly starting at 41 weeks	
Previous fetal demise or stillbirth	Weekly starting at time of intrauterine fetal death (IUFD) or 32 weeks	Weekly starting at time of IUFD or 32 weeks	
Placenta previa	Weekly starting at 34 weeks	Weekly starting at 34 weeks	

Table 58·2	Protocols for Various Fetal Complications		
FETAL COMPLICATION	**NON-STRESS TESTING**	**AMNIOTIC FLUID INDEX**	**ULTRASOUND**
Intrauterine growth retardation (IUGR)	Biweekly from time of diagnosis (>28 weeks)	Biweekly from time of diagnosis (>28 weeks)	Monthly from time of diagnosis
Multiple gestation	Weekly starting at 28–32 weeks	Weekly starting at 28–32 weeks	Monthly starting at 28 weeks
Rh isoimmunization	Weekly starting at 28 weeks	Weekly starting at 28 weeks	Monthly starting at 28 weeks
Polyhydramnios (amniotic fluid index >20)	Weekly starting at 32 weeks	Weekly starting at 32 weeks	
Oligohydramnios (Amniotic fluid index <5)	Biweekly starting at 28 weeks	Biweekly starting at 28 weeks	

- Measure the amniotic fluid in the four quadrants at the deepest, unobstructed, vertical pocket of fluid.
- Add the results from each quadrant together.
- Interpretation of results:
  - Normal—8 to 18 cm
  - <5 to 6 cm is considered oligohydramnios.
  - >20 to 24 cm is considered polyhydramnios.

Client Instructions

No prior preparation is needed.

BIBLIOGRAPHY

Amniotic Fluid. PregMed Web site. http://www.pregmed.org/amniotic-fluid.htm. August 19, 2013.

Fetal Testing Indications. Family Practice Notebook Web site. http://www.fpnotebook.com/legacy/OB/Fetus/FtlTstngIndctns.htm. July 4, 2019.

Wing DA, Fishman A, Gonzalez C, Paul RH. How frequently should the amniotic fluid index be performed during the course of antepartum testing? *Am J Obstet Gynecol.* 1996;174(1 pt 1):33–36. http://www.ncbi.nlm.nih.gov/pubmed/8572030

Chapter **59**

Leopold's Maneuver

Margaret R. Colyar

CPT Code
   None

Leopold's maneuver is performed starting at approximately 24 weeks by palpating the uterus through the abdomen in order to determine the lie and presentation of the fetus.

OVERVIEW

- Usually performed with all pregnancies
- Assess fundal height (see Chapter 60)
- Assess fetal lie
  - Longitudinal (normal)
  - Transverse
  - Oblique
- Assess fetal presentation
  - Breech presentation
  - Cephalic presentation

RATIONALE

- To evaluate fetal lie and fetal presentation

CONTRAINDICATIONS

None

EQUIPMENT

None

PROCEDURE

- See Figure 59.1.
- Have the patient empty her bladder.

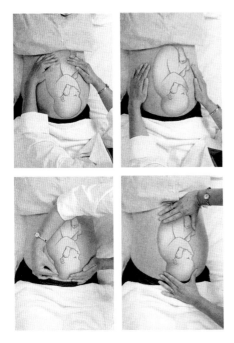

Figure 59.1 Leopold's maneuver.

- Position the woman in the supine position, knees flexed with pillow under her head.
- Warm hands to avoid contraction of abdominal muscles.
- Use a gentle but firm touch.
- Step 1: Fundal grip—Face the woman's head.
  - Used to determine lie or presenting part of the fetus
    - Using the palms of both hands, palpate the top of the fundus.
      - Head or buttocks palpated = vertical lie
      - No head or buttocks palpated = transverse lie
- Step 2: Umbilical grip—Face the woman's head.
  - Used to establish the location of the spine and extremities
    - Using the palm of one hand, apply firm pressure to the right side of the abdomen and palpate the left side with the palm of the other hand.
    - Next, firm pressure is applied to the left side of the abdomen, and the right side is palpated.
- Step 3: Pawlick's grip—Face the woman's feet.
  - Used to establish whether the presenting part is engaged
  - Use the thumb and fingers of one hand to grasp the lower abdomen just above the pubic symphysis.
    - If not engaged, a movable body part will be felt or the presenting part moves upward so the examiner's hands can be pressed together.

- Step 4: Pelvic grip—Face the maternal feet.
  - Used to determine fetal descent
  - Slide the tips of the fingers of each hand toward the pubis over the side of the pregnant woman's fundus.
    - If the head presents, one hand is arrested sooner than the other by a rounded cephalic prominence while the other hand descends deeply into the pelvis.
      - Vertex presentation (normal—full flexion)—The cephalic prominence is on the same side as the small parts.
      - Face presentation (abnormal—head extends)—The cephalic prominence is on the same side as the back.

Client Instructions

- Explain to the mother the lie and presentation of her fetus.

BIBLIOGRAPHY

Leopold's Maneuvers. Family Practice Notebook Web site. http://www.fpnotebook.com/legacy/OB/Exam/LpldsMnvrs.htm. July 4, 2019.
Leopold Maneuvers. RegisteredNurseRN.com Web site. http://www.registerednursern.com/leopold-maneuvers-how-to-correctly-perform-leopold-maneuvers-clinical-nursing-skills/

Chapter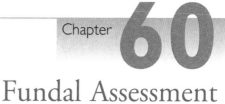

Fundal Assessment

Margaret R. Colyar

CPT Code
   None

Fundal height assessment, also known as McDonald's rule, is measured starting at approximately 12 to 16 weeks' gestation to evaluate the fetus's gestational age. Fundal height measurements offer reassurance of a baby's steady growth and is fairly accurate for singleton births but is not accurate for multiple births. It is measured in centimeters from the top of the symphysis pubis to the top of the fundus (Table 60.1 and Fig. 60.1). Shorter or longer measurements than expected can be due to a number of issues (Table 60.2).

Table 60·1 | Fundal Height Measurement

WEEKS	EXPECTED MEASUREMENT OF FUNDUS
16	Fundus is halfway between the symphysis pubis and the umbilicus
20–22	Fundus will be at the umbilicus
36	Fundus is at the xyphoid process

Note: Between weeks 18 and 30, fundal height in centimeters approximates the fetus's age in weeks plus or minus 2 centimeters.

Table 60·2 | Unexpected Measurements

SHORTER THAN EXPECTED	LONGER THAN EXPECTED
2–4 weeks before delivery	Twins or other multiple births
Error in estimated date of pregnancy	Error in the date of conception
Fetus is healthy, but physically small	Fetus is healthy, but physically large—gestational diabetes, causing a larger baby
Oligohydramnios	Polyhydramnios
Small for gestational age	Large for gestational age

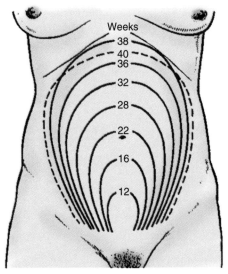

Figure 60.1 Measure from the symphysis pubic to the top of the fundus.

RATIONALE

• To evaluate the growth of the fetus and amniotic fluid development
• To determine steady fetal growth

CONTRAINDICATIONS

None

PROCEDURE

Fundal Assessment

Equipment

* Cloth tape or plastic tape that measures in centimeters

Procedure

* Have pregnant woman empty her bladder.
* Place the pregnant woman in the supine position.
* Place the end of the tape measure at the level of the symphysis pubis.
* Stretch the tape to the top of the uterine fundus.
* Record the measurement.

Client Instructions

* Inform mother of the measurement results and what it indicates.

BIBLIOGRAPHY ▆▆▆▆▆▆▆▆▆▆▆▆▆▆▆▆▆▆▆▆▆▆▆▆▆▆▆▆▆▆

Fundal Height. Wikipedia Web site. http://en.wikipedia.org/wiki/Fundal_height. Last updated July 29, 2018.

Healthy Lifestyle. Pregnancy Week by Week. Mayo Clinic Web site. http://www.mayoclinic.com/health/fundal-height/AN01628.

Morse K, Williams A, Gardosi J. Fetal growth screening by fundal height measurement. *Best Pract Res Clin Obstet Gynaecol.* 2009;23(6):809–818.

White LJ, Lee SJ, Stepniewska K, et al. Estimation of gestational age from fundal height: A solution for resource-poor settings. *J R Soc Interface.* 2012;9(68):503–510.

Healthy Lifestyle. Pregnancy Week by Week. Mayo Clinic Web site. http://www.mayoclinic.com/health/fundal-height/AN01628.

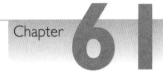

Chapter **61**

Obstetric Ultrasound

Margaret R. Colyar

CPT Code
76801   Diagnostic ultrasound procedures of the pelvis, obstetrical

Obstetric ultrasound uses a small transducer or probe and ultrasound gel to produce pictures of the inside of the body with the use of high-frequency sound waves. The ultrasound images are captured in real time and show structure and movement inside the body in addition to blood flow within blood vessels.

OVERVIEW

- There are four distinct gestational zones during pregnancy in which obstetric ultrasound scans are performed based on different objectives (Table 61.1).
- For benefits of the obstetric ultrasound see Table 61.2.

RATIONALE

- To diagnose and confirm pregnancy/multiple pregnancies
- To evaluate vaginal bleeding in early pregnancy
- To determine gestational age
- To assess fetal size
- To assess fetal viability
- To determine placental placement
- To determine hydramnios and oligohydramnios
- To determine chromosomal anomalies (Table 61.3)

LIMITATIONS

- Cannot identify all fetal abnormalities

CONTRAINDICATIONS

- Allergy to transducer gel
- *Informed consent required*

Table 61·1 | Ultrasound Scans Based on Gestational Ages

SCANS DONE	INDICATION
Before 11 weeks	To verify maternal health, site and number of gestational sac(s), and viability of the pregnancy
11–14 weeks	To screen for chromosomal anomalies—mainly Down syndrome
18–24 weeks	To screen for structural anomalies and fetal well-being
After 28 weeks until term	To determine fetal presentation, position, and fetal well-being/distress (hypoxia and/or acidosis)

Table 61·2 | Benefits of the Obstetric Ultrasound

- Noninvasive
- Extremely safe
- No ionizing radiation such as x-ray used
- Widely available
- Easy to use
- Less expensive than other imaging methods
- Not harmful to the patient, embryo, or fetus
- Clear picture of soft tissues not well shown on x-ray
- Provides much information about the pregnancy
- Temporary discomfort only; almost never painful

Table 61·3	Chromosomal Abnormalities Seen on Obstetric Ultrasound
WHEN	**TYPE**
By 20 weeks	• Hydrocephalus
	• Anencephaly
	• Myelomeningocele
	• Achondroplasia and other dwarfism
	• Spina bifida
	• Exomphalos
	• Gastroschisis
	• Duodenal atresia
	• Fetal hydrops
	• Cleft lip/palate
	• Congenital cardiac abnormalities
By 11–14 weeks—seen in Down syndrome	• Absence of fetal nasal bone
	• Increased fetal nuchal skinfold
	• Tricuspid regurgitation

PROCEDURE

Abdominal Obstetric Ultrasound

Equipment

- Gloves—nonsterile
- Transducer gel
- Ultrasound equipment

Procedure

- Instruct the patient to have a full bladder prior to the procedure.
- Place the patient in a supine position with the abdomen exposed.
- Apply the transducer gel.
- Put on gloves.
- Move the transducer over the area of interest.
- The image of the amniotic sac, the fetus, and the cord can be seen on screen.
- See Table 61.4 for areas to be evaluated during obstetric ultrasound.

Transvaginal Obstetric Ultrasound

Procedure

- Have patient empty bladder prior to the procedure.
- Position the patient supine with feet in stirrups.
- Insert a small amount of gel inside the latex sheath of the transducer.
- Apply the cover to the transducer and remove air.
- Apply gel on the outside of the cover.

Table 61·4	Areas to Be Evaluated During Obstetric Ultrasound
AREA TO BE EVALUATED	**WHEN/WHAT**
Always Measure	
• Crown–rump length	7 to 13 weeks: Very accurate estimation of the gestational age.
• Biparietal diameter—diameter between the sides of the head	After 13 weeks: Increases from about 2.4 cm at 13 weeks to about 9.5 cm at term. Dating in later part of pregnancy is considered unreliable.
• Femur length	14 weeks: Increases from about 1.5 cm at 14 weeks to about 7.8 cm at term. Dating in later part of pregnancy is considered unreliable.
Other	
• Abdominal circumference	Late in pregnancy: Reflects fetal size and weight rather than age.
• Gestational sac	By 4.5 weeks: Increases by about 1 mm per day; not accurate for dating a pregnancy.
• Yolk sac diameter	Between 7 and 11 weeks: Reaches a diameter of up to 7 mm, then decreases in size. If greater than 5.6 mm before 10 weeks, abnormal fetal outcome. Absence of the yolk sac in the presence of an embryo is abnormal and is associated with fetal demise.
• Nuchal skinfold	Between 10 and 13 weeks: The fold is less than 3 mm normally. After 16 weeks, should not exceed 6 to 7 mm. Increased nuchal fold occurs in Turner's syndrome, Down syndrome, and other chromosomal abnormalities.

- Insert the transducer straight into the vagina.
- Tilt clockwise, counterclockwise, upward, and downward to visualize all the structures and bring the fetus into focus.
- Remove the transducer and dispose of the sheath.

Client Instructions

- Full bladder with abdominal ultrasound
- Empty bladder with transvaginal ultrasound

BIBLIOGRAPHY

Obstetric Ultrasound. RadiologyInfo.org Web site. http://www.radiologyinfo.org/en/info.cfm?pg=obstetricus. January 23, 2019.
Pelvic Ultrasound. Health–Johns Hopkins Medicine Web site. http://www.hopkinsmedicine.org/healthlibrary/test_procedures/gynecology/pelvic_ultrasound_92,P07784/
https://www.youtube.com/watch?v=yysllCFyfus
Ultrasound Scan Lectures. Obstetrics and Gynecology Lectures. www.obstetric-ultrasound.com/
Woo J. A Comprehensive Guide. Obstetric Ultrasound Web site. http://www.ob-ultrasound.net/

Chapter **62**

Emergency Delivery

Margaret R. Colyar

CPT Code
59409 Vaginal delivery only
59414 Delivery of placenta

If upon evaluation of a pregnant female the cervix is dilated (to 10 cm) and/or effaced (thinned to about 1 mm) and the baby is crowning, an emergency delivery will need to be performed.

INDICATIONS

- Cervix is dilated to 10 cm.
- Cervix is effaced to about 1 mm.
- Presenting part of fetus is crowning.
- Mother insists she needs to push.
- There is no time to transport the mother to the labor and delivery area.
- Face, foot or feet, hand or arm, and breech presentations are obvious on palpation.

Document the Apgar score (Table 62.1) to provide a rough estimate of the baby's immediate adaption to extrauterine life at 1, 5, and 10 minutes. If the 5-minute score is less than 7, continue scoring every 5 minutes for 20 minutes.

RATIONALE

- To control the eminent delivery of a fetus

CONTRAINDICATIONS

- None

PROCEDURE

Emergency Delivery

Equipment

- Povidone-iodine or antiseptic soap
- 4 × 4 gauze or washcloth
- Towels
- Sheet

Table 62·1	**Apgar Scoring**		
ITEM TO SCORE	**0**	**1**	**2**
Appearance	Blue or pale	Pink body, limbs blue	Pink all over
Pulse	Absent	Less than 100/min	Greater than 100/min
Grimace	No response	Some motion	Crying
Activity	Limp	Weak motion	Active

- Gloves
- Blanket

Procedure

The general procedure for delivery when infant is in the caudal position is as follows:

- Put on gloves.
- Position the patient supine with knees bent and outward.
- Drape with a sheet.
- Swab the perineum with povidone-iodine or antiseptic soap.
- Drape the perineum with towels.
- Usually, the amniotic sac has broken; if not, break the sac with your finger.
  - Note the color and consistency of the amniotic fluid.
- Gently stretch the vaginal opening by pushing outward with your fingers. This will help to widen the opening.
- Once the head emerges, suction the mouth and nose. Control the baby's head with the nondominant hand.
- Check the neonate's neck for the umbilical cord.
  - If it is wrapped around the neck, pull it gently over the head.
  - If this is not possible (either it is too tight or has too many loops), double clamp the cord and divide the cord between the clamps.
- To assist delivery of the anterior shoulder, apply gentle traction toward the mother's posterior.
  - If this is unsuccessful, try pressing down over the mother's bladder to move the anterior shoulder posteriorly.
  - If this is unsuccessful, deliver the posterior shoulder, rotating the anterior shoulder posteriorly, and then deliver that shoulder.
- Once the shoulders are out, the rest of the baby slips out quickly.
- Keep the nondominant hand in place, control the baby's head, and slide the dominant hand under and along the baby as it emerges.
- Once the feet are out, rotate the baby 180 degrees into a football hold.
- Suction the nose and mouth.
- Double clamp the cord 7 to 10 cm from the baby, and cut the cord between the clamps.
- If the child starts breathing and moving and appears to be in good health, turn the baby over to nursing personnel.

- If the birth is complicated by thick meconium (amniotic fluid that is thick and pea green), do not stimulate the baby to cry.
  - Use a 3.0 endotracheal tube, intubate the trachea, and suction it; then stimulate the baby's breathing.
- Do not unclamp the mother's side of the placenta until it is clear that only one fetus is present.
- Palpate the uterus. If it is almost in the pelvis, probably only one fetus exists.
- Let the cord drain, collecting a clot tube for laboratory studies.
  - Feel gently for a pulse. After about 10 minutes, the cord will stop pulsing. Do not cut it before then.
- Allow the third stage of labor, delivery of the placenta, to proceed slowly.
  - Do not pull on the cord.
  - Guide the placenta out as it is expelled.
  - Inspect the placenta to ensure that it is entirely expelled.
- Massage the woman's uterus just below the umbilicus until the uterus feels like a grapefruit low in the abdomen.
- Perform any vaginal or perineal repairs.

Breech Presentation

- Have the mother sit at the edge of a bed and pull her legs to her chest.
- Place pillows or blankets where the baby is likely to fall.
- *Do not* touch the baby until the head is delivered because your touch could stimulate the baby to gasp while the head is still submerged in amniotic fluid.
- The infant's back and bottom will hang down.
- Once the head is delivered, grab the baby under the arms and bring it up to the mother.
- If the head doesn't come out in the push after the arms come out, have the mother squat and push.

Client Instructions

- Keep the mother and baby warm and comfortable. Cover them both in blankets when they're cold, and encourage the mother to keep the baby on her chest. Replace any wet or dirty bedding, and move them to a clean, dry area.
- Keep an ice pack on the vaginal area for the first 24 hours to ease soreness and pain.
- Take Tylenol or Ibuprofen as needed.
- Pour warm water over the vaginal area every time you go to the bathroom to keep clean and prevent infection.
- Have a light meal (crackers and cheese, or peanut butter and jelly sandwich) and a drink.

BIBLIOGRAPHY

Bensoni TE. Labor and Delivery in the Emergency Department Treatment & Management. Medscape. http://emedicine.medscape.com/article/796379-treatment#a1126. Updated July 26, 2017.

63 Chapter

Teaching Breastfeeding

Margaret R. Colyar

CPT Code
None

The first year of an infant's nutrition is critical to future health. The American Academy of Pediatrics recommends that all infants be breastfed exclusively for the first 6 months of life and that feeding with breast milk continue until 12 months of age. Benefits include lower rate of mortality and sudden infant death syndrome in infants and toddlers, along with lower incidence of type 1 and type 2 diabetes, hematological cancers, overweight and obesity, hypercholesterolemia, and asthma as older children and adults.

OVERVIEW

- All healthy full-term infants are born with reflexes that enable them to obtain milk from the mother's breasts (see Table 63.1).
- Breastfeeding is a learned art. Important elements include
  - Facilitating proper latch
  - Facilitating proper positioning
  - Teaching breast massage
  - Teaching hand milk expression
  - Dealing with engorgement
  - Dealing with sore nipples
  - Alleviating concerns about low milk supply
  - Instructions on how to handle a fussy baby
- Realize the child will have growth spurts and will need an increase in feeding. These occur at ages
  - 8 to 12 days
  - 3 to 4 weeks
  - 3 months
- Guidelines for safe handling, storage, and thawing of expressed breast milk are shown in Table 63.2.

RATIONALE

- To facilitate proper techniques of breastfeeding
- To identify problems with breastfeeding usually encountered in the first 6 weeks postpartum

Table 63·1	Reflexes Infants Are Born With
REFLEX	**HOW IT HELPS BREASTFEEDING**
Rooting	Touching the nipple to the infant's mouth causes the mouth to open wide and take in the nipple. Helps with attachment to the breast.
Suckling	The infant's mouth rhythmically compresses the nipple and part of the areola between the tongue and hard palate.
Swallowing	Milk is passed along the esophagus in a wave of peristalsis and into the stomach.

Table 63·2	Guidelines for Safe Handling and Storage of Expressed Breast Milk

Safe Handling

- Practice good hand washing technique.
- Wash containers and breast pump equipment in hot, soapy water and rinse well.
  - Wash in dishwasher or boil.
- Chill same-day milk for 1 hour in a refrigerator, then add to previously chilled milk expressed that same day.
  - Do not add fresh milk to previously frozen milk.

Storage

- Label the container with date.
- Store in 2-oz to 4-oz portions. Avoid ordinary plastic storage bags or formula bottle bags.
- Can remain in the following conditions for the times designated
  - Table or countertop (covered): Less than 77°F for 6 to 8 hours
  - Insulated cooler bag with ice packs in contact with milk: 5°F to 39°F for 24 hours
  - Refrigerator: 39°F for 5 days
  - Freezer
    - 5°F for 2 weeks
    - 0°F for 3 to 6 months
    - –4°F for 6 to 12 months

Thawing

- Transfer milk from freezer to refrigerator OR
- Swirl container of milk in a bowl of warm water.
- Do NOT thaw in a microwave.
  - Destroys nutrient quality
  - Does not heat liquids evenly
- Do NOT heat bottles of breast milk.
- Do NOT refreeze.

CONTRAINDICATIONS

- Serious illness of mother
- Mother taking medications that will affect the infant negatively

PROCEDURE

Teaching Breastfeeding

Facilitate Proper Latch and Positioning

- Mother should sit up straight in a chair and cradle the baby in the curve of the upper arm.
- Align the infant. Infant should be on his side with tummy and knees touching the opposite breast. Infant's ear, shoulder, and hip should be aligned. Infant's head shouldn't be tilted up or to the side.
- Cup the hand in the shape of the letter C and place it under the breast for support. Fingers are under the breast, thumb on top.
- Gently massage the nipple with the thumb to express a small amount of milk.
- Tickle or gently rub the infant's lips with the breast to stimulate the rooting reflex.
  - The baby should root toward the nipple and open his mouth wide.
- Aim the nipple at the baby's nose.
- Once the infant's mouth is open, place the nipple on the infant's tongue with as much areola in his mouth as possible.
  - Lips should curl outward.
- If you hear a sucking sound, the baby's mouth is not correctly positioned and is sucking air between the breast and their mouth. Reposition.
- If the infant seems nervous or excessively sleepy, strip the infant down to his diaper and place him against the mother's skin. This is calming, but also keeps the infant more alert.
  - Drape a light blanket on the mother and infant to prevent chilling.

Teach Massage—Stimulate the Let-Down Reflex

- Start with the palm of the hand on the upper chest near the collar bone.
- Begin a downward massage toward the nipple with firm gentle strokes.
- Divide the breast into quadrants and repeat the massage going around the breast.
- At the armpit quadrant, place your opposite hand over the hand doing the massage and continue toward the nipple in a firm and gentle manner.
- Repeat the procedure on the other breast.

Teach Hand Expression—Stimulate the Let-Down Reflex

- Without touching the nipple or areola, press the fingers together gently over the breast in a milking motion.
- Let the fingers slide toward the nipple.
- Be careful not to touch the nipple or the areola; this will give the mother sore nipples.

Teach How to Deal With Engorgement

- Usually occurs 2 to 7 days posthospital because of milk coming in and vascular congestion in the breast.
- Instruct the mother to place warm compresses on the breast or take warm showers for 10 minutes before nursing.
- Then use hand expression to initiate the let-down reflex.
- Feed the infant every 2 to 2.5 hours for 10 to 15 minutes on each breast.
- If still uncomfortable after feeding infant, hand express or pump enough milk to relieve pressure.
- Ice packs between feedings help reduce swelling.

Teach How to Deal With Sore Nipples

- Reinforce correct positioning and latch.
- Warm soaks to the breast
- Hand expression to initiate let-down reflex
- Air-dry the nipples.
  - Wear a soft shirt or pajama top and leave bra flaps down on a nursing bra.
- Apply pure lanolin on the nipple after nursing. There is no need to remove it for the next feeding. It absorbs into the skin.
- Change infant's position for nursing. Try the football hold.
  - Cradle infant under the arm with the hand behind his head. His legs will be around the mother's back.
  - Place the free hand under the breast for support.

Alleviate Concerns About Low Milk Supply—Usually Perceived, NOT Actual

- Encourage the mother to nurse frequently, every 2 to 2.5 hours, for 10 to 15 minutes on each breast to increase milk supply.
- Encourage an 8-ounce glass of water every time the child is picked up to feed.
  - Encourage extra juice, milk, herbal tea, and ginger ale in addition to water.
  - Avoid too many caffeinated beverages.
- Encourage warm compresses and hand expression to help initiate the let-down reflex.
- Check the infant's diaper—should have 6 to 8 wet diapers in 24 hours.
- Infant should regain his birth weight by his 2-week checkup.
- Infant should gain 2 pounds by the 2-month checkup.

Instruct on How to Handle a Fussy Baby

- Try changing the diaper.
- Try burping.
- Try repositioning the infant in his crib.
- Try rocking the child.
- Limit overstimulation.
  - Too much handling
  - Too much noise
- When in doubt, nurse.

BIBLIOGRAPHY

J Trop Pediatr. http://www.oxfordjournals.org/our_journals//tropej/online/chap10_presentation_bk2.pdf.

Murry N. Safety first in infant feeding: Counseling parents on the avoidance of feeding-associated infections. *Clin Advisor.* September 2013.

Schanler RJ, Enger, L. Patient education: Breastfeeding guide (beyond the basics). UpToDate Web site. https://www.uptodate.com/contents/breastfeeding-guide-beyond-the-basics.

Teaching Breastfeeding. Lactation Education Resources Web site. https://www.lactationtraining.com/resources/educational-materials/handouts-professionals/teaching-breastfeeding.

Head: Eyes, Ears, Nose, and Mouth

Chapter **64**

Audiometry Testing
Margaret Colyar

CPT Code
92551   Screening examination, pure-tone only

The **audiogram** is an objective assessment tool for the detection of hearing problems or loss in most age groups older than 6 months. The **audiogram** is not effective with children younger than 4 months of age. Hearing loss results in delayed speech and language development in infants and toddlers and poor academic progress in preschool-age and school-age children. Hearing loss in adults can be the cause of deterioration in interpersonal behaviors and social interactions.

OVERVIEW

- Incidence of hearing loss
  - Approximately 1 in every 15 (16 million) Americans
  - Infants—1 in 1,000
- Average age of onset of hearing loss
  - 55 to 75 years
- Suggested topics to discuss with the client
  - Epidemiology of the cause of the dysfunction or hearing loss
- Environmental variables that contribute to the dysfunction (including allergies and smoking)
- Intervention variables that can improve the outcome of the problem

HEALTH PROMOTION/PREVENTION
Adults, Children, and Adolescents

- Avoid potential environmental circumstances that would produce severe loud sounds such as
  - High-volume music with or without earphones

- Explosions
- Loud machinery
- Restrict agents that have ototoxic effects.
- Use decibel-reducing earplugs.

Infants and Toddlers

- Prevent factors such as
  - Prenatal infections (cytomegalovirus, rubella, syphilis, human immunodeficiency virus [HIV], herpes)
  - Maternal drug and alcohol abuse
  - Low birth weight
  - Newborn jaundice
  - Meningitis
  - Head trauma
  - Exposure to loud noises

RATIONALE

- To detect hearing problems or loss
- To prevent delayed speech and language development

INDICATIONS

- Evaluation of hearing loss
- Routine screening for infants and children
- Routine adult well-care screening
- Occupational screening for individuals in noisy work settings
- Speech and language development delays in infants and children
- Poor academic progress in school-age children
- High-risk infants for preexisting hearing deficit
- Deterioration in interpersonal skills in home or work environment for the adult
- Unexplained behavior changes in the geriatric individual
- Complaints of tinnitus (ringing in the ears)

CONTRAINDICATIONS

- Cerumen obstruction
- Otitis externa
- Younger than 6 months (inaccurate readings)

PROCEDURE

Audiometry Testing

Equipment

- Audiometry tool with the recommended features (Fig. 64.1)
- Decibel frequencies 500 to 4,000 Hz
- Correct size earpiece to ensure a good seal over the external canal opening
- Quiet room

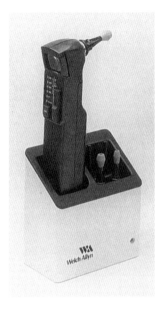

Figure 64.1 AudioScope 3. *(Courtesy of Welch Allyn, Inc.)*

Procedure

- Position the client in a comfortable sitting position.
- Ask the client to indicate hearing a tone by raising his or her hand.
- Inspect the ear canal for infection or cerumen obstruction.
- If using a handheld model, select the proper ear probe for good seal of external canal.
  - Activate probe.
- If using a handheld model, gently grasp the pinna and pull back (for children) or up and back (for adults) to obtain a good seal.
- If using an earphone or earplug model, position the equipment so that it covers the entire external os with a good seal.
- Begin testing as directed by the instrument manual.
- Record the results.
- Interpret the results (examples in Fig. 64.2 are from the AudioScope 3 by Welch Allyn).
  - Note normal hearing screening range.
- If not within normal limits, suggest repeating at another time.
- If results are persistently not in normal range of screening (two or three testings), REFER to an audiologist for further testing.
- Review the results and implications of their interpretation in the management of the client's health problems with the client and/or parents. Suggested topics include
  - Epidemiology of the cause of the dysfunction
  - Environmental variables that contribute to the dysfunction (including allergies and smoking)
  - Intervention variables that can improve outcome of the problem

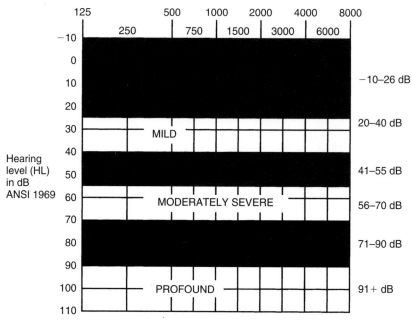

Figure 64.2 Normal hearing screening range. *(Courtesy of Welch Allyn, Inc.)*

- Referral to certified audiologist who can perform more detailed evaluation of hearing loss and recommend appropriate devices that can amplify sound and reduce hearing loss

Client Instructions

- Your hearing loss is caused by _____.
- Some environmental variables that contribute to your hearing loss include
  - Allergies
  - Smoking
  - Loud music
- To improve the outcome of your problem, do not allow smoking in the house.
- You should see a certified audiologist who can perform more detailed evaluation of hearing loss and recommend appropriate devices to amplify sound and reduce hearing loss.

MANUFACTURING COMPANIES

Micro Audiometrics
Maico Hearing Instruments
Welch Allyn, Inc.

BIBLIOGRAPHY ▉▉▉▉▉▉▉▉▉▉▉

Buttross SL, Gearhart JG, Peck JE, et al. Early identification and management of hearing impairment. *Am Fam Physician.* 1995;51(6);1437–1446, 1451–1452.

Pfenninger JL, Fowler GC. *Procedures for Primary Care Physicians.* St. Louis, MO: Mosby; 2019.

Welch Allyn. *AudioScope 3: Instructions Manual for Portable Audiometer Instrument.* Skaneateles Falls, NY: Welch Allyn; 2007.

Chapter **65**

Tympanometry

Cynthia R. Ehrhardt

CPT Code
92567 Tympanometry (impedance testing)
92568 Tympanometry with acoustic reflex

Tympanometry is an objective assessment tool for the mobility of the tympanic membrane, pressure within the middle ear, and volume of the external canal. This tool is used to measure resolution of otitis media and serous otitis media, determine the presence of eustachian tube dysfunction problems, and screen for causes of developmental delays.

RATIONALE

- To assess mobility of the tympanic membrane, pressure in the middle ear, and eustachian tube dysfunction
- To determine causes of developmental delay

INDICATIONS

- Evaluation of hearing loss
- Evaluation of ear pain
- Establishing mobility of the tympanic membrane
- Detection of tympanic membrane perforation
- Assessment of middle ear function when audiometry is not possible
- Documentation of absence or presence of effusions of the middle ear
- Monitoring of effusions of the middle ear
- Evaluation of the effectiveness of pressure-equalization tubes
- Unexplained developmental delays in infants and children

CONTRAINDICATIONS

- Cerumen obstruction
- Otitis externa
- Younger than 4 months—leads to inaccurate readings

PROCEDURE

Tympanometry

Equipment

- Tympanometry tool with the recommended features (Fig. 65.1)
- 226-Hz probe tone
- Ear tips of various sizes that ensure a good seal over the external canal opening
- Air pressure range of 400 daPa (decaPascals) to +200 daPa (1.02 mm H^2O equals 1.0 daPa)
- Easy-to-use buttons to activate tool
- Readable numbers
- Printable results—optional

Procedure

Inspect the ear canal for infection or cerumen obstruction.

- Adjust tympanometer device for altitude (usually not needed below 1,280 feet) (Table 65.1).
- Position the client in a comfortable sitting position.
- Explain the procedure, including how the client will indicate hearing the tone.
- Select the proper ear tip for good seal of external canal.

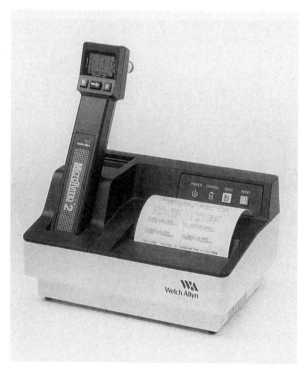

Figure 65.1 MicroTymp 2, portable tympanometric instrument. *(Photo courtesy of Welch Allyn, Inc.)*

Table 65·1 **Altitude Adjustments**				
ALTITUDE, ft	**ADJUST-MENT FOR 0.5 mL (mL)**	**ADJUST-MENT FOR 1.0 mL (mL)**	**ADJUST-MENT FOR 1.5 mL (mL)**	**ADJUST-MENT FOR 2.0 mL (mL)**
1,280	0.0	0.0	0.0	0.0
2,530	0.0	0.1	0.1	0.2
3,220	0.0	0.1	0.2	0.3
4,770	0.1	0.2	0.3	0.4

- Activate.
- Gently grasp the pinna and pull back (for children) or up and back (for adults) to obtain a good seal.
- Apply the probe to the external canal with a good seal.
- When a good seal is achieved (machine indicates this), activate the test switch.
- Record the reading as directed by the instrument manual.
- Print out the results.
- Interpret the tympanogram results (examples are from the MicroTymp 2 by Welch Allyn).
  - Normal tympanogram (Fig. 65.2)
  - Too much artifact (Fig. 65.3)
  - Ear canal occlusion (Fig. 65.4)
  - Otitis media with effusion (Fig. 65.5)
  - Oncoming or resolving otitis media with effusion (Fig. 65.6)
  - Tympanic membrane abnormalities or ossicular disruption (Fig. 65.7)
  - Negative middle ear pressure (Fig. 65.8)
  - Patent **tympanostomy** tube or perforated tympanic membrane (Fig. 65.9)
- Review the results and their interpretation in the management of the client's health problems with the client and/or parents. Suggested topics include
  - Epidemiology of the cause of the dysfunction
  - Environmental variables that contribute to the dysfunction (including allergies, smoking, loud noises)
  - Intervention variables that can improve outcome of the problem

Client Instructions

- You have the following problems: _____.
- Stay away from factors in the environment that cause your allergies to flare.
- No smoking is permitted in the house.

MANUFACTURING COMPANIES

- Grason-Stadler, Inc.
- Maico Hearing Instruments
- Micro Audiometrics
- American Electromedics Corporation
- Welch Allyn, Inc.

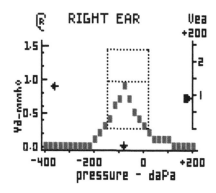

* Produces tympanogram within normal limits
A   relative to height and width

Tympanometric Measurement	Child's Ear (Under Age 10) 90% Range	Adult's Ear (Over Age 10) 90% range
Peak Ya	0.2 to 0.9 mmho	0.3 to 1.4 mmho
Gradient (GR) (Tympanometric Width)	60 to 150 daPa	50 to 110 daPa
Tympanometric Peak Pressure (TPP)	-139 to +11 daPa	-83 to 0 daPa
Equivalent Ear Canal Volume (Vea)	0.4 to 1.0 cc	0.6 to 1.5 cc

NOTE: For purposes of tympanometric norms, an adult is defined as a person 10 years of age or older, and a child as under age 10.
Normative data are taken from a study by Margolis and Heller (1987), and from the "Guidelines for Screening for Hearing Impairments and Middle
B   Ear Disorders" ASHA (1990).

Figure 65.2 The normal ear. (A) Tympanogram from a normal ear. (B) Normative tympanometric data. *(Photo courtesy of Welch Allyn, Inc.)*

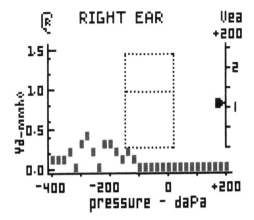

Tympanogram with Too Much Artifact
- Caused by patient or practitioner movement
- Requires repeating measurement

Figure 65.3 Conditions that cause too much artifact. *(Photo courtesy of Welch Allyn, Inc.)*

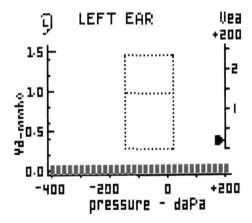

Ear Canal Occlusion
- Can produce flat tympanogram with ear canal volume lower than expected
- May also produce BLOCK message
- Requires repeating measurement

Figure 65.4 Conditions that artificially flatten the tympanogram. *(Photo courtesy of Welch Allyn, Inc.)*

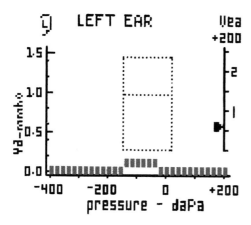

• Produces low static admittance (low peak height) tympanogram
• Tympanogram is also typical of tympanosclerosis, cholesteatoma, and middle ear tumor

Figure 65.5 Otitis media with effusion. *(Photo courtesy of Welch Allyn, Inc.)*

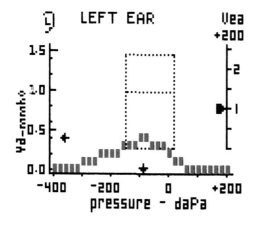

• Produces normal peak height, but tympanogram that is too wide
• Tympanogram is also typical of tympanosclerosis

Figure 65.6 Oncoming or resolving otitis media with effusion. *(Photo courtesy of Welch Allyn, Inc.)*

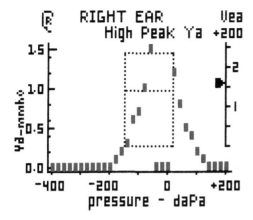

• Produces high static admittance (high peak height) tympanogram

Figure 65.7 Tympanic membrane abnormalities or ossicular disruption. *(Photo courtesy of Welch Allyn, Inc.)*

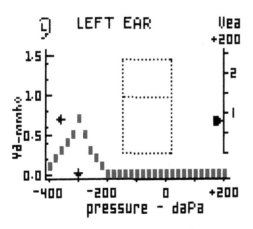

• Produces negative Tympanometric Peak Pressure (TPP) tympanogram
• Usually not associated with effusion when Peak Ya is normal
• Also associated with eustachian tube dysfunction, cold, or allergies

Figure 65.8 Negative middle ear pressure. *(Photo courtesy of Welch Allyn, Inc.)*

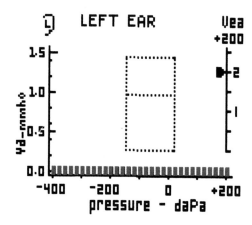

• Can produce flat tympanogram with ear canal volume higher than expected
• May also produce OPEN message

Figure 65.9 Patent tympanotomy tube or perforated tympanic membrane. *(Photo courtesy of Welch Allyn, Inc.)*

BIBLIOGRAPHY

Bredfeldt R. An introduction to tympanometry. *Am Fam Physician.* 1991;44(6): 2113–2117.

Buttross SL, Gearhart JG, Peck JE. Early identification and management of hearing impairment. *Am Fam Physician.* 1995;51(6):1437–1446, 1451–1452.

Isaacson JE, Vora NM. Differential diagnosis and treatment of hearing loss. *Am Fam Physician.* 2003;68(6):1125–1132.

Pfenninger JL, Fowler GC. *Procedures for Primary Care Physicians.* St. Louis, MO: Mosby; 2019.

Robb P, Watson A. *ENT in Primary Care.* London: Rila Publication Ltd.; 2007.

Welch Allyn. *AudioScope 3: Instructions Manual for Portable Audiometer Instrument.* Skaneateles Falls, NY: Welch Allyn; 2007.

Chapter **66**

Visual Function Evaluation
Snellen, Illiterate E, Pictorial
Margaret R. Colyar

CPT Code
None: Included in the office visit

Evaluation of visual function includes the testing of visual acuity, visual field defects, **strabismus**, and color vision. Visual acuity is tested using the Snellen eye chart. If the client is young or unable to read, the Illiterate E or the Pictorial chart should be used. Visual field defects are tested by performing **confrontation**. Strabismus (squint, crossed eye) is tested in the ambulatory care setting using the cover/uncover test, corneal light reflex, and extraocular muscle movement tests. Color vision is tested using the Ishihara's or Hardy Rand Rittler's **polychromatic** cards.

OVERVIEW

- Incidence
  - All yearly examinations and if an eye disorder is suspected
- The main causes of decreased visual acuity
  - Diabetes mellitus
  - Hypertension
  - Cataracts
  - Glaucoma
  - Retinal detachment
- The main causes of visual field defects
  - Glaucoma
  - Retinitis
  - Intracerebral tumors
  - Detached retina
- The main causes of strabismus
  - Hyperthyroidism
  - Myasthenia gravis
  - Cranial artery aneurysms
  - Multiple sclerosis
  - Neurological disease
  - Orbital disease
  - **Amblyopia**

Eight percent of white males and 4% of black males inherit the recessive X-linked trait for color blindness. Although not disabling, a deficit in color vision may cause problems in learning and the ability to assess traffic lights.

RATIONALE

- To evaluate visual function
- To determine the presence of visual defects

INDICATIONS

- Children
- Clients with visual complaints
- Ocular trauma
- Screening for school and employment
- Headache

CONTRAINDICATIONS

- None

PROCEDURE

Visual Examination

Equipment

- Penlight
- Snellen, Illiterate E, or Pictorial eye chart (Fig. 66.1)
- 20-foot hall
- Color vision book—Ishihara or Hardy Rand Rittler set
- Near-vision chart or newspaper

Procedure

VISUAL ACUITY

- Have the client stand 20 feet from the chart.
  - Use the Snellen letter test, Illiterate E, or Pictorial test.
- Cover one of the client's eyes and have the client read the smallest line. Do the same with the alternate eye. Then test with both eyes open.
  - If there is a difference of two or more levels between the eyes, suspect amblyopia. REFER to an ophthalmologist.
- Record the results.
  - The first number indicates how far the client was standing from the eye chart. The second number indicates how far the person with normal sight could read the letters of a particular height.
  - A measurement of 20/40 means the client can read at 20 feet what a normally sighted person can read at 40 feet.
  - Always indicate if this measurement is with or without glasses.
  - If the client is aged 40 or older, check near vision by having the client read at a distance of 14 inches.

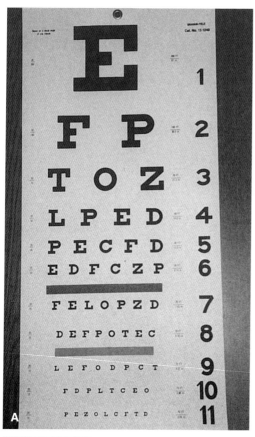

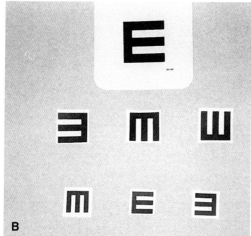

Figure 66.1 (A) Snellen and (B) Illiterate E eye charts.

VISUAL FIELDS—CONFRONTATION
- Stand 2 feet from the client.
  - Have the client cover one eye with his or her hand and stare into your eye. The examiner also must cover the same eye.
  - Hold an object (pencil, penlight) in each of the visual fields.
  - Have the client indicate when he or she can see the object in each of the visual fields.
  - The client's peripheral vision should match the vision of the examiner.
- Record the results.
  - Document where a deficit occurs by using time on a clock or blackened circles (Fig. 66.2).

STRABISMUS
If discovered, REFER to an ophthalmologist.
- Observe both eyes to detect the deviation of one eye.
  - Exotropia—lateral deviation
  - Esotropia—nasal deviation
- To differentiate between paralytic and nonparalytic strabismus, check extraocular movement 2 to 3 feet away. Document deviation of the eyes.

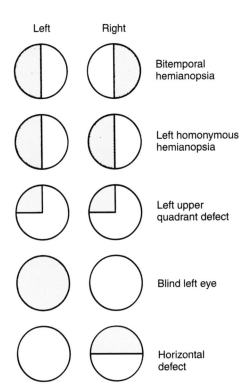

Left   Right

Bitemporal
hemianopsia

Left homonymous
hemianopsia

Left upper
quadrant defect

Blind left eye

Horizontal
defect

Figure 66.2 One method to document where a deficit occurs is to use blackened circles.

- Perform corneal light reflex test.
  - Have the person look at a light.
  - Observe where light falls on the cornea.
  - With strabismus, the light falls on different parts of the cornea.
- Perform cover/uncover test.
  - Cover one of the person's eyes.
  - Have the person stare straight ahead.
  - Uncover the eye and observe.
  - With strabismus, the covered eye wanders and may or may not return to its position when uncovered.

COLOR VISION
- Using a color vision book, have the client read the numbers on each page of the book.
- Record on the chart the numbers that the client cannot read.
- Use the interpretive guidelines provided by the color vision book.

Client Instructions
- Based on the tests done in the office/clinic today, we observed the following problems:_____.
  - An examination by an ophthalmologist is needed/not needed.
  - Please make an appointment with your ophthalmologist within the next day/week/month for evaluation.

BIBLIOGRAPHY

Bickley LS. *Bates' Guide to Physical Examination and History-Taking.* 11th ed. Philadelphia, PA: Lippincott-Raven; 2016.
Jarvis C. *Physical Examination and Health Assessment.* Philadelphia, PA: Saunders; 2015.

Chapter

67

Corneal Abrasion and Foreign Body Removal
Eye
Margaret R. Colyar

CPT Code
65205 Removal of foreign body; external eye, conjunctival, superficial
65210 Removal of foreign body; external eye, conjunctival, embedded
65220 Removal of foreign body; external eye, corneal without slit lamp
99070 Eye tray: Supplies and material provided by physician over and above what usually is included in office visit

---

Corneal abrasions occur because of trauma to the anterior globe of the eye with or without penetration by a foreign object. Corneal foreign bodies result from superficial penetration by a foreign object to the anterior globe of the eye. The practitioner should attempt to remove only foreign bodies that are superficial.

Protective eyewear is recommended for all ages while participating in sports, when working around any machinery, and to protect the eye against excessive and prolonged light exposure.

OVERVIEW

- Incidence
  - 93% of injuries to the eye are nonperforating in nature.
  - 67% involve the anterior chamber.
  - 65% of injuries in children result from falls or sports.
  - 5% of injuries to the eye are superficially perforating in nature.
- Always perform an eye examination prior to any eye procedure.
  - Document visual acuity with the use of the Snellen chart or eye card.
  - Visually inspect the eye and orbit region.
  - Inspect and palpate orbit rim for instability.
  - Verify equivocal sensation to orbit rim.
  - Verify presence or absence of corneal reflex (cotton wisp test).
  - Verify pupillary response.
  - Verify conjunctival status.
    - Absence or presence of subconjunctival hemorrhage
    - Injection
    - Chemosis

- Note the location of any visible foreign body.
- Note whether the foreign body is superficially embedded or not.
- Perform an ophthalmic examination.
  - Inspect anterior globe for
    - Clarity
    - Presence or absence of hyphema
    - Red reflex
    - Lens opacities
    - Vitreous appearance
    - Optic disc appearance
    - Retinal abnormalities (papilledema, vessel occlusion)

OPTIONS

- Corneal abrasion
- Removal of foreign body—eye

RATIONALE

- To diminish discomfort
- To promote healing
- To prevent loss of vision

INDICATIONS

- Onset of irritation and/or pain to the eye with a history of trauma
- Unilateral sensation of a foreign body present in the eye
- History of exposure to ultraviolet light, prolonged sunlight, or tanning bed use
- History of wearing contact lens
- Mild chemical exposure
- Red eye
- In neonates and infants with unexplained crying, photosensitivity, unilateral tearing, and conjunctival inflammation

CONTRAINDICATIONS

- Emergent—REFER immediately to an ophthalmologist.
  - Chemical acid or alkali exposure
    - *If not in the office*—Instruct the client to wash the eyes out immediately with water for a full 15 minutes, then go to the nearest emergency department for further treatment. Alkali chemicals have a more delayed presentation than acid chemicals.
    - *If in the office*—Apply ophthalmic anesthetic, and begin vigorous irrigation using standard intravenous tubing and 0.9% sodium chloride solution or lactated Ringer's solution for 15 minutes or 2 L, whichever comes first.
  - History of high-velocity injury
    - *If not in office*—Close the eyelid, and apply a nonpressure clean dressing to the eye and place sunglasses on.
    - *If in the office*—Apply a nonpressure eye patch and shield.

- Ruptured globe
- Corneal or sclera lacerations
- Lid lacerations
- Conjunctival lacerations
- Corneal ulceration
- Deeply embedded foreign object
- Unsuccessful removal of foreign body
- Uncooperative patient (adult, child, or infant) who requires sedation
- Urgent—REFER within 48 hours to an ophthalmologist.
  - Onset of corneal opacities
  - Presence of a "rust ring" at the former location of embedded foreign body
  - Increasing pain
  - Loss of vision
  - Nonresolution of corneal abrasion
  - Onset of preseptal cellulitis with periorbital cellulitis
  - All children

▶ *Informed consent required*

PROCEDURE

Corneal Abrasion and Foreign Body Removal—Eye

Equipment

CORNEAL ABRASION AND FOREIGN BODY REMOVAL—EYE
- Penlight
- Direct ophthalmoscope
- Gloves—nonsterile
- Fluorescein strips
  - Use individually packaged strips—multivial drops increase the risk of infection.
- Cobalt blue light **(Wood's light)**
- Eye patches
- Adhesive tape
- Intravenous tubing with sterile 0.9% sodium chloride or lactated Ringer's solution
- Tissue or 4 × 4 gauze—nonsterile
- Ophthalmic medication (Table 67.1)

FOREIGN BODY REMOVAL—EYE ONLY
- Cotton-tipped applicators—nonsterile
- 27- or 25-gauge, ½- or 1-inch needle

Procedure

CORNEAL ABRASION
- Cover the lateral corner of the face with a drape or facial tissue to prevent drainage of dye onto another area of the face because dye can cause permanent stain to clothing.

- Provide tissue for client to wipe drips.
- Instill one to two drops of ophthalmic anesthetic or cycloplegic if no contraindications.
- Moisten strips with two to three drops of sterile 0.9% sodium chloride.
- Retract the lower lid and touch the moistened strip to the base of the globe until there is good fill.
- Allow the client to blink several times to disperse the dye.
- Turn off the overhead light and turn on cobalt blue light (Wood's light).
  - Abrasions to the cornea are seen as bright yellow or yellow-green.
- Note the size, shape, and location of the abrasion.
- *If close to the central line of vision, consider REFERRING to an ophthalmologist because of a high incidence of permanent scarring in this area.*
- When completed, initiate a vigorous irrigation with 0.9% sodium chloride to remove all dye from the eye to lessen any further irritation. Always apply topical ophthalmic antibiotic of choice if an abrasion is found because of the avascular character of the cornea.
- Document—may be pictorial or description of location of abrasion.
- Apply a single or double eye patch (Fig. 67.1).
- Use of a patch should be considered in children older than age 5 years.
- The use of a single or double eye patch for all adults with corneal abrasion depends on the comfort of the client.
  - Contraindicated in cases of conjunctivitis

Table 67·1	Ophthalmic Drops That Can Be Used to Treat Corneal Abrasion and Foreign Body Removal	
TYPE OF MEDICATION		**ONSET/DURATION**
Anesthetic Ophthalmic Drops		
Tetracaine (Pontocaine) 0.5%		25 sec/15 min or longer
Proparacaine (Ophthaine) 0.5%		20 sec/10–15 min
Mydriatics		
Phenylephrine (Neo-Synephrine) 2.5% and 10% drops		5 min/2–3 hr
Cycloplegics/Mydriatics		
Cyclopentolate (Cyclogyl) 1%		5 min/24 hr
Tropicamide (Tropicacyl) 0.5% and 1%		5 min/6 hr
Homatropine (Homatrine) 2% and 5%		5 min/10–48 hr
Scopolamine (Isopto Hyoscine) 0.25%		5 min/3–5 days
Ophthalmic Antibiotics		
Erythromycin ophthalmic ointment Gentamicin (Garamycin) 3 mg/mL solution Tobramycin (Tobrex) 3 mg/mL solution or 3 mg/g ointment Sulfacetamide (Sodium Sulamyd)—10% and 30% solution or 10% ointment		

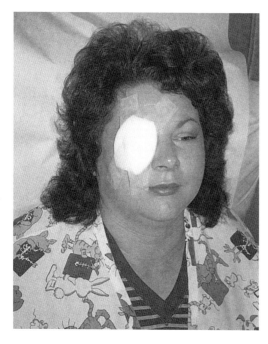

Figure 67.1 Apply an eye patch after the antibiotic is instilled in the eye.

REMOVAL OF FOREIGN BODY—EYE

- Have the client lie in a comfortable supine position.
- Put on gloves.
- Instill one to two drops of ophthalmic anesthetic.
- Spread the eyelids apart with the thumb and index finger.
- Have head positioned so that the foreign body is at the highest point on eye globe.
- Instruct the client to fix a gaze toward a certain point.
- *If not embedded,* use moistened sterile cotton-tipped applicator with gentle rolling motion to remove.
- *If embedded,* use a 27- or 25-gauge needle bevel side up (Fig. 67.2) with pencil grip.
  - Rest your lateral hand on side of the client's cheek for more stability in movement.
- Approach at a 90-degree angle to eye globe.
- Gently apply pressure across the surface to dislodge foreign body.
- After several unsuccessful attempts, apply antibiotic ointment, apply nonpressure patch, and REFER to an ophthalmologist.
- After removal of the foreign body, proceed to check for a corneal abrasion with fluorescein stain and patching.

Client Instructions

- *Do not drive yourself home.*
- Prolonged use of an eye patch greater than 48 hours increases the risk of **amblyopia** for the client (especially children).

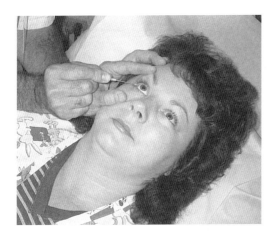

Figure 67.2 Remove the embedded foreign body using a 25- to 27-gauge needle.

- Tetanus booster: Needed if not received within 5 years.
- To relieve pain—use acetaminophen with codeine (Tylenol No. 3) every 4 to 6 hours as needed for the first 24 hours. Then use plain or extra-strength acetaminophen (Tylenol) every 4 hours as needed.
  - If the pain persists, call the office.
- *Avoid all topical ophthalmic anesthetics* because retardation in healing can occur.
- Avoid nonsteroidal therapy for 48 hours because retardation in healing can occur.
- Avoid removing the eye patch and rubbing the eye because this can slow the healing process.
- Return to the office in 24 and 48 hours to affirm that the healing process is occurring.
  - The *absence* of pain does not guarantee complete resolution of the corneal injury.
- Return to the office sooner if there is
  - Increasing pain without relief with medication
  - Purulent (yellow or green) drainage from eye
  - Loss of vision

BIBLIOGRAPHY

Jones N. Eye injury in sport. *Sports Med.* 1989;7:163–181.
Murtagh J. *Practice Tips.* 7th ed. New York, NY: McGraw-Hill; 2017.
Pfenninger JL, Fowler GC. *Procedures for Primary Care Physicians.* St. Louis, MO: Mosby; 2019.
Porte RS. *The Merck Manual.* Rahway, NJ: Merck; 2018.
Silverman H, Nunez L, Feller DB. Treatment of common eye injuries. *Am Fam Physician.* 1992;45(5):449–456.

68 Chapter

Eye Drop Insertion

Margaret R. Colyar

CPT Code
None

Eye medications are administered for various medical problems. It is necessary to understand the actions of the medication and how to avoid and identify possible adverse effects (Table 68.1).

OVERVIEW

- If both eye drops and ointment are ordered, instill the eye drops first and then the ointment.

RATIONALE

- To treat infection and inflammation
- To treat allergy symptoms
- To treat glaucoma

CONTRAINDICATIONS

- If acute-angle-closure glaucoma is suspected, this is a medical emergency. Refer to an ophthalmologist immediately.

PROCEDURE

Eye Drop Insertion

Equipment

- Bottle of eye drops or ointment
- Gloves—nonsterile
- Tissue

Procedure

EYE DROPS

- Wash your hands with soap and water and dry.
- Put on gloves.
- Remove any crusting or drainage with a wet cotton ball.

Table 68·1 **Eye Medication**

TYPE	DOSAGE	DISEASE PROCESS
Antiviral		
Acyclovir 3% ointment (Zovirax)	1-cm ribbon 5 × per day for 3 days	Herpes simplex
Antibacterial		
Ciprofloxacin 0.3% drops (Ciloxan) • Don't use in children under 1 y.o.	1 gtt tid for 3 to 5 days	Keratitis (corneal ulcers) Conjunctivitis Blepharitis
Gentamicin 0.3% drops (Genoptic) • Use with caution in pregnancy	1 to 2 gtt tid for 3 to 5 days	Keratitis (corneal ulcers) Conjunctivitis Blepharitis
Tobramycin 0.3% drops (Tobrex)	1 gtt tid for 3 to 5 days	Keratitis (corneal ulcers) Conjunctivitis Blepharitis
Corticosteroid Drops and Ointment		
Dexamethasone 0.1% (Maxidex)	1 gtt 4 to 6× per day prn	Allergic conditions Noninfectious inflammation
Fluorometholone 0.1% drops (Flucon)	1 gtt 2 to 4× per day prn	Inflammation
Prednisolone drops 1.0%, 0.12%, or 0.5% (Pred Forte)	1 gtt 2 to 4× per day prn	Inflammation
NSAID Drops		
Diclofenac sodium 0.1% (Voltaren) • Do not use in third trimester because of premature closure of ductus arteriosus	1 gtt 4 to 6 hours	Decreases inflammatory response in cataracts, squint, and trabecular surgeries Relieves pain and photophobia after corneal surgery or trauma
Intraocular Pressure Reducers		
Topical beta blockers • Betaxolol • Levobunolol • Timolol	1 to 2 gtt bid	Decreases intraocular HTN and chronic open-angle glaucoma

Continued

Table 68-1	**Eye Medication—cont'd**	
TYPE	**DOSAGE**	**DISEASE PROCESS**
Use with caution in patients with bradycardia, heart block, cardiac failure, airway disease, or history of anaphylaxis. Can mask hypoglycemia in diabetes and symptoms of thyrotoxicosis. Avoid in pregnancy near delivery because of fetal/neonatal bradycardia.	1 to 2 gtt bid	Decreases intraocular HTN and chronic open-angle glaucoma
Betaxolol (Betoptic 0.5% and 0.25%)	1 gtt bid	Lowers intraocular pressure within 30 minutes
Levobunolol (Betagan 0.5% & 0.25%)	1 gtt bid	Lowers intraocular pressure within 1 hour
Timolol (Timpotic 0.1%, 0.25%)	1 gtt daily	Lowers intraocular pressure within 20 minutes
Carbonic Anhydrase Inhibitors		
Dorzolamide 2% (Trusopt)	1 gtt bid–tid	Lowers intraocular pressure by reducing aqueous production in the ciliary body
Alpha-2 Agonists		
Brimonidine 0.2% (Alphagan) Use with caution with severe cardiovascular or cerebrovascular disease, pregnancy, and lactation.	1 gtt tid	Decreases production of aqueous in ciliary body by vasoconstriction of afferent ciliary blood vessels
Direct-Acting Parasympathomimetics		
Pilocarpine 2% Use with caution with asthma, pregnancy, and lactation.	1 to 2 gtt 2 to 4 per day	Contraction of the ciliary muscle stretches the trabecular meshwork and improves the outflow of aqueous

- Shake the eye drops container gently.
- Remove the cap of the bottle and place it on its side on a clean tissue.
- Do not touch the medication bottle tip with your hand or any object.
- Turn the bottle upside down.
- Have patient open both eyes and tilt his or her head backward.
- Pull the lower lid down gently to form a pocket for the drop.
- Position the tip of the eye drop bottle so that it does not come closer than ¾ inch above the lower lid.
- Squeeze the bottle lightly to allow the drop to fall into the pocket.
- Have the patient close his or her eyes without squeezing them.
- Gently blot the eyes with a clean tissue.
- Gently press on the inner part of the eye for 30 seconds.

Note: If the patient blinks too much, use the thumb of one hand to hold the upper lid lashes against the eyebrow and a finger from the other hand to simultaneously hold the lower lid while instilling the drops.

EYE OINTMENT

- Wash your hands with soap and water and dry.
- Put on gloves.
- Remove any crusting or drainage with a wet cotton ball.
- Have patient open both eyes and tilt his or her head backward.
- Pull the lower lid down gently to form a pocket for the ointment.
- Position the tip of the eye ointment tube so that it does not come closer than ¾ inch above the lower lid.
- Squeeze the tube lightly to allow the ointment to fall into the pocket.
- Have the patient close his or her eyes without squeezing them.
- Gently remove excess ointment from the eyes with a clean tissue.

Client Instructions

- Do not put any medication into your eyes unless the label says "ophthalmic."
- Do not wear contacts while using eye medication.
- If you have both eye drops and ointment to put in the eye:
  - Instill the eye drops first, then apply the ointment.
- Avoid touching the eyedropper with your fingers, your eye, lashes, or eyelid.
- Point your fingernail away from your eye to avoid accidentally scratching your eye.
- Open both eyes, tilt your head back, and focus on the ceiling to avoid blinking.
- Avoid squeezing or blinking your eyes after putting in drops.
- To blot excess eye drops from the eyes, use a clean, separate tissue for each eye.
- Wait at least 5 minutes between putting in each drop.
- Check the bottle's expiration date—throw it away if it is outdated.
- Do not leave eye drops in direct sunlight.

BIBLIOGRAPHY

Eye Drop Tips. Glaucoma Research Foundation Web site. https://www.glaucoma.org/treatment/eyedrop-tips.php

How to Use Eye Drops Properly. SafeMedication Web site. http://www.safemedication.com/safemed/MedicationTipsTools/HowtoAdminister/HowtoUseEyeDropsProperly.aspx

69 Chapter

Eye Irrigation

Cynthia R. Ehrhardt

CPT Code
None—Billed as part of the office visit

Irrigation of the eye is a procedure done to rid the eye of irritants from chemical exposure. Strong precautions should be taken when working with acid and alkali chemicals because they are strong chemical irritants. Exposure to *alkali chemicals,* such as lye, lime, mortar, cement, plaster, and liquid ammonia, is highly damaging to the eye and *constitutes an ocular emergency.* Seek immediate emergency care.

Prevention is focused on eliminating situations that can result in the incidence of chemical splashing. Use of safety glasses is recommended.

OVERVIEW

- Causes
  - Accidental exposure by splashing of alkali or acid liquids into the eye
- Complicating factors
  - Corneal injury
  - Temporary or permanent loss of vision
  - Delayed irrigation of alkali chemicals has a higher incidence of permanent vision loss.
  - All alkali burns should be followed up by an ophthalmologist because of the high incidence of permanent injury to the cornea.
  - A signed statement by the client indicating understanding of the importance of follow-up should be obtained because a high percentage of injuries caused by alkali burns have a delayed presentation.

RATIONALE

- To preserve vision

INDICATIONS

- Reported history of chemical splash injury to the eye

CONTRAINDICATIONS

- Suspected globe penetration or rupture injury

PROCEDURE

Eye Irrigation

Equipment

- Snellen chart
- Penlight
- Ophthalmoscope
- 9% Sodium chloride, lactated Ringer's, or water—2 L
- Intravenous tubing
- Gloves—sterile
- 4 × 4 gauze—sterile
- Towels or absorbent pads
- Catch basin
- Eye irrigation kit—optional
  - Several companies offer an apparatus to insert into the eye for irrigation in place of intravenous tubing
  - Intravenous stand or hook to hang intravenous fluids
  - Ophthalmic anesthesia/antibiotics (Table 69.1)

Procedure

- Secure the client in a comfortable position.
- Perform an ophthalmic examination to ensure no globe perforation.
  - Although a thorough examination of the eye for defects should be undertaken, this should not unnecessarily delay the implementation of eye irrigation.
  - *Do not perform fluorescein examination until eye irrigation has been completed.*
- Administer ophthalmic anesthesia to the affected eye.

Table 69·1	**Ophthalmic Anesthesia and Antibiotics**
Ophthalmic Anesthesia*	
• Tetracaine (Pontocaine) 0.5%	
• Onset of action within 25 sec	
• Duration 15 min or longer	
• Proparacaine (Ophthaine) 0.5%	
• Onset of action within 20 sec	
• Duration of 10 to 15 min	
Ophthalmic Antibiotics*	
• Erythromycin ophthalmic ointment	
• Gentamicin (Garamycin) 3 mg/mL solution	
• Tobramycin (Tobrex) 3 mg/mL solution or 3 mg/g ointment	
• Sulfacetamide (Sodium Sulamyd) 10% and 30% solution or 10% ointment	

*To avoid allergic conjunctivitis, single-agent drops are suggested.

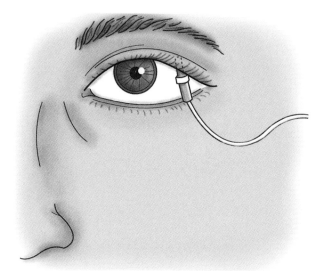

Figure 69.1 Insert the tip of the irrigation tube into the eye space, and allow the eyelid to hold the intravenous tubing tip in place.

- Prepare the irrigation solution and hang the bag from the intravenous stand approximately 3 feet above the head of the client.
- Wrap protective garb (towels or absorbent pads) around the client.
- Position the catch basin to capture the used irrigation solution.
- Put on gloves.
- Gently retract the upper eyelid, and insert the tip of the irrigation tube into eye space (Fig. 69.1). Allow the eyelid to hold the intravenous tubing tip in place.
- Turn on the solution and administer at a rate of continuous flow for the irrigation to be completed in 15 to 20 minutes.
- Remove the irrigation tip on completion of irrigation.
- Perform a fluorescein stain examination (see Chapter 67).

Client Instructions

- *Do not drive yourself home.*
- Take acetaminophen or Tylenol No. 3 every 4 to 6 hours as needed for pain.
- Avoid topical ophthalmic anesthetics because they retard healing.
- Avoid nonsteroidal therapy for 48 hours because retardation in healing can occur.
- Antibiotics usually are not required. They may be used in the presence of corneal abrasion.
- Follow-up care
  - In alkali splashes, a follow-up appointment with the ophthalmologist is scheduled for _____.
  - If corneal abrasion is present and eye patch applied, avoid removing the eye patch and rubbing the eye because this can slow the healing process.

- Must keep follow-up appointments at 24 and 48 hours to affirm the healing process is occurring; if not, REFER to ophthalmologist.
- Return to the office sooner if
  - Eye pain increasing without medication relief
  - Purulent drainage from eye
  - Loss of vision

BIBLIOGRAPHY

Garcia G. Management of ocular emergencies and urgent eye problems. *Am Fam Physician.* 1996:53(2):347–356.
Hodge C, Lawless M. Ocular emergencies. *Am Fam Physician.* 2008;37(7):506–509.
Muth CC. Eye emergencies. *JAMA.* 2017;318(7):676.
Patel PS. Top 10 eye emergencies. Slide show. https://www.aao.org/young-ophthalmologists/yo-info/article/top-10-eye-emergencies. May 24, 2016.
Silverman H, Nunez L, Feller DB. Treatment of common eye injuries. *Am Fam Physician.* 1992;45(5):449–456.

Chapter **70**

Eye Trauma Stabilization

Cynthia R. Ehrhardt

CPT Code
None—part of the office visit

Eye trauma includes blunt or penetration injuries to the globe of the eye and is usually associated with blunt trauma, such as physical assault, or with situations that precipitate objects becoming projectiles, such as archery arrows and BB-gun pellets.

Prevention is focused on eliminating situations that can result in the incidence of blunt trauma and penetration wounds. Prevention includes the promotion of safety awareness habits, safety habits in gun and hunting situations, protection against projectile objects with the use of safety glasses, and avoidance of situations that produce projectile objects.

OVERVIEW

- Complications
  - Fractures of the facial bones
  - Loss of sight in the affected eye

- Thoroughly examine the region for anatomical defects.
  - If possible, establish visual acuity.
  - *Avoid any pressure to the eyelid and the globe of the eye because it may precipitate a spontaneous and premature rupture and loss of the **vitreous humor**. Loss of vitreous humor results in permanent blindness.*
- Inspect for disruption in the sclera.
  - Rotate the globe in an upward and downward motion.
  - This is important because when the eyelid closes, the globe automatically rotates upward.
- Funduscopic examination
  - Note any iritis injection.
  - Note the absence of the anterior chamber.
  - Note wrinkling of anterior chamber (represents rupture of the chamber).
  - Note the presence or absence of macular edema.
  - Check the vitreous humor for clouding (represents hemorrhage).
  - Note the presence or absence of retinal detachment (i.e., changes in the color and shape of the retinal eye backgrounds compared with the uninjured eye).
- Inspect the maxillary structures for loss of integrity.
- Inspect the orbit structures for loss of integrity.
- Perform a neurological examination to exclude accompanying head injury.

RATIONALE

- To preserve eye function

INDICATIONS

- Visual inspection of the globe of the eye reveals laceration
- Projectile object embedded in the globe of the eye
- History of the injury suggests potential for eye globe injury

CONTRAINDICATIONS

- None

PROCEDURE

Eye Trauma Stabilization

Equipment

- Snellen or other visual acuity chart
- Ophthalmoscope
- Slit lamp—optional
- Plastic or Styrofoam cup or large eye shield
- Two rolls—4-inch gauze wrap
- Ophthalmic antibiotic ointment
- Eye patch
- Adhesive tape (1 or 2 inches)

Procedure

Do not perform the procedure for corneal abrasion (fluorescein stain) if a globe injury is suspected.

- Position the client in a comfortable position with the eye easily accessible.
- Make a donut ring using the 4-inch gauze wrap.
  - Wrap loosely around the hand six to eight times in an approximate diameter to cover the eye (Fig. 70.1).
  - Then, in a continuous motion, wrap the other 4-inch gauze wrap in a circular fashion around the loose gauze until a firm donut forms (Fig. 70.2).
  - Cut and use tape to anchor edge of the gauze.
- Apply ophthalmic antibiotic ointment to the injured eye.
- Apply the gauze donut over the orbit of the eye without coming in contact with the globe (Fig. 70.3).
- Place the plastic or Styrofoam cup or eye shield on the gauze donut (Fig. 70.4).

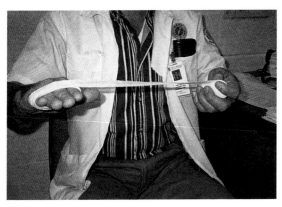

Figure 70.1 Wrap gauze loosely around the hand six to eight times.

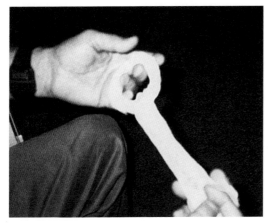

Figure 70.2 Wrap gauze in a circular fashion around the loose gauze until a firm donut forms.

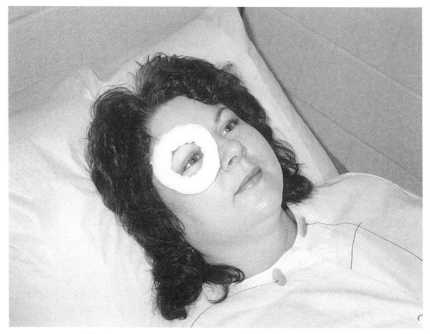

Figure 70.3 Apply the gauze donut over the orbit of the eye.

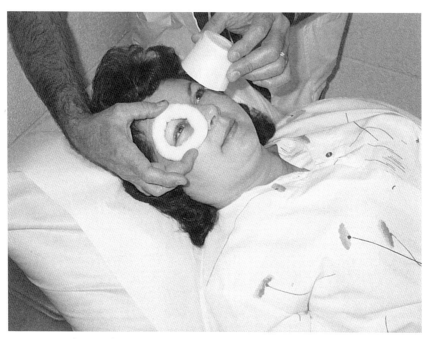

Figure 70.4 Place a plastic or Styrofoam cup or eye shield on the gauze donut.

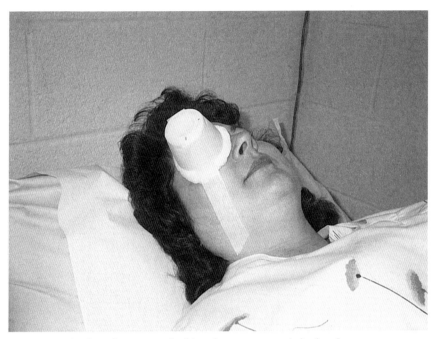

Figure 70.5 Anchor the cup or shield with gauze around the head.

- Anchor the cup or shield with 4-inch gauze around the head with several wraps (Fig. 70.5).
- Apply a double eye-patch dressing to the unaffected eye, and continue wrapping the head to anchor both of the eye dressings (Fig. 70.6).
- Transport to the nearest emergency department in a slightly upright position for further evaluation by an ophthalmologist.

Client Instructions

- To prevent eye movement and further eye damage, it is necessary for both eyes to be covered.
- Try not to cough, sneeze, or breathe deeply.

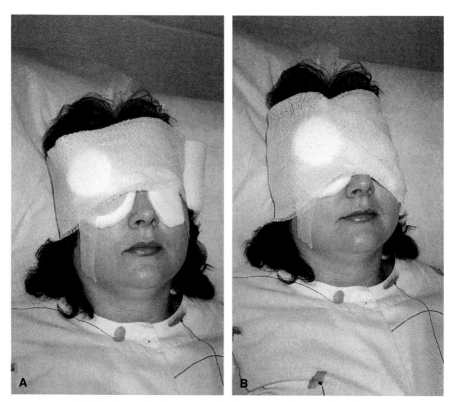

Figure 70.6 (A) Apply a double eye-patch dressing to the unaffected eye, and (B) continue wrapping the head with gauze.

BIBLIOGRAPHY

Garcia G. Management of ocular emergencies and urgent eye problems. *Am Fam Physician.* 1996;53(2):347–356.
Hodge C, Lawless M. Ocular emergencies. *Am Fam Physician.* 2008;37(7):506–509.
Pfenninger JL, Fowler GC. *Procedures for Primary Care Physicians.* St. Louis, MO: Mosby; 2019.
Pokhrel PK. Ocular emergencies. *Am Fam Physician.* 2008;76(6):829–836.

Chapter **71**

Eyebrow Laceration Repair

Cynthia R. Ehrhardt

CPT Code
12011   Simple repair of superficial wounds of face, ears, eyelids, nose, lips, or mucous membranes—2.5 cm or less
12013–18 Simple repair of superficial wounds of face, ears, eyelids, nose, lips, or mucous membranes—2.5 cm or greater

---

Eyebrow laceration repair may be required when there is trauma to the eyebrow. These lacerations most commonly are caused by blunt injury to the supraorbital area.

Prevention includes elimination of situations that can result in laceration of the eyebrow, promoting safety habits when playing organized contact sports, use of safety devices such as protective headgear, and prevention of falls.

OVERVIEW
- Incidence
  - Usually associated with falls, contact sports, and other trauma
- Complications
  - Fractures of the orbit and facial bones
  - Globe injuries to the eye
- General principles
  - Use contrasting suture material to allow easier removal of the sutures.
  - Suturing beyond the ideal time of 6 hours postlaceration is considered because of cosmetic implications.
  - Lacerations above and below the eyebrow may be closed with **Steri-strips** if the wound is less than 0.25 cm in length and there is enough room to anchor the tape. This is generally not recommended, however, because of poorer cosmetic healing.
- *Never shave the eyebrow.*

RATIONALE
- To promote healing of the laceration and prevent cosmetic complications

INDICATIONS
- Eyebrow laceration of greater than 0.25 cm
- Gaping eyebrow laceration

CONTRAINDICATIONS

- Multiple lacerations with involvement of the intramarginal lid of the eye
- Greater than 12 hours since the laceration occurred
- Suspected serious injuries, such as globe penetration and orbit fractures
- ▶ *Informed consent required*

PROCEDURE

Eyebrow Laceration Repair

Equipment

- Antiseptic skin cleanser
- Towels (fenestrated and nonfenestrated)—sterile
- Gloves—sterile
- 0.9% sodium chloride—sterile 3-mL syringe
- 25- to 27-gauge, ½- to 1½-inch needle for anesthesia administration
- Syringe—30 or 60 mL without needle for irrigation
- Lidocaine 1% or 2% with or without epinephrine
- 5-0 or 6-0 Ethicon suture material—contrasting color
- Topical antibiotic ointment (Bactroban, Bacitracin, or Polysporin)
- Sterile suture kit (prepackaged or self-made) should include
  - Curved and straight **hemostats**
  - Needle holders (4½ and 6 inch)
  - **Forceps** with teeth
  - Iris scissors
  - Cup to hold sterile 0.9% sodium chloride solution
  - Cup to hold povidone-iodine (Betadine) solution
  - 4 × 4 in sterile gauze

Procedure

- Thoroughly inspect the region.
  - Anatomical defects to nasolacrimal duct and lacrimal canaliculus region
  - Extraocular movements
  - Orbit rim
  - Eye for foreign bodies (see Chapter 67), hyphema, and globe injuries
- Drape the area to prevent any solution from draining into the eye.
- Infiltrate the borders of the laceration without accentuation of the margins (Fig. 71.1).
- Gently cleanse the skin around the wound with antiseptic skin cleanser, being careful to avoid getting the solution into the eye.
- Gently irrigate the wound with 30 to 60 mL of sterile 0.9% sodium chloride solution, being careful to avoid getting the solution into the eye.
- Carefully align the eyebrow margins (Fig. 71.2).
- If moderate maceration of the laceration, excise tissue in a parallel fashion to attain better margin alignment (Fig. 71.3).
- Use the suture technique of your choice (usually simple or running suture) (see Chapter 22).

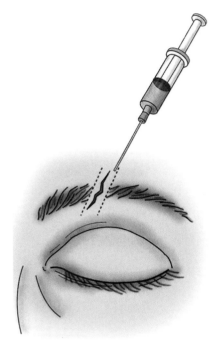

Figure 71.1 Infiltrate the borders of the laceration without accentuation of the margins.

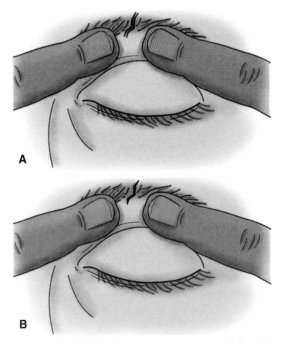

Figure 71.2 Align the eyebrow margins carefully. (A) Incorrect alignment; (B) correct alignment.

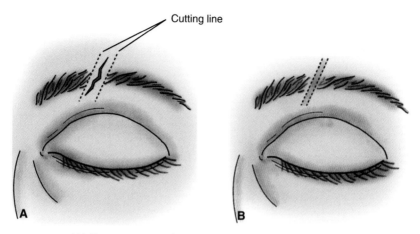

Figure 71.3 (A) Excise macerated tissue in a parallel fashion to (B) attain better margin alignment.

- Apply topical antibiotic.
- Apply light pressure dressing for 1 to 2 hours.

Client Instructions

- Apply an ice pack to decrease pain and swelling to the area.
- Keep the area clean and dry for 24 hours.
- Take the dressing off in 24 hours.
  - Continuous covering of wound increases risk of infection.
- If a crust develops over the site, cleanse by gently rolling a cotton-tipped applicator saturated with hydrogen peroxide over the site. Gently rinse the area with warm water, and blot dry with clean towel or cotton gauze.
- Observe for signs and symptoms of infection, such as
  - Increase in pain after 24 hours
  - Increase in temperature
  - Redness or swelling
  - Yellow or greenish drainage
  - Foul odor
- If any signs or symptoms of infection are found, return to the office.
- Bruising below the eye may occur in 24 to 48 hours.
- *Optional*—Return to the office in 48 hours for wound recheck.
- Return to the office in 3 to 5 days for removal of sutures (children and adults).
- Take acetaminophen every 4 to 6 hours as needed for pain.
- Tylenol No. 3 for pain is rarely needed.
- **Antibiotics generally are not recommended. Topical antibiotic ointment may be applied to the wound, however, to lessen scab formation.**

BIBLIOGRAPHY

Pfenninger JL, Fowler GC. *Procedures for Primary Care Physicians*. St. Louis, MO: Mosby; 2019.

Trott A. *Wounds and Lacerations: Emergency Care and Closure*. St. Louis, MO: Mosby; 2012.

Chapter **72**

Eyelid Eversion

Margaret R. Colyar

CPT Code
None

Eversion of the eyelid is a technique used to inspect the conjunctiva of the upper eyelid.

OVERVIEW
- Used to check for foreign bodies in the eye

RATIONALE
- To inspect the upper palpebral conjunctiva for
  - Change in color
  - Swelling
  - Lesion
  - Foreign body

INDICATIONS
- Eye trauma
- Complaints of eye irritation

CONTRAINDICATIONS
- Foreign body protruding through the eyelid
- Eyelid laceration
- Uncooperative client

PROCEDURE
Eyelid Eversion

Equipment
- Cotton-tipped applicator—nonsterile

Procedure
- Instruct the client to look downward.
- Get the client to relax the eye.
- Grasp the upper eyelashes between the thumb and forefinger and pull down and forward gently (Fig. 72.1).

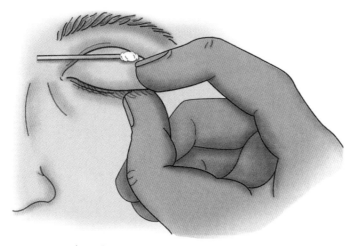

Figure 72.1 Place the tip of a cotton-tipped applicator on the upper eyelid. Grasp the upper eyelashes between the thumb and forefinger. Pull down and forward gently.

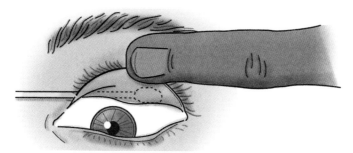

Figure 72.2 Push downward with the cotton-tipped applicator. Lift the lashes upward gently. The lid turns inside out.

- With the other hand, place the tip of the cotton-tipped applicator on the upper lid approximately 1 cm above the lid margin.
- Push down with the cotton-tipped applicator, and lift the lashes up gently. The lid turns inside out. Do not put pressure on the eyeball (Fig. 72.2).
- After inspection, gently pull the lashes outward as the client looks up. Eyelid returns to normal position.

BIBLIOGRAPHY

Bickley L. *Bates' Guide to Physical Examination and History-Taking.* 11th ed. Philadelphia, PA: Lippincott-Raven; 2012.

Jarvis C. *Physical Examination and Health Assessment.* Philadelphia, PA: Saunders; 2016.

Mayhew MS. *Procedures for Primary Care Practitioners.* St. Louis, MO: Mosby; 2016.

Chapter **73**

Auricular Hematoma Evacuation

Margaret R. Colyar

CPT Code
69000 Draining external ear; abscess or hematoma, simple
69005 Draining external ear; abscess or hematoma, complicated

An **auricular** hematoma is the accumulation of blood and serum between auricular cartilage and **perichondrium** (Fig. 73.1). Application of ice to ear intermittently for 24 hours after trauma helps decrease the chance of hematoma formation.

OVERVIEW

- Causes
  - Direct blow to the external ear
  - Indirect blow to the external ear

RATIONALE

- To prevent
  - Aseptic necrosis
  - Loss of cartilage
  - Secondary infection
  - Perichondritis
  - Cauliflower ear

INDICATIONS

- Local pressure
- Blood supply to ear decreased

CONTRAINDICATIONS

- Auricular laceration producing a hematoma
- *Informed consent required*

PROCEDURE

Auricular Hematoma Evacuation

Equipment

- Antiseptic skin cleanser
- Drape—sterile

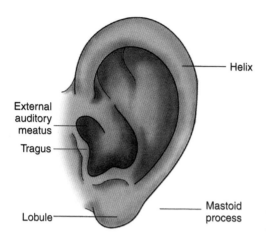

Figure 73.1 Anatomy of the external ear.

- Gloves—sterile
- Two syringes, 3 mL
- Two needles—27 to 30 gauge, 1½ inch, and 18 to 20 gauge, 1½ inch
- 1% lidocaine
- No. 15 scalpel or scissors—sterile
- Curved **hemostat**—sterile
- **Forceps**—sterile
- Goggles
- 4 × 4 gauze—sterile
- Topical antibiotic ointment (Bactroban, Bacitracin, or Polysporin)
- 2-inch gauze roll
- Suture—4-0 or 5-0 nylon

Procedure

- Position the client for comfort with the injured ear easily accessible.
- Cleanse the ear with topical skin cleanser.
- Drape the patient with the ear exposed.
- Put on gloves.
- Inject anterior and posterior to the hematoma using 1% lidocaine and a 27- to 30-gauge needle.
- Insert the syringe with an 18- to 20-gauge needle into the hematoma.
- Aspirate the hematoma.
- If the hematoma cannot be aspirated, incise the hematoma with the No. 15 scalpel.
- Using curved hemostats and digital pressure, explore the wound to remove remaining clots.
- Apply topical antibiotic.
- Roll 2-inch gauze into 1½-inch-diameter pressure rolls.
- Apply a pressure roll over incision on each side of the ear and tape securely.

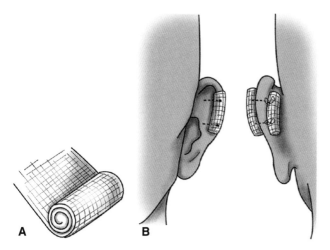

Figure 73.2 (A) Roll 2-inch gauze into ½-inch-diameter pressure rolls; (B) apply the pressure rolls on both sides of the ear directly over the expressed hematoma and suture in place.

- If you cannot apply the pressure roll as described, using 4-0 or 5-0 nylon suture, insert the suture through one end of the roll, through the ear, into gauze roll on the posterior side of the ear, and back through the ear and anterior gauze (Fig. 73.2). Tie securely.

Client Instructions

- Take cephalexin (Keflex), 500 mg twice a day for 5 to 7 days.
- Observe for signs and symptoms of infection and perichondritis, such as
  - Increase in pain after 24 hours
  - Increase in temperature
  - Redness or swelling
  - Yellow or greenish drainage
  - Foul odor
- If any signs or symptoms of infection are found, return to the office.
- To relieve pain
  - Take Tylenol No. 3 every 4 to 6 hours for 24 hours.
  - Take acetaminophen or ibuprofen every 4 to 6 hours for mild pain relief.
- Bleeding and oozing are normal for the first 24 hours. Apply an ice pack intermittently to the ear for 24 hours.
- Return to the office in 1 week for dressing removal.

BIBLIOGRAPHY

Kellerman RD, Rakel D. *Conn's Current Therapy 2019*. Philadelphia, PA: Elsevier; 2019.
Pfenninger JL, Fowler GC. *Procedures for Primary Care Physicians*. St. Louis, MO: Mosby; 2019.
Stone CKI, Humphries RL. *Current Emergency Diagnosis and Treatment*. Norwalk, CT: Appleton & Lange; 2019.

74 Chapter

Cerumen Impaction Removal
Irrigation of the Ear and Curette Technique

Margaret R. Colyar

CPT Code
69210   Removal impacted cerumen, one or both ears

Cerumen impaction is the buildup of earwax in the auditory canal. Normal cerumen is sticky and honey-colored, hard and brown, or dry and scaly. Accumulation of cerumen can lead to pain and hearing difficulties. Irrigation of the ear is a technique used to cleanse the ear of large amounts of excess cerumen. To remove small amounts of cerumen, the curette technique can be used.

OVERVIEW

- Need for removal of cerumen must be weighed against possible complications of
  - Tympanic membrane perforation
  - Vertigo
  - Tinnitus
  - Abrasions of the external canal
  - Decreased or loss of hearing

HEALTH PROMOTION/PREVENTION

- Use earwax softeners periodically.

OPTIONS

- *Method 1*—Curette technique
  - Used for small amounts of cerumen that are easily visible
- *Method 2*—Irrigation of the ear canal
  - Used for cerumen impactions that occlude visualization of the tympanic membrane

RATIONALE

- To remove wax buildup
- To remove foreign bodies from the ear

- To reduce hearing impairment from occlusion of the ear canal
- To diminish pain

INDICATIONS

- Otalgia
- Hearing difficulty
- Unable to visualize the tympanic membrane

CONTRAINDICATIONS

- Drainage from the ear—yellow, green, or bloody exudate
- Tympanic membrane disrupted

PROCEDURE

Cerumen Impaction Removal

Equipment

- Methods 1 and 2
  - Gloves—nonsterile
  - Basin—nonsterile
  - Absorbent drapes or towels
  - Cotton-tipped applicators—nonsterile
  - Alcohol
- Method 1 only
  - Ear curette
- Method 2 only
  - 60-mL syringe or Waterpik
  - Hydrogen peroxide OR vinegar and water mixture 1:1

Procedure

METHOD 1—CURETTE TECHNIQUE

- Position the client sitting or lying with ear exposed.
- Drape client with absorbent pad or towels to protect clothing.
- Put on gloves.
- Grasp the pinna and straighten the ear canal.
  - Down and back for children younger than 6 years old
  - Up and back for individuals older than 6 years old
- Using an otoscope, visualize the position of the cerumen.
- Carefully insert the curette through the otoscope, and gently dislodge and remove the cerumen (Fig. 74.1).
- After the cerumen is dislodged, there may be slight bleeding in the ear canal. Cleanse the ear canal with alcohol applied to a cotton-tipped applicator.

METHOD 2—IRRIGATION OF THE EAR CANAL

- Position the client sitting up with ear to be irrigated tilted slightly downward.
- Mix hydrogen peroxide or vinegar and water in basin or Waterpik basin at room temperature. Cold or excessively warm fluid may cause vertigo.

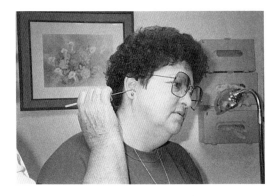

Figure 74.1 Curette technique.

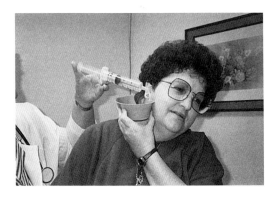

Figure 74.2 Irrigation with a 60-mL syringe.

- Drape the client with absorbent pad or towels to protect clothing.
- Put on gloves.
- Hold basin snugly under the ear to be irrigated.
- Grasp the pinna and straighten the ear canal.
  - Down and back for children younger than 6 years old
  - Up and back for individuals older than 6 years old
- If using the 60-mL syringe to irrigate
  - Aspirate the hydrogen peroxide or vinegar and water mixture into the syringe, and inject the mixture into the ear. The stream should be directed toward the ear canal, not the tympanic membrane.
  - Gentle but vigorous irrigation may be necessary.
- Attaching a short section of intravenous tubing to the syringe allows you to reach farther into the ear to irrigate (Fig. 74.2).
- If you are using the Waterpik for irrigation (Fig. 74.3)
  - Insert the irrigation wand into the ear.
  - Start the Waterpik using low pressure.
  - Increase the water pressure as tolerated.
  - Direct the water stream into the ear canal but not directly at the tympanic membrane.
- After the cerumen is dislodged, dry the ear canal with alcohol applied to a cotton-tipped applicator.

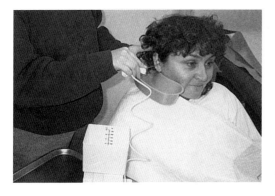

Figure 74.3 Irrigation with a Waterpik.

Client Instructions

- If cerumen was not dislodged, instill two drops of warmed glycerin, mineral oil, 0.5% acetic acid, or over-the-counter preparation four times per day for 4 days to soften the cerumen, then return to the office for a repeat irrigation.
- If dizziness, pain in the ear, or drainage from the ear occurs, return to the office for evaluation.

BIBLIOGRAPHY

Cheever KK, Hinkle JL. *Brunner and Suddarth's Textbook of Medical-Surgical Nursing.* Philadelphia, PA: Lippincott-Raven; 2017.
Ignatavicius DD, Workman ML, Rebar CR. *Medical-Surgical Nursing: Patient-Centered Collaborative Care.* 9th ed. Philadelphia, PA: Saunders; 2012.

Chapter **75**

Epistaxis Control

Cynthia R. Ehrhardt

CPT Code
30901   Control nasal hemorrhage, anterior, simple (limited cautery and/or packing); any method
30903   Control nasal hemorrhage, anterior, complex (extensive cautery and/or packing); any method. Control nasal hemorrhage, posterior, single; any method

Epistaxis is the onset of nasal hemorrhage with or without trauma. Because of potential complications, any client older than 40 years with a positive history of cardiovascular, pulmonary, hepatic, or renal disorder may receive anterior packing as a temporary stabilizing measure but should be referred to an emergency department as soon as possible.

Prevention of epistaxis is focused on the causes. Minimizing exposure to known allergens and increasing humidity through the use of humidifiers and normal saline nose drops applied to each nostril on a regular basis are very helpful. Also treating all nasal and sinus bacterial infections, minimizing the use of nasally administered chemicals, and avoiding the use of medicines that produce coagulopathies, such as aspirin and nonsteroidal medications, along with avoidance of tobacco and secondhand smoke, can cut down on incidence of epistaxis. Lastly, limit children from having unsupervised contact with small items such as beads, round seeds, and marbles.

OVERVIEW

- Causes
  - Physical trauma to the nose
  - Nasal mucosal irritation
    - Allergic rhinitis irritations
    - Bacterial infections
    - Chemical irritation
    - Climate (low humidity)
    - Drug induced (legal or illegal)
    - Foreign bodies (mostly with children)
    - Coagulopathies (aspirin, nonsteroidal drugs, warfarin)
    - Rhinoviruses
    - Tobacco smoking
  - Disease pathology
    - Hypertension
    - Non–drug-induced coagulation disorders
    - Liver disorders (including alcohol abuse)
    - Cardiovascular disorders
    - Diabetes
- Location
  - Anterior epistaxis
    - 90% frequency
    - Most common between 3 and 40 years of age
    - Low incidence of underlying abnormal pathology
    - Rarely require REFERRAL to ears, nose, and throat (ENT) specialist for consultation
    - Hospitalization rarely required
  - Posterior epistaxis
    - 10% frequency
    - If in individuals older than age 40, must consider evaluation of local or systemic disease process
    - More difficult to control bleeding with packing
    - Usually requires ENT consultation
    - Higher incidence of hospitalization

- Complications include
  - Rhinitis
  - Sinusitis
  - Otitis media
  - Pressure necrosis of the nasal membranes from the packing
  - Iatrogenic sleep apnea
  - Hemotympanum
  - Bacteremia with possible toxic shock presentation
  - Respiratory distress
  - Cardiac arrhythmia
  - Rupture of the balloon with aspiration of saline if posterior packing is used

OPTIONS

- *Method 1*—Cotton applicator technique
  - Used for superficial anterior bleed
- *Method 2*—Dental/tonsillar packing technique
  - Used for superficial anterior bleed
- *Method 3*—Anterior nasal packing technique
  - Used for heavy anterior hemorrhaging
- *Method 4*—Posterior nasal packing technique
  - Used for heavy posterior hemorrhaging

RATIONALE

- To control nasal hemorrhage
- To prevent hypovolemia

INDICATIONS

- Nontraumatic epistaxis not controlled by simple pressure to the nostril for 5 to 10 minutes

CONTRAINDICATIONS

- History of clotting disorder
- History of chronic obstructive pulmonary disease
- Suspected trauma
- Suspected foreign body
- Positive cardiovascular history
▶ *Informed consent required*

PROCEDURE

Epistaxis Control

Equipment

- Methods 1, 2, 3, and 4
  - Good light source (head lamp with magnifying lens is ideal)
  - Gloves—nonsterile
  - Pharyngeal mirror

- Nasal **speculums** (small, medium, large)—sterile
- Cotton applicators—sterile
- Suction machine with No. 5 Fraser tip
- Methods 2, 3, and 4 only
  - Bayonet **forceps**—sterile
  - Emesis basin—sterile
  - Tongue blades
  - Topical vasoconstrictor agent
- Methods 3 and 4 only
  - Gloves—sterile
  - Fenestrated sheets—sterile
- Method 2 only
  - Dental/tonsil packing and expandable nasal packing—sterile
- Method 3 only
  - Impregnated petrolatum and antibiotic (usually triple antibiotic ointment) gauze packings (prepackaged as ½ inch × 72 inches)
- Method 4 only
  - Iris scissors—sterile
  - No. 14 Fr catheter (with 10- to 30-mL bulb)—sterile
  - 30-mL syringe—sterile
  - 0.9% sodium chloride—sterile
  - Triple antibiotic ointment
  - Portable pulse oximeter

Procedure

METHOD 1—COTTON APPLICATOR TECHNIQUE

- Secure the client in a comfortable position.
- Put on gloves.
- Locate the source of the bleed by using a nasal speculum to expand the nares.
- Gently suction the site clean.
- Dry the site with a cotton-tipped applicator.
- Select a vasoconstrictive agent.
- Saturate a cotton-tipped applicator with the vasoconstriction agent.
  - In the case of silver nitrate, applicators are prepackaged.
- Place the applicator gently on the bleeding site for 5 minutes (Fig. 75.1).
  - Caution should be taken not to damage any of the surrounding tissue; otherwise there is an increase in tissue necrosis. This is especially common with the use of silver nitrate sticks.
- Keep the client upright for an additional 5 minutes.
- Inspect the site to ensure bleeding has halted.

METHOD 2—DENTAL/TONSILLAR PACKING TECHNIQUE

- Secure the client in a comfortable position.
- Put on gloves.
- Locate the source of the bleed by using a nasal speculum to expand the nares.
- Gently suction the site clean.

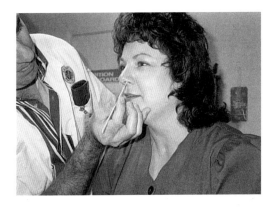

Figure 75.1 Method 1. Place the vasoconstriction agent gently on the bleeding site for 5 minutes.

Table 75·1	Topical Vasoconstrictor Agents

- Topical 4% lidocaine mixed with 1:1000 epinephrine in a 1:1 ratio
- Topical tetracaine
- Topical phenylephrine hydrochloride (Neo-Synephrine) 0.05% to 1%
- Benzocaine spray
- Silver nitrate sticks
- Petrolatum jelly

- Dry the site with a cotton-tipped applicator.
- Select a vasoconstrictive agent (Table 75.1).
- Saturate the packing with the vasoconstriction agent of choice.
  - *Silver nitrate cannot be used with this technique.*
- Insert the packing into nostril using the bayonet forceps through the nasal speculum.
- Have the client pinch his or her nose and hold for 5 to 10 minutes.
- Remove the packing, and inspect site to verify bleeding has halted.

METHOD 3—ANTERIOR NASAL PACKING TECHNIQUE
- Secure the client in a comfortable position.
- Put on nonsterile gloves.
- Locate the source of the bleed using a nasal speculum to expand the nares.
- Gently suction the site clean.
- Dry the site with cotton-tipped applicator.
- Select a vasoconstrictive agent.
- Apply the fenestrated drape.
- Put on sterile gloves.
- Prepare nasal packing by removing the ½-inch impregnated petrolatum and antibiotic from packaging and folding it in half.
- Stabilize the nasal speculum with one hand resting on cheek, and expand the nares to visualize site (Fig. 75.2).

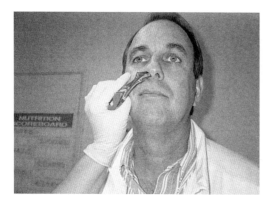

Figure 75.2 Expand the nares with the nasal speculum.

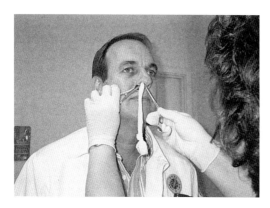

Figure 75.3 Insert the impregnated packing as far as possible into the anterior chamber.

- Take the packing at the folded end and insert as far into the anterior chamber floor as possible using bayonet forceps (Fig. 75.3).
  - Repeat the procedure in a layered fashion until no further packing can be inserted.
- Tie a large knot in the packing protruding from the nares to prevent a dislocation of the anterior packing (Fig. 75.4).
- Recheck vital signs after 5 to 10 minutes (especially pulse oximetry).
- Remove packing after 48 hours.

METHOD 4—POSTERIOR NASAL PACKING TECHNIQUE
- Secure the client in a comfortable position.
- Monitor with pulse oximetry if available.
- Put on nonsterile gloves.
- Locate the source of the bleed using a nasal speculum to expand the nares.
- Identify the presence of posterior hemorrhage using the pharyngeal mirror.
- Gently suction the site clean.
- Spray the postpharyngeal wall with benzocaine.
  - Advise the client about possible choking sensation and hoarseness from the medication.
- Apply the fenestrated drape.

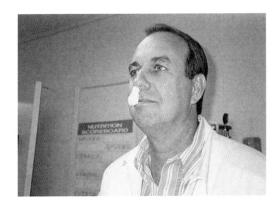

Figure 75.4 Tie a large knot in the packing to prevent dislocation.

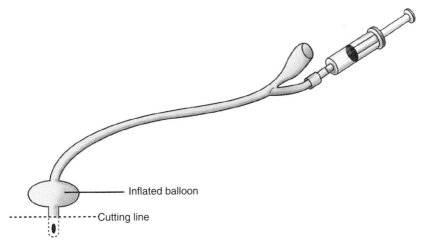

— Inflated balloon

—Cutting line

Figure 75.5 Verify an intact bulb of the no. 14 Fr catheter. Sever the distal tip without losing balloon function.

- Put on sterile gloves.
- Verify an intact bulb of the no. 14 Fr catheter by expanding the balloon, then deflating it.
- Sever the tip distal of the no. 14 Fr catheter without losing balloon function (Fig. 75.5).
- Lubricate the catheter liberally with antibiotic ointment.
- Introduce the catheter until it contacts the choana (Fig. 75.6).
  - Ask the client to open his or her mouth; visualize the catheter with a pharyngeal mirror.
- Inflate the balloon gently with 5 mL 0.9% sodium chloride.
- Inflate the balloon with a total of 10 to 15 mL 0.9% sodium chloride once proper position has been verified (Fig. 75.7).
- Stabilize the catheter with tape.
- Begin insertion of anterior packing to stabilize the catheter.

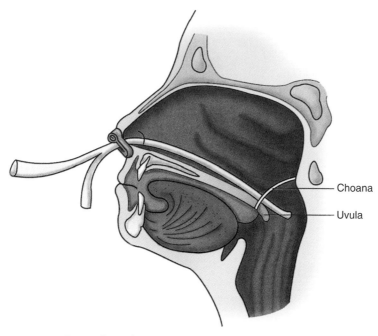

Choana

Uvula

Figure 75.6 Insert the catheter into the nares until the choana is reached.

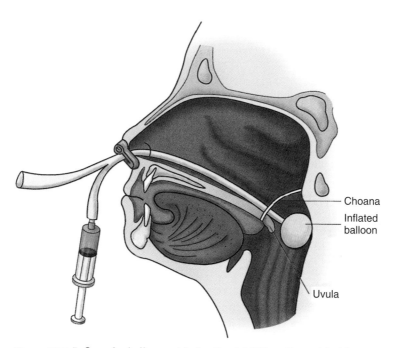

Choana

Inflated
balloon

Uvula

Figure 75.7 Inflate the balloon with 5 mL of 0.9% sodium chloride.

- Recheck in 5 to 10 minutes with the pharyngeal mirror to verify cessation of bleeding.
- Deflate the balloon, and reverify absence of bleeding.
- Leave catheter in place for 12 hours in case of recurrence of hemorrhage.
- Transport to ENT physician or emergency department for follow-up care and possible hospitalization.

Client Instructions

- Activities
  - Avoid strenuous exercise and bending and lifting for 5 days.
- Hygiene
  - Avoid sneezing, blowing nose, and rubbing nose.
  - Do not insert anything into nose.
  - Humidification may be used in low-humidity environments.
- Drugs to be avoided include aspirin, alcohol, and nonsteroidals for 5 days.
  - Minimal amount of decongestant or antihistamines may be used to control severe nasal drainage.
- Avoid factors that led to the hemorrhage.
  - Use either normal saline drops (three drops each nostril three to four times a day) or petroleum jelly to nares (three to four times a day) to decrease friable nasal mucosa.
  - If hemorrhage should recur, initiate pressure to the nares.
- If no relief has occurred, return for more aggressive treatment.
- *Anterior nasal packing*—as above except avoid sneezing or pulling packing out.
- Observe for signs and symptoms of infection and complications including
  - Fever greater than 99.5°F
  - Increased frequency of headaches
  - Facial pain (especially below the eye)
  - Malodorous breath or nasal discharge
  - Change in level of consciousness (especially children)
  - Increasing breathing difficulty
  - Unexplained bleeding and/or bruising
  - Recurrence of nasal bleeding
- Antibiotics
  - Required with nasal packing to prevent stasis sinusitis.
  - Drug of choice should be a broad-spectrum antibiotic that covers the flora normally found in the nasopharyngeal chamber.
  - Frequently used are amoxicillin, amoxicillin with clavulanic acid (Augmentin), erythromycin, or second-generation cephalosporins.
  - Give acetaminophen for appropriate age and/or weight for pain.
  - Occasional use of Tylenol No. 3 can be considered in moderate and severe pain.
- Avoid nonsteroidal medication for 5 days.
- Children should not take ibuprofen.
- Decongestants and antihistamines may be used sparingly if excessive nasal drainage occurs.

- Return to the office before scheduled visit if bleeding recurs.
- Return to the office
  - *Anterior packing*—in 48 hours and recheck in 5 days
  - *Posterior packing*—requires immediate transport to hospital or ENT office for further evaluation and may be followed up if further diagnostic workup is required

BIBLIOGRAPHY

Bamimore O. Acute epistaxis. Medscape Web site. https://emedicine.medscape.com/article/764719-overview. Updated April 22, 2019.

Kucik CJ, Clenney T. Management of epistaxis. *Am Fam Physician.* 2005;71(2):305–311.

Pfenninger JL, Fowler GC. *Procedures for Primary Care Physicians.* St. Louis, MO: Mosby; 2019.

Randall D, Freema S. Management of anterior and posterior epistaxis. *Am Fam Physician.* 1991;43(6):214–221.

76 Chapter

Laryngoscopy
Indirect and Direct Flexible
Margaret R. Colyar

CPT Code

31575 Laryngoscopy—Flexible fiberoptic, diagnostic
31576 Laryngoscopy—Flexible fiberoptic, with biopsy
31577 Laryngoscopy—Flexible fiberoptic, with removal of foreign body
31578 Laryngoscopy—Flexible fiberoptic, with removal of lesion

---

Laryngoscopy is an examination performed at the back of the throat, the larynx, and vocal cords to determine the cause of voice problems, throat and ear pain, and trouble swallowing. It can also be used to check for injuries to the throat, narrowing of the throat, or blockages in the airway.

OVERVIEW

- There are two types of laryngoscopy
  - Indirect: done in the physician's office

Table 76·1	Common Reasons for Performing Laryngoscopy

Use indirect and flexible laryngoscopy for
- Chronic bad breath
- Chronic cough
- Chronic shortness of breath
- Chronic throat pain
- Chronic voice problems lasting more than 3 weeks
  - Hoarseness
  - Weak voice
  - Raspy voice
  - No voice
- Coughing up blood
- Difficult or unable to swallow
- Ear pain that does not go away
- Feeling that something is stuck in the throat
- Long-term smoker
- Noisy breathing (stridor)
- Mass in the head or neck area with signs of cancer

Use direct rigid laryngoscopy for
- Biopsy
- Foreign body removal

- Direct (transnasal flexible and rigid).
  - Direct transnasal flexible laryngoscopy: done in the office
  - Rigid laryngoscopy: done in surgery
- Table 76.1 summarizes common reasons for performing laryngoscopy.

RATIONALE

- To diagnose different conditions involving the throat, larynx, and vocal cords

CONTRAINDICATIONS

- Partially blocked airway
  - Tumors, polyps, or severe inflammation of the tissues at the back of the throat
▶ *Informed consent required*

PROCEDURE

Laryngoscopy—Indirect and Direct Flexible

Equipment

BOTH METHODS
- Topical anesthesia spray
  - Lidocaine with phenylephrine—0.5 mL for each nostril

- Chair
- Gloves—nonsterile

INDIRECT LARYNGOSCOPY
- Gauze
- Head mirror
- Light

DIRECT—FLEXIBLE METHOD
- Flexible laryngoscopy instrument

Procedure

INDIRECT LARYNGOSCOPY
- Position the patient upright in a chair.
- Instruct the patient to stick out the tongue as far as he or she can.
- Put on gloves.
- Hold the tongue down with gauze.
- Spray throat with anesthesia spray.
- Hold a mirror at the back of the throat and shine a light into the mouth.
- Instruct the patient to say "e-e-e-e" sound or "a-a-a-a" to visualize the vocal cord mobility.

DIRECT—FLEXIBLE
- Position patient upright in a chair.
- Inform the patient that there will be a gagging sensation, but it will pass.
- Spray nostrils and back of throat with anesthesia, if needed (optional).
- Put on gloves.
- Stand behind the patient.
- Insert the tube in the patient's nose, avoiding the septum.
- Instruct the patient to breathe through the nose. Ask the patient to keep the lips together.
- Gently advance the laryngoscope downward into the throat.
- When the laryngoscope is past the soft palate, instruct the patient to stick out his or her tongue to better visualize the base of the tongue and vallecula (depression just behind the root of the tongue between the folds in the throat).
- Instruct the patient to say "e-e-e-e" or "a-a-a-a" to visualize the vocal cord mobility.
- Instruct the patient to sniff to visualize the subglottis.

BOTH METHODS—RESULTS
- **Normal**
  - Larynx does not have swelling, masses, leukoplakia, polyps, erythema, edema, injury, narrowing, or foreign bodies.
  - Vocal cords do not have scar tissue, growths (tumors), or signs of not moving correctly (paralysis).

- **Abnormal**
  - Larynx has inflammation, injury, strictures, tumors, or foreign bodies.
  - Vocal cords have scar tissue or signs of paralysis.

Client Instructions

- 1 to 2 hours postprocedure—Nasal and throat spray wears off.
- 2 hours postprocedure—Do not eat or drink anything until you are able to swallow without choking.
  - Start with sips of water; then proceed to a normal diet.
- Do not clear your throat or cough hard for several hours.
- Speak in your normal tone of voice.
  - Do not talk for very long.
  - Whispering or shouting can strain your vocal cords.
- If your vocal cords were affected during the procedure, rest your voice completely for 3 days.

BIBLIOGRAPHY ▬▬▬▬▬▬▬▬▬▬

Healthwise staff. Laryngoscopy. Cigna Web site. http://www.cigna.com/ individualandfamilies/health-and-well-being/hw/medical-tests/laryngoscopy -hw232056.html

Pfenninger JL, ed. *Pfenninger and Fowler's Procedures for Primary Care*. Philadelphia, PA: Mosby Elsevier; 2019.

Chapter *77*

Nasal Lavage (Irrigation)
Margaret R. Colyar

CPT Code
None

In the bones of the skull there are four pairs of air-filled mucus-lined passages (sinuses) that drain the two nasal passages that filter air. When the nasal passages become inflamed, they swell and block the sinuses from draining. When the membranes swell, the cilia cannot do their job. Nasal lavage or irrigation uses an isotonic or hypertonic saline solution (Table 77.1) to loosen, thin, and flush out excess mucus and debris from the nose and sinuses and functions as an antibacterial irrigant.

Table 77·1	**Irrigation Solutions**

Do not use: Tap water is not isotonic or hypertonic
- Causes irritation of mucous membranes

Use: Isotonic/hypertonic solution with buffering (baking soda)
- Decreases pH of the irrigation solution to that of the body so there is no irritation of the mucous membranes

Recipe: I Quart

Mix together
I to 2 tsp pickling, canning, or kosher salt
½ to I tsp baking soda
I quart distilled, sterile, or boiled water

Recipe: I Cup

Mix together
3 tsp salt
I tsp baking soda
Then add I tsp of dry ingredients to I cup distilled, sterile, or boiled water

OVERVIEW

- Three methods of nasal lavage/irrigation are:
  - Squeeze bottle
  - Neti pot
  - Syringe

RATIONALE

- To relieve the nasal cavity and sinuses of irritation and infectious agents
- To relieve sinus symptoms
- To relieve allergy symptoms
- To ease inflammation and swelling in the sinuses and nasal passages

INDICATIONS

- Done for chronic sinus symptoms, nasal allergies, acute sinusitis, and colds

CONTRAINDICATIONS

- Tap water may be contaminated with amoeba *(Naegleria fowleri),* which could cause meningoencephalitis.
- Ear infection
- Nostril is plugged and hard to breathe through.
- Incompletely healed facial trauma

PROCEDURE
Nasal Lavage (Irrigation)

Equipment
- Methods 1, 2, and 3
  - Hypertonic saline solution with buffering
  - A small basin or sink
- Method 1
  - Squeeze bottle
- Method 2
  - Neti pot
- Method 3
  - A bulb syringe

Procedure

METHOD 1—SQUEEZE BOTTLE

See Figure 77.1A.
- Fill the squeeze bottle with isotonic/hypertonic solution.
- Have the patient bend over the sink, leaning head at a 45-degree angle.
- Instruct the patient to breathe through the mouth.
- Gently insert the tip of the squeeze bottle snuggly into the nose.
- Slowly squeeze the bottle so that the liquid gently squirts into the nose.
- Let the solution drain from the nostril. It may exit from the other nostril or from the mouth.
- When the squeeze bottle is empty, have the patient exhale gently through both nostrils to clear excess solution and mucus.
- Repeat in the other nostril.
- Use one full bottle in each nostril.

METHOD 2—NETI POT

See Figure 77.1B.
- Fill the neti pot with the isotonic/hypertonic solution.
- Have the patient lean over the sink (about 45 degrees), so that one nostril is above the other.
- Gently insert the spout of the neti pot into the uppermost nostril to form a comfortable seal. Do not press the spout against the septum of the nose.
- Instruct the patient to breathe through the mouth.
- Raise the handle of the filled neti pot so that the solution enters the upper nostril.
- The solution will begin to drain from the lower nostril.
- When the neti pot is empty, have the patient exhale gently through both nostrils to clear excess solution and mucus.
- Repeat in the other nostril.

METHOD 3—SYRINGE

See Figure 77.1C.
- Squeeze the air from the syringe and draw as much saline as possible from the basin.

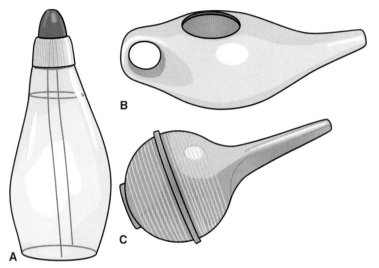

Figure 77.1 (A) Irrigation with squeeze bottle; (B) irrigation with neti pot; (C) irrigation with syringe.

- Turn the syringe upright, squeeze to remove any remaining air, and again draw the saline to completely fill the syringe.
- Have the patient bend over the sink, leaning head at a 45-degree angle.
- Instruct the patient to breathe through the mouth.
- Gently insert the tip of the syringe into the nose the width of the fingertip.
- Angle the tip of the syringe toward the outer corner of the eye; then slowly squeeze the bulb so that the liquid gently squirts into the nose.
- Let the solution drain from the nostril. It may exit from the other nostril or from the mouth.
- When the syringe is empty, have the patient exhale gently through both nostrils to clear excess solution and mucus.
- Repeat in the other nostril.
- Use two full syringes in each nostril.

Client Instructions

- Teach patient to irrigate three times per week to prevent symptoms.
- Teach patient to irrigate three times per day when sinus symptoms are present.
- If solution is irritating to the nostrils, decrease the salt by one-half teaspoon.

BIBLIOGRAPHY

Health and Wellness. UW Health Web site. https://www.uwhealth.org/news/nasal-irrigation
-helps-control-sinus-problems/20447. April 8, 2019.

Rabago D, Zgierska A. Saline nasal irrigation for upper respiratory infections. *Am Fam Physician.* 2009;80(10):1117–1119.

Rabago D, Zgierska A, Mundt M, Barrett B, Bobula J, Maberry R. Efficacy of daily hypertonic nasal irrigation among patients with sinusitis: a randomized controlled trial. *J Fam Pract.* 2002:51(12):1049–1055.

Chapter **78**

Removal of Foreign Body
Ear and Nose
Margaret R. Colyar

CPT Code
69200 Removal of foreign body from external auditory canal without
general anesthesia
30300 Removal of foreign body, intranasal; office-type procedure

Foreign bodies, such as vegetation, small solid objects, and insects, are found commonly in the external auditory canal and nose in young children.

OVERVIEW
- Objects commonly found in ears and nose include
  - Vegetation—beans, nuts, seeds, popcorn, paper balls, fabric, modeling clay
  - Solid objects—beads, small toys, money, watch batteries, rocks
  - Insects—roaches, flies, ticks, spiders

OPTIONS
- *Method 1*—Irrigation technique
  - Used for small solid objects, vegetation, and dead insects
- *Method 2*—Light technique
  - Used for live insects

RATIONALE
- To relieve pain
- To remove foreign bodies from the ears and nose
- To prevent infection

INDICATIONS
- Foreign body seen in ear or nose

CONTRAINDICATIONS
- Hard vegetation that has become swollen
- Foreign body in inner third of auditory canal in which easy access is occluded—REFER to a pediatrician or ENT specialist
- Child uncooperative—REFER to a pediatrician

PROCEDURE

Removal of Foreign Body—Ear and Nose

Equipment

- Methods 1 and 2
  - Ear and nasal **speculum**
  - Topical ear anesthetic (Auralgan or Otocain)
  - 0.9% sodium chloride for irrigation
  - Gloves—nonsterile
  - Drape or towel—nonsterile
  - Cotton-tipped applicator—nonsterile
  - Alcohol
- Method 1 only
  - Foreign body extraction tools (Fig. 78.1)
    - Nasal **forceps**
    - Alligator forceps
    - Ear **curettes** with hook
- Method 2 only
  - Flashlight or penlight

Procedure

METHOD 1—IRRIGATION TECHNIQUE

- Position the client for comfort.
- Apply a drape or towel to protect clothing.
- Put on gloves.
- Instill topical anesthesia into the ear canal or nose.
- Insert the speculum.
- Insert the appropriate tool through the speculum, grasp the object, and gently remove.
  - If the auditory canal or nasal passage is only partially occluded, try the hooked curette.
  - If the object is hard, try alligator forceps or nasal forceps.

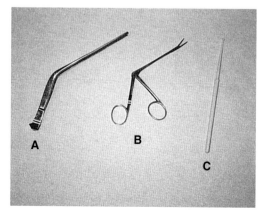

Figure 78.1 Foreign body extraction tools include (A) nasal forceps, (B) alligator forceps, and (C) ear curettes.

- Irrigate the orifice with 0.9% sodium chloride to remove remaining debris.
- If there is bleeding present, cleanse the orifice with a cotton-tipped applicator saturated with alcohol.

METHOD 2—LIGHT TECHNIQUE
- Position the client for comfort.
- Apply a drape or towel to protect clothing.
- Put on gloves.
- Instill topical anesthesia into the ear canal or nose.
- Insert the speculum.
- Turn on flashlight or penlight, and shine the light into the ear canal or nasal passage.
  - Many times the insect follows the light source and walks out of the orifice.
- Irrigate the orifice with 0.9% sodium chloride to remove remaining debris.
- If there is bleeding present, cleanse the orifice with a cotton-tipped applicator saturated with alcohol.

Client Instructions

- Take acetaminophen or ibuprofen every 4 to 6 hours for pain.
  - If pain continues after 24 hours, notify the practitioner.
  - Although slight, there is a chance of infection. Observe for signs and symptoms of infection, such as
    - Increase in pain after 24 hours
    - Increase in temperature
    - Yellow or greenish drainage
    - Foul odor
- If any of the signs and symptoms of infection are found, return to the office.

BIBLIOGRAPHY

Cheever KJ, Hinkle JL. *Brunner and Suddarth's Textbook of Medical-Surgical Nursing.* Philadelphia, PA: Lippincott-Raven; 2017.
Ignatavicius DD, Workman ML. *Medical-Surgical Nursing: Patient-Centered Collaborative Care.* 8th ed. Philadelphia, PA: Saunders; 2016.

79

Chapter

Frenotomy for Ankyloglossia

Cynthia R. Ehrhardt

CPT Code
41010 Incision of a lingual frenulum

Frenotomy is a procedure used to release an abnormal attachment of **frenulum** to the tongue. This abnormal attachment is known as **ankyloglossia**. It can lead to poor feeding in infants and speech impairment in older children.

OVERVIEW

- Causes unknown
  - Hereditary predisposition suggested

RATIONALE

- To release the tongue and provide full range of motion for essential growth and development

INDICATIONS

- Difficulty sucking
- Difficulty breastfeeding
- Difficulty chewing
- Inhibits tongue protrusion
- Abnormal dentofacial growth and development
- Speech impairment

CONTRAINDICATIONS

- Severe ankyloglossia that interferes with lingual function should be REFERRED to a surgeon, dentist, or otolaryngologist.

PROCEDURE

Frenotomy

Equipment

- 3-mL syringe
- 25- to 27-gauge, ½-inch needle
- 1% lidocaine with epinephrine
- Topical 20% benzocaine
- Tongue retractor

- Hemostat—sterile
- Gloves—sterile
- Iris scissors—sterile
- 4 × 4 gauze—nonsterile
- Cotton-tipped applicators—nonsterile
- Adequate light source

Procedure

- Position the client in a comfortable position with easy access to the mouth.
- Locate the frenulum.
- Apply a cotton-tipped applicator saturated with benzocaine to the lingual frenulum (Fig. 79.1).
- Retract and stabilize the tongue (Fig. 79.2).
- Using the tip of the **hemostat,** grasp the area of the frenulum that is to be ligated, then clamp and crush to the depth required (Fig. 79.3).
  - After a few seconds, release and remove the hemostat.
- Using the iris scissors, snip the tissue crushed by the hemostat.
- Apply pressure with a clean cotton-tipped applicator.
  - If bleeding continues, apply a cotton-tipped applicator saturated with 1% lidocaine with epinephrine until bleeding is halted.

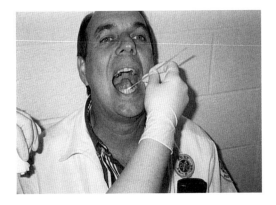

Figure 79.1 Anesthetize the lingual frenulum with benzocaine.

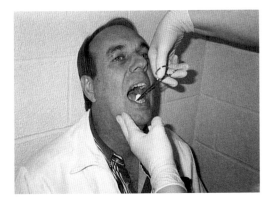

Figure 79.2 Retract and stabilize the tongue.

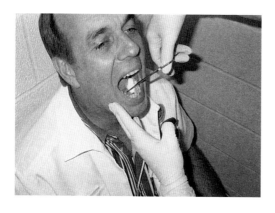

Figure 79.3 Clamp and crush the frenulum to the depth planned for ligation.

Client Instructions

- Infant may begin feeding immediately.
- Observe for signs and symptoms of infection, such as
  - Increase in pain after 24 hours
  - Increase in temperature
  - Redness or swelling
  - Yellow or greenish drainage
  - Foul odor
  - Decreased feeding
- If any signs or symptoms of infection are found, return to the office.
- Antibiotics generally are not required unless secondary infection occurs.
- To relieve pain
  - Take acetaminophen every 4 to 6 hours as needed.
  - No children's ibuprofen should be used.
- Return to the office in 2 weeks for recheck.

BIBLIOGRAPHY

Chaubal TV, Dixit MB. Ankyloglossia and its management. *J Indian Soc Peridontol.* 2011;15(3):270–272.

Paradise J. Evaluation and treatment of ankyloglossia. *JAMA.* 1990;263:2371–2374.

Pfenninger JL, Fowler GC. *Procedures for Primary Care Physicians.* St. Louis, MO: Mosby; 2019.

Lip Laceration Repair

Cynthia R. Ehrhardt

CPT Code
40650   Repair lip, full thickness; vermilion only
40652   Repair lip, full thickness; vermilion only—up to half vertical
           height
40654   Repair lip, full thickness; vermilion only—over one half vertical
           height, or complex

Lip lacerations usually are caused by trauma to the perioral area of the face resulting from blunt injury or falls. Suturing beyond the ideal time of 6 hours after laceration is considered because of the cosmetic implications.

Prevention includes elimination of situations that can result in laceration of the lip and promotion of safety habits and use of protective mouth gear when playing organized contact sports.

OVERVIEW

- Incidence unknown; usually associated with falls and contact sports
- Complications
  - Fractures of the facial bones

RATIONALE

- To promote healing
- To promote esthetics

INDICATIONS

- Lip laceration of greater than 0.25 cm
- Gaping lacerations

CONTRAINDICATIONS

- Suspected injury of the orbicularis oris muscle
- Suspected facial bone fracture
- Need for extensive revision and/or debridement to the lip
- Laceration through the margin of the lip
- Vertical through-and-through laceration
- If more than 12 hours since the laceration has occurred, the patient should be referred to a plastic surgeon for evaluation.

PROCEDURE
Lip Laceration Repair
Equipment

- Gloves—sterile
- Towels (fenestrated and nonfenestrated)—sterile
- 3-mL syringe
- 25- to 27-gauge, ½-inch needle for anesthesia administration
- Syringes—30 or 60 mL without needle for irrigation
- 1% or 2% lidocaine without epinephrine
- No. 6-0 Ethicon suture material
- 0.9% sodium chloride—sterile
- Topical antibiotic ointment (Bactroban, Bacitracin, or Polysporin)
- Cotton-tipped applicators—nonsterile
- Sterile suture kit (prepackaged or self-made) should include
  - Curved and straight **hemostats**
  - Needle holders (4½ inch and 6 inch)
  - **Forceps** with teeth
  - Iris scissors
  - Cup to hold sterile normal saline solution
  - 4 × 4 sterile gauze

Procedure

- Thorough inspection for anatomical defects to the following areas
  - Lip region to determine whether the laceration is through the margin
  - Structural defect in the musculature, including injury to the orbicularis oris muscle, by examination of the symmetry of the smile
  - Maxillary structures for loss of integrity
  - Mandible structure for loss of integrity and range of motion of the temporomandibular joint
  - Teeth for stability
- Drape the area to prevent any solution from draining into mouth.
- Infiltrate the borders of the laceration, but avoid as much as possible distortion of the lip margins.
- *Do not* clean the wound with povidone-iodine.
- Gently irrigate the wound with 30 to 60 mL of sterile normal saline solution, being careful to avoid getting the solution into the mouth.
- Carefully align the lip margins (Fig. 80.1).
- Suture the wound.
- Apply topical antibiotic.

Client Instructions

- Apply an ice pack to decrease pain and swelling to the area.
- Keep the area as clean as possible.
- If a crust develops over the site, cleanse by gently rolling a cotton-tipped applicator saturated with hydrogen peroxide over the site. Then gently rinse the area with warm water and blot dry with clean towel or cotton gauze.

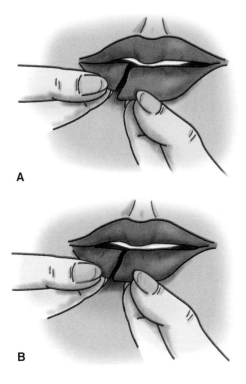

A

B

Figure 80.1 Align lip margins. (A) Incorrect alignment; (B) correct alignment.

- Eat a clear liquid diet for the first 24 hours, then soft diet for 3 to 4 days.
- No sucking or straw usage until sutures are removed.
- To lessen the discomfort, avoid citrus or acidic foods.
- Observe for signs and symptoms of infection, such as
  - Increase in pain after 24 hours
  - Increase in temperature
  - Redness or swelling
  - Yellow or greenish drainage
  - Foul odor
- If any signs or symptoms of infection are found, return to the office.
- Return to the office in 3 to 5 days (children and adults) for suture removal.
- To relieve pain, take acetaminophen every 4 to 6 hours as needed.
  - Tylenol No. 3 is rarely needed.
- Antibiotics generally are not recommended.

BIBLIOGRAPHY

Pfenninger JL, Fowler GC. *Procedures for Primary Care Physicians.* St. Louis, MO: Mosby; 2019.

Trott A. *Wounds and Lacerations: Emergency Care and Closure.* St. Louis, MO: Mosby; 2012.

Tongue Laceration Repair

Cynthia R. Ehrhardt

CPT Code
41250 Repair of laceration 2.5 cm or less; floor of mouth and/or anterior two-thirds of tongue
41251 Repair of laceration 2.5 cm or less; posterior one-third of tongue

---

Tongue laceration most commonly is caused by biting. Trauma to the face rarely involves fractured teeth except in instances of blunt trauma to the face.

OVERVIEW

- Usually associated with falls and contact sports

HEALTH PROMOTION/PREVENTION

- Eliminate situations that can result in laceration of the tongue.
  - Promote safety habits when playing organized contact sports, such as
    - Use of tooth guards
    - Prevention of falls

RATIONALE

- To promote healing

INDICATIONS

- Tongue laceration of greater than 1 cm
- Gaping tongue lacerations

CONTRAINDICATIONS

- If laceration is less than 1 cm and/or not gaping, suturing is not recommended.
- Through-and-through laceration should be sutured only on dorsal surface.

PROCEDURE

Tongue Laceration Repair

Equipment

- Gloves—sterile
- Towels (fenestrated and nonfenestrated)—sterile
- 3-mL syringe

- 25-gauge, 1½-inch needle
- 30- or 60-mL syringe without needle for irrigation
- 1% or 2% lidocaine
- No. 5-0 chromic (Vicryl) suture
- No. 2-0 Ethicon suture—optional
- 0.9% sodium chloride—sterile
- Two bite blocks
- Sterile suture kit (prepackaged or self-made) should include
  - Curved and straight **hemostats**
  - Needle holders (4½ and 6 inch)
  - **Forceps** with teeth
  - Iris scissors
  - Cup to hold sterile 0.9% sodium chloride solution
  - 4 × 4 sterile gauze

Procedure

- Insert bite blocks on each side of the mouth to prevent accidental biting by the client during the procedure.
- Stabilization of the tongue by either of the following methods is necessary for proper suturing of the tongue:
  - Have the assistant grasp the distal one-third of the tongue with 4 × 4 gauze and extend until the laceration can be easily accessed.
  - Locally anesthetize with lidocaine the area of the tongue where two No. 2-0 Ethicon sutures can be placed temporarily to facilitate extension of the tongue by the assistant to expose the laceration (Fig. 81.1).
- Anesthetize the area by local infiltration of the laceration borders.
- Avoid vigorous irrigation of the laceration. Use gentle irrigation with 30 to 60 mL of 0.9% sodium chloride.
- Insert chromic (Vicryl) sutures for good approximation of the lacerated edges using a simple suture (see Chapter 22).
- Avoid long suture tails because they create increased irritation.

Client Instructions

- Do not eat or drink until the anesthetic has worn off (usually about 1 hour).
- Apply cool compresses (e.g., ice or Popsicle) to the tongue to decrease pain and swelling.
- Eat a clear liquid diet for the first meal after the suturing, then soft diet for 3 to 4 days.
- Use a mixture of one-half hydrogen peroxide and one-half water as a mouth rinse as needed for 3 to 4 days (swish and spit).
- To relieve pain, take acetaminophen or Tylenol No. 3 every 4 to 6 hours as needed for pain.
- Antibiotics generally are not recommended.
- Observe for signs and symptoms of infection, such as
  - Increase in pain after 24 hours
  - Increase in temperature

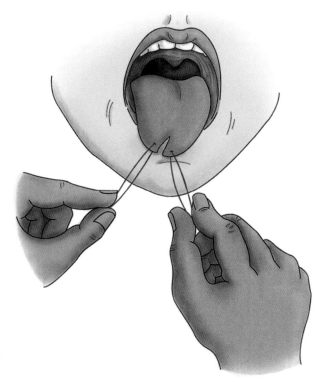

Figure 81.1 Insert two sutures for an assistant to expose the laceration.

- Redness or swelling
- Yellow or greenish drainage
- Foul odor
- If any signs or symptoms of infection are found, return to the office.
- Suture removal is not required because the sutures are absorbable.

BIBLIOGRAPHY

Pfenninger JL, Fowler GC. *Procedures for Primary Care Physicians.* St. Louis, MO: Mosby; 2019.

Trott A. *Wounds and Lacerations: Emergency Care and Closure.* St. Louis, MO: Mosby; 2012.

Chapter **82**

Tooth Avulsion and Fracture

Cynthia Ehrhardt

CPT Code
None

Tooth fracture is caused by trauma to the tooth with or without **avulsion** or **exarticulation** from the socket. Tooth avulsion is caused by trauma to a tooth resulting in complete displacement (avulsion or exarticulation) from the socket.

Promotion of safety habits when playing organized contact sports and use of tooth guards are good methods of prevention.

OVERVIEW
- Causes
  - Contact sports
  - Blows to the face
  - Poor dental hygiene
  - Chewing hard objects (e.g., ice, hard candy, hard-shelled food, inanimate objects)
- Complications
  - Laceration of the gum
  - Partial or complete avulsion of the tooth
  - Trauma and/or fracture of the facial bones
- General principles
  - Key to successful preservation and restoration of the tooth is REFERRAL to the dentist for evaluation of the extent of the injury.
  - If the fractured or avulsed tooth is found, preservation in transport medium should be undertaken.
  - Time is the major factor in tooth preservation.

RATIONALE
- To preserve the tooth and its function

INDICATIONS
- Presence of abnormal-appearing tooth after an incident, with or without pain
- Visualization of the fracture with or without partial displacement of tooth (permanent or immature) from the socket
- Total displacement of an intact tooth (permanent or immature) from the socket

CONTRAINDICATIONS

- Suspected facial fractures
- Laceration to the socket

PROCEDURE

Tooth Avulsion and Fracture

Equipment

- Transfer medium if unable to reinsert tooth (order of preference)
  - Hank's balanced salt solution (from local pharmacy)
  - Milk
  - 0.9% sodium chloride—sterile
  - Saliva
  - Water
- *Do not transport in tissue or towel because it will dry out the tooth cells.*

Procedure

- For fractured tooth with avulsion and less than 1 hour after injury
  - Locate the tooth and its fragments.
  - Inspect the tooth.
  - If tooth pulpal (root) appears totally intact and is not contaminated
    - Irrigate the tooth socket with 0.9% sodium chloride or water to ensure that any clot has been removed.
    - Grasp tooth at distal tip.
    - Gently rinse with 10 to 30 mL of 0.9% sodium chloride.
    - Gently set the tooth back into socket.
  - If tooth pulpal (root) has been contaminated
    - Irrigate the tooth socket with 0.9% sodium chloride or water to ensure that any clot has been removed.
    - Grasp tooth at distal tip.
    - Gently rinse with 10 to 30 mL of 0.9% sodium chloride or water.
    - Gently set tooth back into socket.
    - Consult with a dentist.
- For fractured tooth with avulsion and more than 1 hour after injury
  - Locate tooth and its fragments.
  - Inspect tooth.
  - Follow reimplantation instructions as given for injuries less than 1 hour old.
  - If not possible to re-implant, place the fractured tooth in the transport medium.
  - Contact dentist or endodontist as soon as possible for treatment.

Client Instructions

- If reimplantation is successful, do not dislodge the tooth from the socket.
- Gently clench the teeth. This may allow support of the tooth.

- Minimize activities such as talking, drinking, or chewing to prevent further trauma to the injured tooth and decrease the risk of dislodging from the socket.
- Seek dental attention (dentist or endodontist) as soon as possible. Delay in restoration can result in complete loss of the tooth.

BIBLIOGRAPHY

Decision Trees for Management of an Avulsed Permanent Tooth. American's Pediatric Dentists Web site. www.aapd.org—Decision trees for management of an avulsed permanent tooth.

Pfenninger JL, Fowler GC. *Procedures for Primary Care Physicians*. St. Louis, MO: Mosby; 2019.

Cardiovascular Procedures

Chapter 83

Doppler Technique

Margaret R. Colyar

CPT Code
93922 Noninvasive physiologic studies of upper or lower extremity arteries, single-level, bilateral (e.g., ankle/brachial indices, Doppler waveform analysis, volume plethysmography, transcutaneous oxygen tension measurement)

Doppler technique is the examination of artery function with an instrument that ultrasonically detects arterial blood flow. A good understanding of the anatomy of the arterial system is necessary (Fig. 83.1).

RATIONALE

- To examine arterial function

INDICATIONS

- Extremity cool, edematous, pale, or cyanotic
- Arterial pulsation cannot be palpated in the extremity
- Determine placement for an arterial stick
- Assist in Allen's test

CONTRAINDICATIONS

- None

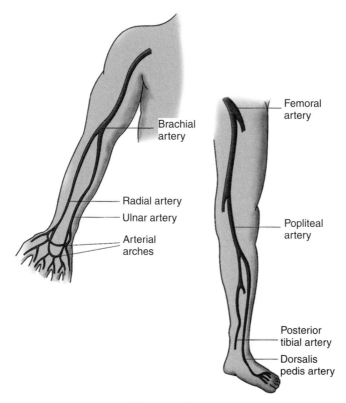

Figure 83.1 Anatomy of the arterial system in the extremities.

PROCEDURE

Doppler Technique

Equipment

* Ultrasound lubricant
* Doppler (Fig. 83.2)
* Marking pen

Procedure

* Position the client with the area to be assessed easily accessible.
* Apply ultrasound lubricant.
* Turn Doppler on.
* Apply Doppler probe to the area of expected arterial pulse (Fig. 83.3).
* Gently move the Doppler probe until the pulse is detected.
* Mark the area of pulse with a marking pen.

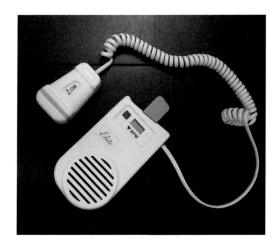

Figure 83.2 Doppler.

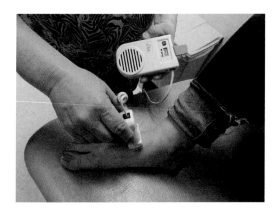

Figure 83.3 Apply the Doppler probe to the lubricated area of expected arterial pulse. Move the probe until the pulse is detected.

BIBLIOGRAPHY

Pfenninger JL, Fowler GC. *Procedures for Primary Care Physicians*. St. Louis, MO: Mosby; 2019.
Potter PA, Perry AG. *Clinical Nursing Skills and Techniques*. St. Louis, MO: Mosby; 2018.

84

Electrocardiogram (EKG) Interpretation

Margaret R. Colyar

CPT Code
93000   Electrocardiogram (EKG) complete
93005   ECG technical component

The **EKG** is a unique tool used to assist the clinician in diagnosing or ruling out myocardial **infarction** (MI); potential life-threatening arrhythmias; and many cardiac problems caused by medications, electrolyte imbalance, or disease processes. Interpreting an EKG is not difficult. After learning the basic rules, you can understand and apply them easily.

OVERVIEW

- Performed on almost every client presenting to the emergency department or ambulatory health-care facility with chest pain

RATIONALE

- To diagnose and rule out cardiac problems

INDICATIONS

- Chest pain
- Recent or remote MI follow-up
- Differential diagnosis of cardiac problems
- Baseline data if client is at risk for cardiac problems
- Preoperative workup
- Client starting an exercise program

CONTRAINDICATIONS

- None

PROCEDURE

EKG Interpretation

Basic Cardiac Information Needed

- **Depolarization**—electrical stimulation of the heart muscle causing the heart cells to contract

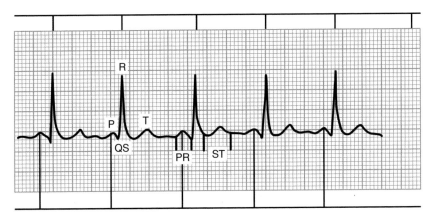

Figure 84.1 EKG components.

- **Repolarization**—resting or relaxation phase of the heart muscle
- EKG components
  - **P wave**—depicts atrial stimulation or depolarization
  - **PR interval**—depicts the time it takes atrial stimulation to reach the atrioventricular (AV) node
    - During this time, blood flows from the atria through the AV valves into the ventricles. Normal time for this to occur is less than 0.2 second (Fig. 84.1).
  - **QRS complex**—depicts the beginning of ventricular contraction or depolarization; normal time for this to occur is less than 0.12 second
    - **Q wave**—the first downward deflection of the QRS complex
      - You may notice that sometimes the Q wave is absent from the QRS complex. *Don't be alarmed.* This is a physiological variation and may happen occasionally.
    - **R wave**—the first upward deflection of the QRS complex
    - **S wave**—any downward deflection that first is preceded by an upward deflection of the QRS complex
    - **ST segment**—the pause after the QRS complex
      - The line should be flat. If it is elevated or depressed, there is a major problem.
    - **T wave**—depicts ventricular repolarization or relaxation
- EKG paper
  - One small square is 1 mm long and wide (0.04 second)
  - One large square (from one heavy line to the next heavy line) is 5 mm long and wide (0.2 second)
- Baseline EKG tracing—first tracing done on which further EKG changes are based
- Limb leads are measured in the frontal plane (Table 84.1). A pair of **electrodes** (one is + and one is −) forms a **limb lead**.
- Chest leads are measured in the horizontal plane (Fig. 84.2). The chest leads normally produce a positive deflection in a progressive manner. The placement of the chest leads correlates with the area of the heart measured.

Table 84·1	Lead EKG Tracing: Limb Lead Titles, Location, and Normal	
LEAD	**PLACEMENT**	**WHAT IS MEASURED?**
V1	Fourth intercostal space (ICS) right of sterna border (RSB)	Right side of the heart
V2	Fourth ICS left of sterna border (LSB)	Right side of the heart
V3	Halfway between V2 and V4	Intraventricular septum
V4	Fifth ICS midclavicular line	Intraventricular septum
V5	Anterior axillary line lateral to V4	Left side of the heart
V6	Midaxillary line lateral to V5	Left side of the heart

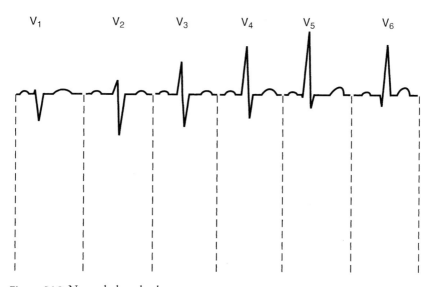

Figure 84.2 Normal chest leads.

METHODOLOGICAL INTERPRETATION

There are five general areas—rate, rhythm, axis, **hypertrophy**, and infarction.

- Rate—The following is the best method for measuring rate or beats per minute (beats/min) on the 12-lead EKG because it is based on 3 seconds of tracing (Fig. 84.3). Other methods are easier for measuring rate on a rhythm strip.
  - Look at the EKG paper and measure from one R wave to the next R wave.
    - First heavy black line to the next heavy black line (1/300 minute) = 300 beats/min.
    - Then = 150 beats/min (2 heavy lines = 2/300 or 1/150)
    - Then = 100 beats/min (3 heavy lines = 3/300 or 1/100)
    - Then = 75 beats/min (4 heavy lines = 4/300 or 1/75)
    - Then = 60 beats/min (5 heavy lines = 5/300 or 1/60)
    - Then = 50 beats/min (6 heavy lines = 6/300 or 1/50)

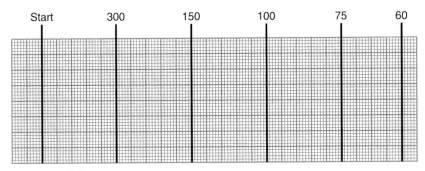

Figure 84.3 Measure rate.

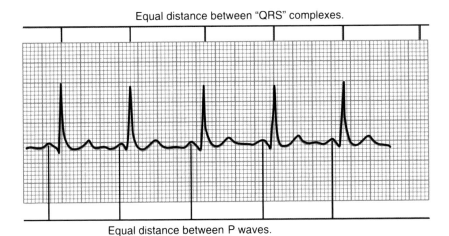

Figure 84.4 Normal sinus rhythm.

- Within a 6-second strip, count cycles from R wave to R wave and multiply by 10 (the number of 6-second intervals in 1 minute = cycles/min).
  - Bradycardia (slow)—less than 60 cycles/min
  - Tachycardia (fast)—greater than 100 cycles/min
- Rhythm—The pattern of electrical conduction phenomena of the heart as the electrical current passes from the **sinoatrial node** (SA) through the AV node through the **bundle of His, bundle branches,** and the **Purkinje fibers.**
  - Regular—distance between R waves is always equal.
    - Normal sinus rhythm (60 to 100 beats/min) (Fig. 84.4)
  - Irregular—distance between R waves is not always equal.
    - AV blocks (Fig. 84.5)
      - First-degree AV block—P-R interval is greater than 0.2 second on each cycle.
      - Second-degree Wenckebach (type I)—P-R interval gets progressively longer until one P-R interval is finally dropped (not life threatening).
      - Second-degree Mobitz II (type II)—a QRS complex is dropped with no lengthening of P-R interval (can lead to complete heart block).

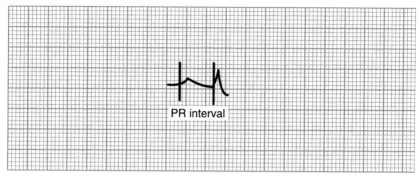

A   PR interval greater than 0.20 mm (5 small blocks)

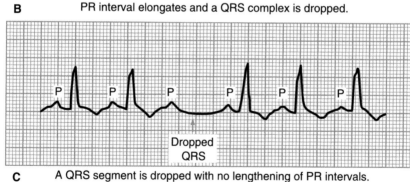

B   PR interval elongates and a QRS complex is dropped.

C   A QRS segment is dropped with no lengthening of PR intervals.

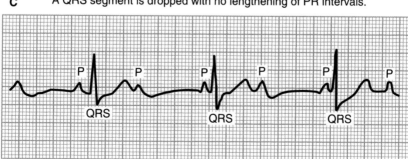

D   PR intervals are unrelated to QRS complexes.

Figure 84.5 AV blocks. (A) First-degree AV block, (B) second-degree Wenckebach (type I), (C) second-degree Mobitz II (type II), and (D) third-degree (complete heart block).

- Third-degree AV block (complete heart block)—none of the P-R intervals are related to a QRS complex.
- The rate lets you know the focus from which it originates.
- Ventricle focus is at a rate of 20 to 40 beats/min.
- A junctional focus is at a rate of 40 to 60 beats/min.
- Bundle-branch block (BBB) (Fig. 84.6)—usually the bundle branches are depolarized simultaneously.
  - A delay of electrical impulse to either the right or the left bundle branches results in one ventricular depolarization slightly later than the other.
  - On the EKG, a "double-peaked" or "joined" widened QRS complex appears.
  - For a right BBB, check chest leads V_1 and V_2 for double-peaked QRS complexes.
  - For a left BBB, check chest leads V_5 and V_6 for double-peaked QRS complexes. These also are known as *hemiblocks* and commonly are associated with MI. MI is hard to diagnose, however, in the presence of a left BBB.

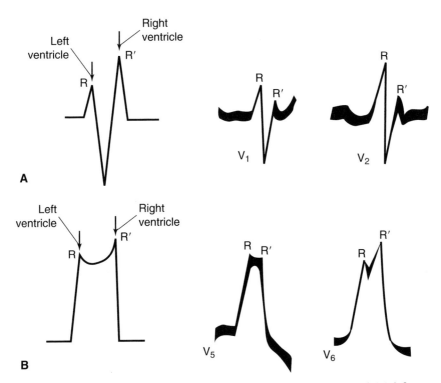

Figure 84.6 Bundle-branch blocks. (A) Right bundle-branch block and (B) left bundle-branch block.

- Ectopic foci—stimulus from an ectopic focus (Fig. 84.7); results in premature beats (short beats) or escape beats (prolonged beats). Included are
- Paroxysmal atrial tachycardia—150 to 250 beats/min
- Supraventricular tachycardia—150 to 250 beats/min
- Ventricular tachycardia—150 to 250 beats/min
- Premature atrial contractions—early SA node contraction
- Premature ventricular contractions (PVCs)—early ventricular firing
  - PVCs can be *unifocal* or *multifocal.*
    - A unifocal PVC comes from an abnormal focus in the *same place* in the ventricle *every* time and looks the same each time.
    - A multifocal PVC comes from *several* abnormal foci in the ventricles and looks different each time. A multifocal PVC is a much worse indicator of more serious heart disease than a unifocal PVC.
- **Flutter**—250 to 300 beats/min
  - Flutter can be atrial or ventricular in origin.
  - A flutter has a regular single ectopic focus. It is sawtoothed in appearance.
- **Fibrillation**—350 to 450 beats/min
  - Fibrillation can be atrial or ventricular in origin.
  - A fibrillatory beat is irregular and comes from multiple foci. It is *irregular* in appearance and is an indicator of much worse heart disease.
- Axis (vector)—direction and magnitude of the electrical stimulus of depolarization starting at the AV node and continuing through the ventricles
  - Axis is measured in degrees.
  - With a normal axis, the mean QRS (+0 to +84 degrees) **vector** points downward and toward the client's left side because that is the way the normal heart lies in the chest (Fig. 84.8). To measure axis, do the following:
    - With the AV node as the center, imagine a circle around the heart measured in degrees positive (+) and negative (−).
      - Positive degrees are measured in the lower half of the heart.
      - Negative degrees are measured in the top half of the heart.
    - In lead I, measure the right and left spheres (halves) of axis (left is +, right is −).
      - A + deflection occurs when the stimulus is moving toward the left (left axis deviation).
      - A − deflection occurs when the electrical stimulus is moving toward the right (right axis deviation).
    - The aVF measures the upper and lower spheres (halves) of axis (upper is −, lower is +).
      - If the deflection is mainly +, the mean QRS vector is downward.
      - If the deflection is mainly −, the mean QRS vector is upward.
    - Chest leads record axis on a horizontal plane.
      - They should be − in leads V_1 and V_2 and + in leads V_5 and V_6.
      - A progression from − in V_1 to + in V_6 is normal.

text continues on page 386

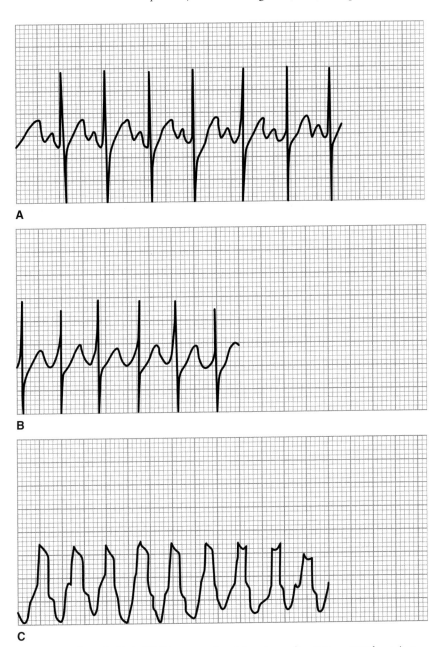

Figure 84.7 Ectopic foci. (A) Paroxysmal atrial tachycardia, 150 to 200 beats/min; (B) supraventricular tachycardia; (C) paroxysmal ventricular tachycardia;

Continued

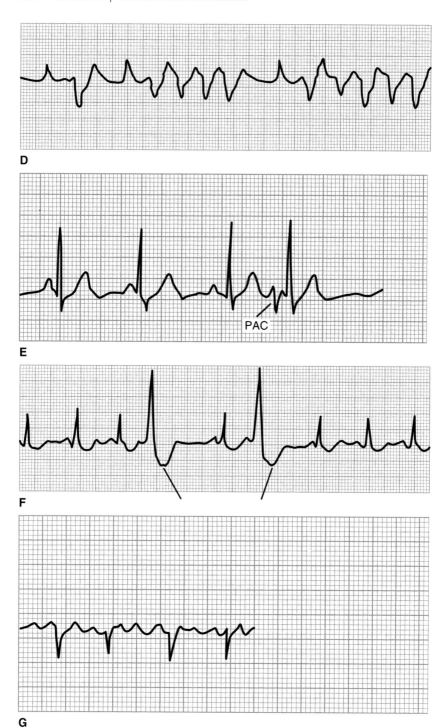

D

E

PAC

F

G

Figure 84.7 cont'd (D) runs of paroxysmal ventricular tachycardia; (E) premature atrial contraction; (F) premature ventricular contractions; (G) atrial flutter;

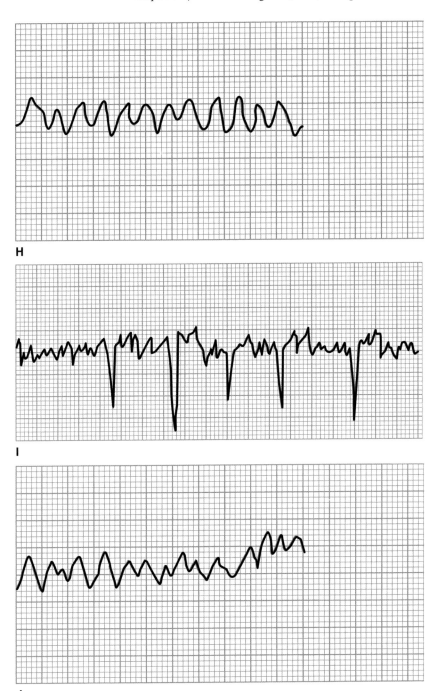

Figure 84.7 cont'd (H) ventricular flutter; (I) atrial fibrillation; and (J) ventricular fibrillation.

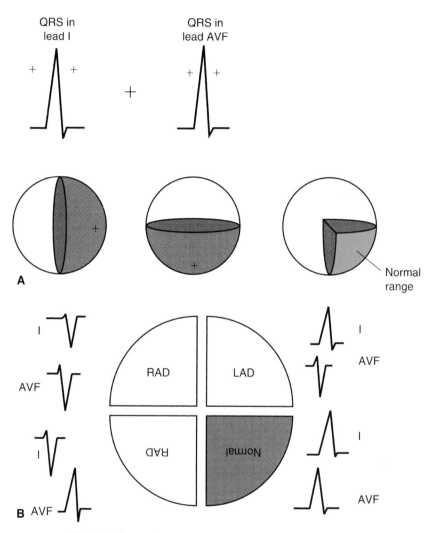

Figure 84.8 Check leads I and AVF to determine (A) normal axis or (B) axis deviation.

- Lead V_2, because of its position, projects through the anterior wall of the heart to the posterior wall of the heart and gives the best information on anterior and posterior wall MIs.

Things That Affect Axis

- Obesity—pushes the heart up, and the mean QRS vector is directed to the left of +0 degrees.
- Infarction—no electrical stimulus goes through dead tissue, and the mean QRS vector *turns away* from the infarcted area of tissue.

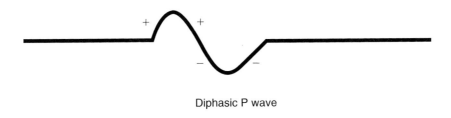

Diphasic P wave

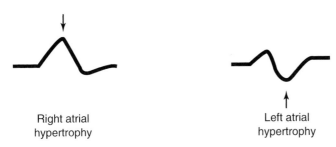

| Right atrial hypertrophy | Left atrial hypertrophy |

Figure 84.9 Atrial hypertrophy.

- Ventricular hypertrophy—has electrical activity, and the mean QRS vector *deviates* toward the enlarged ventricle.
- Hypertrophy—increase in heart size or wall thickness because of an increased volume in the chambers of the heart (Fig. 84.9).
  - Atrial hypertrophy
    - P wave depicts contraction of the atria.
    - Lead V_1 is placed directly over the atria (fourth intercostal space [ICS], right sternal border).
    - Hypertrophy of atria is shown as a diphasic (+ or − deflection) P wave in lead V_1.
    - If right atrial hypertrophy is present, the *beginning* portion of the diphasic wave is larger.
    - If left atrial hypertrophy is present, the *end* portion of the diphasic wave is larger.
  - Ventricular hypertrophy—QRS wave depicts the contraction of the ventricles
    - Lead V_1 tracing is usually negative (small R wave and large S wave) because depolarization is *away* from the right side of the heart toward the thicker left side of the heart.
    - Hypertrophy of the ventricles is shown by the deflection of the QRS in lead V_1 (+ or −) (Fig. 84.10).
      - Right ventricular hypertrophy—V_1 has a + deflected QRS
        - The electrical stimulus is away from the left side toward the thicker right side.

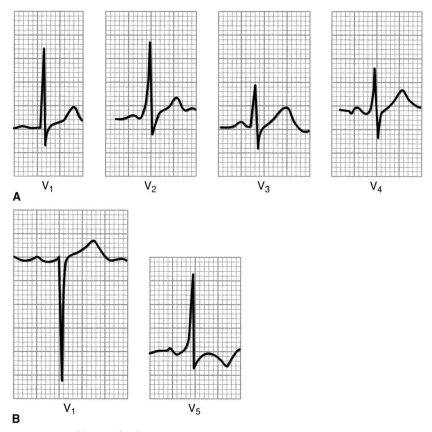

Figure 84.10 Ventricular hypertrophy. (A) Right ventricular hypertrophy; (B) left ventricular hypertrophy.

- Progression of V_1 to V_6 starts with large R waves in V_1 and ends with a small R wave in V_6.
- V_2 is directly over the right ventricle and is the best place to look for right ventricular *strain*.
- Left ventricular hypertrophy—more depolarization toward the left than usual
  - A *small R wave* and *deep S wave* in V_1.
  - Lead V_5 is directly over the left ventricle, so if the left ventricle is enlarged, V_5 has a more + deflection resulting in a *tall R wave*.
  - You must *add* the S wave in V_1 and the R wave in V_5 together in millimeters. If these add up to greater than 35 mm, left ventricular hypertrophy is present.
- T waves also indicate ventricular hypertrophy.
  - V_5 and V_6 are directly over the left ventricle and are the best place to look for left ventricular *strain*.
  - The wave is *inverted* and *asymmetric*.

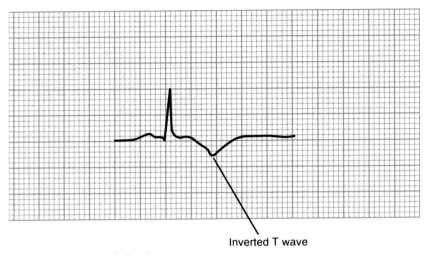

Inverted T wave

Figure 84.11 Myocardial ischemia.

- Hypoxia—occlusion of a coronary artery (by thrombus or arteriosclerotic plaques) producing lack of blood supply to the heart, resulting in decreased oxygenation to the cells
  - Usually only the left ventricle suffers an MI.
  - On the EKG, you can determine if the heart has suffered **ischemia**, *injury*, or *infarction*.
    - Ischemia (decreased blood supply)—"smiley" face (Fig. 84.11)
      - Shown as a T-wave inversion and symmetry
      - In V_2 to V_6, this indicates pathology.
      - In limb leads, this is a normal variation.
    - Injury (acuteness of infarct)—"frowny" face (Fig. 84.12)
      - Shown as elevated ST segment
      - Elevation of ST segment indicates *only* a small acute infarct, pericarditis, or ventricular aneurysm (T wave does *not* return to baseline).
      - Depressed ST segment may indicate a partial-thickness (subendocardial) infarct or digitalis effect.
    - Infarction (Fig. 84.13)—not diagnosable if left BBB is present
      - Check all leads for *significant Q waves*. Q waves that are significant are 0.04 second (one small square) wide *or* one-third amplitude of the entire QRS complex.
      - Q waves (first downward deflection of the QRS) are usually absent in the healthy person.
      - *Tiny Q waves are insignificant* in leads I, II, V_5, and V_6.
      - Anterior infarction (V_1 to V_4)
        - Check all chest leads (V_1 to V_4) for the presence of significant Q waves (0.04 second) and for elevated ST segment. Because all chest leads are anteriorly placed, it makes sense to check these leads.

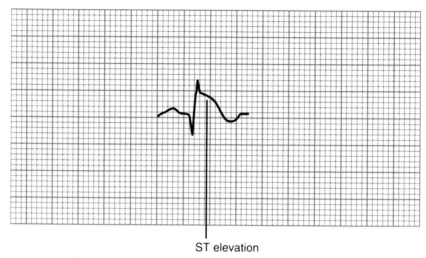

ST elevation

Figure 84.12 Myocardial injury.

- Lateral infarction (aVL, lead I)
  - Check aVL and lead I for significant Q waves and elevated ST segment.
- Inferior infarction (aVF, leads II and III)
- Check aVF and leads II and III for significant Q waves or elevated or depressed ST segments.
- Posterior infarction (V_1 to V_2)
  - Opposite picture from anterior MI. There is a larger R wave and obviously depressed ST segment.
  - Do the mirror test. Turn the EKG upside down and look at it in a mirror. It should look like the classic acute infarct.

QUICK AND EASY INTERPRETATION

- Rate—300, 150, 100, 75, 60, 50
  - If bradycardia, check 6-second strip and multiply by 10.
- Rhythm—regular or irregular? AV block or BBB?
- Axis—Right or left? Positive or negative? If present, think hypertrophy and infarction.
- Hypertrophy
  - Atrial—V_1—diphasic P wave
    - Large *initial* positive deflection—right atrial hypertrophy
    - Large *ending* negative deflection—left atrial hypertrophy
  - Ventricular
    - V_1—positive deflection of QRS—right ventricular hypertrophy
    - V_2—inverted and asymmetric T—right ventricular hypertrophy
    - Check V_1—if deep S wave, measure
    - Check V_5—if large R wave, measure
    - Add V_1 and V_5 together; if greater than 35 mm—left ventricular hypertrophy

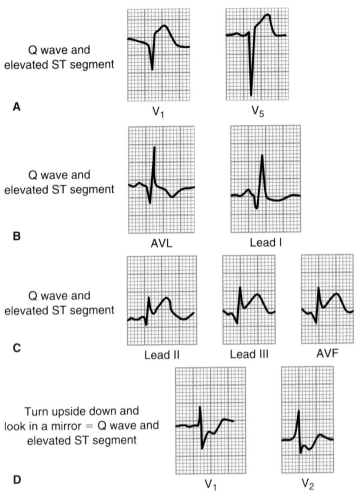

Figure 84.13 Myocardial infarction. (A) Anterior infarction, (B) lateral infarction, (C) inferior infarction, and (D) posterior infarction.

- Check V_5 and V_6—if inverted and asymmetric T wave = left ventricular hypertrophy
- Hypoxia
  - Ischemia—smiley face—T wave inverted and symmetric in V_1 to V_6 only
  - Injury—frowny face—ST segment elevated—acute full-thickness MI
    - Depressed ST segment = partial-thickness MI
  - Infarction
    - Q wave present
    - ST elevation
      - Anterior MI—Q in V_1 to V_4 and ST wave elevation
      - Lateral MI—aVL and lead I—Q wave and ST wave elevation
      - Inferior MI—aVF, leads II and III—Q wave and ST wave elevation

• Posterior MI—opposite of anterior MI; larger R wave with ST wave depression

OTHER HEART PROBLEMS

See Figures 84.14 and 84.15.

• Digitalis effect—downsloping QT segment
• Digitalis toxicity—PVCs (bigeminy or trigeminy), ventricular tachycardia, ventricular fibrillation, atrial fibrillation
• Emphysema—low voltage in leads I, II, and III and right axis deviation (lead I negative, aVF positive)
• Hypercalcemia—short QT segment
• Hypocalcemia—long QT segment

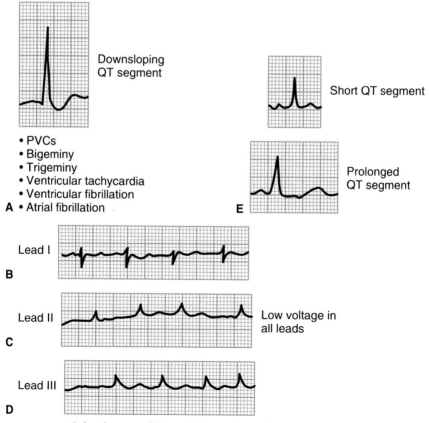

Figure 84.14 Other heart problems. (A) Digitalis effect, (B) digitalis toxicity, (C) emphysema, (D) hypercalcemia, and (E) hypocalcemia.

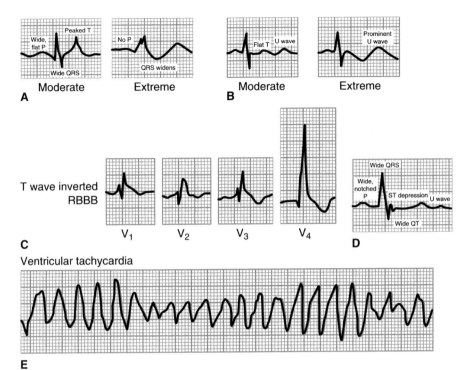

Figure 84.15 Other heart problems. (A) Hyperkalemia, (B) hypokalemia, (C) pulmonary embolus, (D) quinidine effect, and (E) quinidine toxicity.

- Hyperkalemia—peaked T wave, flattened P wave, widened QRS
- Hypokalemia
  - Moderate—flat T wave
  - Extreme—prominent U wave (wave sometimes appearing immediately after the T wave)
- Pulmonary embolus
  - Large S wave in lead I
  - ST segment depression in lead II
  - Large Q wave in lead III with T wave inversion
  - Right BBB and T wave inversion in V_1 to V_4
- Quinidine effect—notched P wave, widened QRS, ST segment depressed, prolonged QT segment, U waves
- Quinidine toxicity—ventricular tachycardia

85

Electrocardiogram (EKG) Lead Placement

Margaret R. Colyar

CPT Code
93000 EKG, routine; with at least 12 leads; with interpretation and report
93005 EKG tracing only; with interpretation and report
93010 EKG interpretation and report only

To ensure an accurate EKG, correct lead placement is vital. Leads that are misplaced can cause potentially dangerous interpretation errors.

OVERVIEW

- Common errors include
  - Placement of leads in wrong anatomical locations
    - Switching one lead with another lead in a comparable area
    - Inaccurate positioning, especially precordial, can create the impression of mirror-image dextrocardia or possible lateral MI.
  - Exchange of two or more precordial leads can produce misleading patterns.
  - Exchange of right and left leg leads—no significant change
  - Exchange of left leg and left arm leads—insignificant Q wave in lead III
  - Exchange of left arm and right leg leads—low voltage in lead III
  - Leg leads placed on abdomen or arm leads placed on upper chest—distortion of pattern
  - Exchange of right and left arm leads—misinterpretation of pattern—lateral MI
  - Exchange of right arm and right or left leg leads—misinterpretation of pattern—inferior wall MI or previous MI, pericardial effusion, emphysema, or thyroid problem
  - When placing electrodes on a *female* client, always place the electrodes under the breast rather than on the breast.

RATIONALE

- To ensure satisfactory EKG tracings
- To promote pertinent EKG readings

INDICATIONS

- Chest pain
- Rule out cardiac involvement

CONTRAINDICATIONS

- None

PROCEDURE

EKG Lead Placement

Equipment

- EKG machine with limb leads, chest leads, and cable
- EKG paper
- Electrodes
- Grounded safe electrical outlet

Procedure

- Position the client supine.
- Plug in machine.
- Enter client identification data into the machine, if required.
- Set speed at 25 mm/sec and size sensitivity at 10 mm/sec.
- Cleanse skin with alcohol if dirty or oily.
- Apply electrodes in proper configuration.
  - Limb leads (Fig. 85.1)
    - Legs—distal third of lower leg on anterior medial surface
    - Arms—volar surface of distal third of forearms
  - Chest leads (Fig. 85.2)
    - V_1—fourth intercostal space (ICS) right sternal border
    - V_2—fourth ICS left sternal border
    - V_3—halfway between V_2 and V_4
    - V_4—fifth ICS midclavicular line
    - V_5—anterior axillary line lateral to V_4
    - V_6—midaxillary line lateral to V_5
- Attach cable to the electrodes.
- Push the record button.
- If an arrhythmia is seen, obtain a rhythm strip (long lead II).
- Remove the electrodes and cleanse the skin if needed.

Client Instructions

- Lie still while the EKG machine is running.
- There will be no electrical shock.

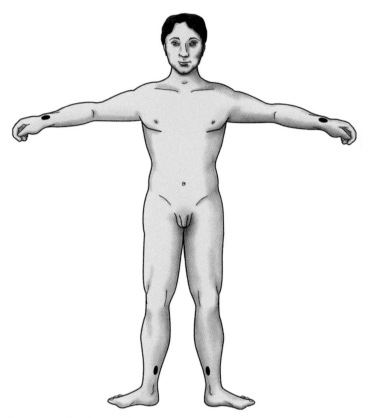

Figure 85.1 Limb lead placement.

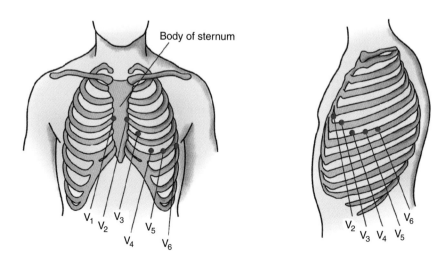

Figure 85.2 Chest lead placement.

BIBLIOGRAPHY ▮▮▮▮▮▮▮▮▮▮▮▮▮▮▮▮▮▮▮▮▮▮▮▮▮▮▮

Batchvarov VN, Malik M, Camm AJ. Incorrect electrode cable connection during electrocardiographic recording. *Europace*. 2007;9:1081–1090. http://europace.oxfordjournals.org/content/9/11/1081.full.pdf.

Edmunds MW. *Procedures for Primary Care Practitioners*. St. Louis, MO: Mosby; 2016.

Peberdy MA, Ornato JP. ECG leads: Misplacement and misdiagnosis. *Emerg Med*. October 1994:37–38.

Chapter **86**

Holter Monitor Application
Continuous 24-Hour Ambulatory Cardiac Monitoring

Margaret R. Colyar

CPT Code
93230–37 EKG monitoring for 24 hours

A Holter monitor is a portable EKG machine with memory. A Holter monitor oversees cardiac activity for 24 hours, usually to detect and evaluate cardiac disease, drug effects, and pacemakers.

OVERVIEW

• During the 24-hour period, the heart has approximately 100,000 cardiac cycles.
• Used to evaluate
  • Arrhythmias
  • Chest pain
  • Poor blood flow (ischemia)
  • Cause of fainting and/or dizziness
  • Effect of antiarrhythmic drug therapy
  • Client status after an acute MI
  • Client status after the implantation of a pacemaker

RATIONALE

• To detect and evaluate cardiac disease, drug effects, and operation of pacemakers

INDICATIONS

- MI
- Pacemaker
- Chest pain
- Cardiac symptoms
- Unexplained fainting

CONTRAINDICATIONS

- None

PROCEDURE

Holter Monitoring

Equipment

- Monitor with new battery
- Case with strap
- Cassette tape
- Electrodes
- Electrode gel
- Cable and lead wires
- Alcohol or **acetone**
- 4 × 4 gauze—nonsterile
- Disposable razor
- Tape
- Diary

Procedure

- Position the client in a seated, upright position.
- Shave the electrode-placement sites.
- Cleanse the electrode sites with alcohol or acetone to remove body oils.
- Apply electrodes. Follow directions for unit being used.
  - Remove paper backing.
  - Press firmly in position.
  - Attach the cables to the electrodes.
- Attach the cables to the monitor.
- Place the monitor strap around the client's neck.
- Place the monitor in the monitor case.
- Run the monitor cables through the front of the client's shirt or blouse and button.
- Ground wire—Place over the left midclavicular line at the first ICS.

DIARY

Log all daily activities (Fig. 86.1). Compare with the Holter recording to determine a correlation between the client's symptoms and cardiac arrhythmias.

- Fill the diary with time and activity whenever you change activity, such as
  - Stair climbing
  - Running

Time	Activity	Symptoms
9 AM	Watching TV	
11:30 AM	Eating lunch	Short of breath
1 PM	Reading	
2 PM	Taking a walk	Dizzy, short of breath
3:30 PM	Went to pick up children	Dizzy, chest pain, sweaty
5 PM	Eating supper	Short of breath
7 PM	Watching TV	
9:30 PM	To bed	Weak
6 AM	Getting ready for work	Short of breath, chest pain
7 AM	At computer at work	Dizzy, weak

Figure 86.1 Example of a daily diary.

- Walking
- Sleeping
- Elimination
- Intercourse
- Emotional upset
  - Note physical symptoms such as
    - Dizziness
    - Palpitations
    - Chest pain
    - Any pain
    - Fatigue
    - Shortness of breath

* Ingestion of medications
* Eating

Client Instructions

* Wear loose-fitting clothes.
* Wear a watch so that you can complete accurately the activity and symptom diary.
* You may take a sponge bath, but avoid wetting the equipment and dislodging the electrodes. If the electrodes become dislodged, do the following:
  * Partially dislodged—Depress the center to reattach.
  * Fully dislodged—Return to the office for lead placement.
* Avoid magnets, metal detectors (e.g., at airports), high-voltage areas, and electric blankets.

BIBLIOGRAPHY

Grauer K, Leytem B. A systemic approach to Holter monitor interpretation. *Am Fam Physician.* 1992;45:1641–1645.

Pfenninger JL, Fowler GC. *Procedures for Primary Care Physicians.* St. Louis, MO: Mosby; 2019.

Thaler MS. *The Only EKG Book You'll Ever Need.* Philadelphia, PA: Lippincott; 2018.

Chapter

87

Stress Testing (Stress EKG)

Margaret R. Colyar

CPT Code
93016 Stress test: Supervision only, without interpretation and report

---

Stress testing shows how the heart works during physical stress and is a useful screening tool for the detection of significant coronary artery disease. It is designed to determine whether one or more of the coronary arteries feeding the heart contains fatty deposits that block a blood vessel by 70% or more. Stress testing is needed for many reasons (Table 87.1).

OVERVIEW

* Two types of stress tests
  * Standard stress test—shows changes in the heart's electrical activity during exercise

Table 87·1	**Reasons for Stress Testing**

To determine whether a person can handle an exercise program after
- Coronary heart disease
- Myocardial infarction

To determine how well treatment relieves symptoms
- Angioplasty—with or without stent placement
- Coronary artery bypass grafting

Other signs of heart problems
- Chest pain
- Rapid heartbeat
- Fluttering in chest
- Feeling faint
- Shortness of breath

- Imaging stress test—shows blood flow throughout the heart, heart valve action, and movement of the heart muscle. Imaging stress tests include
  - Stress echo—uses ultrasound
  - Positron emission tomography (PET)—uses radioactive dye injected intravenously
  - Thallium stress test—uses radioactive dye injected intravenously
- Risks linked with stress testing
  - Irregular heartbeat
  - Low blood pressure
  - Dizziness
  - Fainting
  - Jitteriness
  - Chest pain
  - Wheezing
  - Shortness of breath
- Areas to be evaluated prior to stress testing are shown in Table 87.2.

RATIONALE
- To detect significant coronary artery disease
- To evaluate medical therapy
- To evaluate cardiac rehabilitation following myocardial infarction

CONTRAINDICATIONS
- See absolute and relative contraindications in Table 87.3.

Procedure

STANDARD EXERCISE STRESS TEST
- Explain the procedure to the patient.
- Apply EKG electrodes and connect to EKG monitor.

Table 87·2	**Pertinent Data Needed Before Exercise Stress Testing**

History
- Type, character, direction, and radiation of symptoms
- Medications

Physical Examination
- Cardiac
- Pulmonary
- Vascular
- Musculoskeletal

Laboratory Values
- Complete blood count
- Comprehensive metabolic panel
- Thyroid-stimulating hormone (TSH)
- Free T4
- Cardiac enzymes
- Prothrombin time/international normalized ratio (PT/INR)
- Lipids

Resting EKG

- Apply a blood pressure cuff.
- Record baseline EKG and vital signs—blood pressure, respiratory rate, and heart rate.
- Have the patient get on the treadmill and start walking.
- Inform the patient that the rate will increase and the incline will increase every 3 minutes until the patient reaches his or her target heart rate (220 – patient's age × 0.85 beats/min).
- Monitor and record EKG and vital signs every 3 minutes.
- Stop the test if
  - The patient feels chest pain
  - The patient becomes short of breath
  - The patient becomes dizzy
  - EKG shows ischemia
  - The patient exhibits excessive tiredness
  - The patient experiences leg pain
  - The patient's blood pressure becomes abnormally high or low
- When patient reaches the target heart rate, stop the test and continue monitoring for at least 10 to 15 minutes or until the heart rate returns to baseline.

Interpretation—See Table 87.4 for items included in stress testing interpretation.

Table 87-3 Contraindications for Exercise Stress Testing

- Acute cardiac problems
  - Myocardial infarction
  - Unstable angina
  - Pericarditis
  - Endocarditis
  - Myocarditis
  - Congestive heart failure—severe
  - Ventricular arrhythmias—uncontrolled sustained
  - Supraventricular arrhythmias—symptomatic
  - High-grade AV block
  - Significant aortic stenosis
- Other cardiac conditions
  - Mitral valve prolapse
  - Wolff-Parkinson-White syndrome
- Malignant hypertension (systolic >200 mm Hg or diastolic >110 mm Hg)
- Severe acute medical illness
  - Anemia
  - Hepatic disorder
  - Renal disorder
  - Metabolic disorder
  - Thyroid disorder
- Electrolyte abnormalities
  - Calcium
  - Magnesium
  - Potassium
- Thromboembolic processes
  - Pulmonary embolism
  - Deep vein thrombosis
- Poor candidate for exercise
  - Physical disability
  - Crippling arthritis
  - Extreme obesity, >350 lb
- Medications
  - Digoxin
  - Type I antiarrhythmic agents
  - Tricyclic antidepressants
  - Vasodilators
  - Beta-adrenergic blockers

Table 87·4	Items Included in Interpretation of Exercise Stress Test

- EKG interpretation
- Symptoms reported during testing
- Reason for ending exercise
- Estimate of exercise capacity in metabolic equivalents (METS)
- Blood pressure response
- Presence and frequency of arrhythmias
- Conclusions
  - Positive—development of
    - Exercise-induced hypotension
    - Exercise-induced angina
    - Appearance of S_3, S_4, or heart murmur during exercise
  - Negative
    - No exercise-induced hypotension
    - No exercise-induced angina
    - No appearance of S_3, S_4, or heart murmur during exercise
  - Equivocal—development of
    - Premature ventricular contractions
    - Atrial or junctional tachyarrhythmias
  - Uninterpretable—development of
    - Primary or secondary atrioventricular blocks
    - Bundle-branch blocks
    - Hemiblocks
    - Changing atrioventricular conduction
- Goal achieved
  - Maximal—achieves the target heart rate, exercise level, or time limit established for the patient
  - Submaximal—does not achieve the target heart rate, exercise level, or time limit established for the patient

Client Instructions

- No caffeinated beverages 24 hours before the test.
- No eating or smoking for 3 hours prior to the test.
- Wear comfortable shoes and loose clothing.
- Check with primary care provider regarding medications to be taken or excluded prior to the test.
- Diabetics may be asked to adjust their medications the day of the test—usually no insulin and only a half dosage of oral hypoglycemic agents the day of the test.

BIBLIOGRAPHY ▰▰▰▰▰▰▰▰▰▰▰▰▰▰▰

Darrow MD. Ordering and understanding the exercise stress test. *Am Fam Physician.* 1999;59(2):401–410.

Stress Testing. National Heart, Lung, and Blood Institute Web site. https://www.nhlbi.nih .gov/health-topics/stress-testing

Chapter **88**

Types of Pacemakers

Margaret R. Colyar

CPT Code
None

A pacemaker is a small, battery-operated device that senses the beating of the heart and sends an electrical stimulus to the heart to beat at the correct pace.

OVERVIEW

- Pacemakers can have one, two, or three wires.
  - Single-chamber—one wire to right ventricle
  - Dual-chamber—two wires; one to the right atrium and one to the right ventricle to help coordinate timing of the two chambers' contractions
  - Biventricular—three wires; one to the atrium and two to the ventricles (one to each ventricle)
    - Used in severe heart failure and matches up the beating of both sides of the heart
    - Also used as an implantable cardiac resynchronization therapy (CRT) and cardiac defibrillator (ICD)
- There are two types of pacemaker programming
  - Demand—Sends electrical impulse if the heart is slow or misses a beat.
  - Rate responsive—Speeds up or slows down the heart rate based on activity. Monitors sinus node rate, breathing, and blood temperature.

RATIONALE

- To correctly pace the heart
- To slow the heart
- To correct abnormal rhythm
- To coordinate electrical signaling between the ventricles
- To coordinate electrical signaling between the upper and lower chambers of the heart

INDICATIONS

- Arrhythmias—atrial fibrillation
- Bradycardia
- Certain congenital heart disorders
- Heart failure with ejection fraction less than 35%
- Heart transplants
- History of cardiac arrest
- Long QT syndrome
- Syncope
- Tachycardia

COMPLICATIONS

- Dislodgment of lead—occurs in 2.5% of patients
- Malposition—usually occurs with patients with atrial or ventricular septal defects
- Venous thrombosis—occurs in up to 40% of patients; symptoms include neck discomfort, swelling of the arms, face, and head
- Device problems—conductor failure, insulator failure
- Abnormal heart rhythms
- Bleeding
- Punctured lung
- Infection
- Puncture of the heart

Client Instructions

- Have pacemaker checked every 3 months.
- Battery replacement should occur between 5 and 15 years (average is 6 to 7 years).
- Avoid prolonged contact/exposure with electrical devices or devices with strong magnetic fields such as
  - Cell phones—may have in shirt pocket if cell phone is turned off
  - MP3 players—wear on right arm
  - Microwaves
  - High-tension wires
  - Metal detectors
- Stay 2 feet away from industrial welders and electrical generators.
- No MRI, shock-wave lithotripsy, electrocauterization to stop bleeding during surgery.
- Wear a medical identification tag.
- Avoid full-contact sports.

BIBLIOGRAPHY

Kotsakou M, Kioumis J, Lazaridis G, et al. Pacemaker insertion. *Ann Trans Med*. 2015:3(3):42.
Panicker GK, Desai B, Lokhandwala Y. Choosing pacemakers appropriately. *Heart Asia*. 2009; 1(1):26–30. Available at https://www.ncbi.nlm.nih.gov/pmc/articles/PMC4898486/.

Chapter **89**

Arterial Puncture
Margaret R. Colyar

CPT Code
82803   Gases, blood, any combination of pH, P_{CO_2}, P_{O_2}, CO_2, HCO_3
(including calculated O_2 saturation)

Arterial puncture is performed to determine the client's acid-base balance, oxygenation, and ventilation. Arterial blood gases (ABGs) are a mixture of measured and calculated values. The pH, P_{O_2}, P_{CO_2}, and HCO_3 measurements are used to interpret the meaning of the ABGs. Analysis of ABGs is usually a two-step process. First, the acid-base balance is determined. Second, the oxygenation status is determined. Normal ABG values are given in Table 89.1. Abnormal ABG values with interpretation are given in Table 89.2.

OVERVIEW
- Site selection (Fig. 89.1)
  - First choice—radial artery
    - Less chance of hematoma because of the ease of compression over bones and ligaments of wrist.
    - Do **Allen's test** to check for collateral circulation through the ulnar artery before the stick (Fig. 89.2).
  - Second choice—brachial artery
    - Larger artery but deeper and close to a vein and nerve
  - Third choice—femoral artery
    - Large artery
    - Easily palpated and punctured but poor collateral circulation
    - Increased risk of infection because of the location of the site
    - Palpate just below inguinal ligament
    - From lateral to medial, structures are
      - Nerve
      - Artery
      - Vein

RATIONALE
- To determine acid-base balance, oxygenation, and ventilation

Table 89·1	Normal Values for Arterial Blood Gases		
pH	**PCO$_2$**	**HCO$_3$**	**PO$_2$**
7.35–7.45	35–45 mm Hg	24–28 mEq/L	75–100 mm Hg

Table 89·2	Abnormal (Arterial Blood Gas) Values With Interpretation		
pH	**PCO$_2$**	**HCO$_3$**	**INTERPRETATION**
<7.35	>45	Normal	Respiratory acidosis
<7.35	>45	>28	Respiratory acidosis with metabolic compensation
>7.45	<35	Normal	Respiratory alkalosis
>7.45	<35	<24	Respiratory alkalosis with metabolic compensation
<7.35	Normal	<24	Metabolic acidosis
<7.35	<35	<24	Metabolic acidosis with respiratory compensation
>7.45	Normal	>28	Metabolic alkalosis
>7.45	>45	>28	Metabolic alkalosis with respiratory compensation

INDICATIONS

- Respiratory disorder
- Cardiac failure
- Renal disease
- Drug overdose
- Uncontrolled diabetes mellitus
- Metabolic disorder

CONTRAINDICATIONS

- No collateral circulation

PROCEDURE

Arterial Puncture

Equipment

- Gloves—nonsterile
- Syringe—3 to 5 mL
- 23- to 25-gauge, 1-inch needle
- Heparin (1,000 U/mL), 1 mL
- Alcohol swabs
- Povidone-iodine (Betadine) swabs
- Cup of ice
- Small block of rubber or latex
- 2 × 2 gauze
- Tape

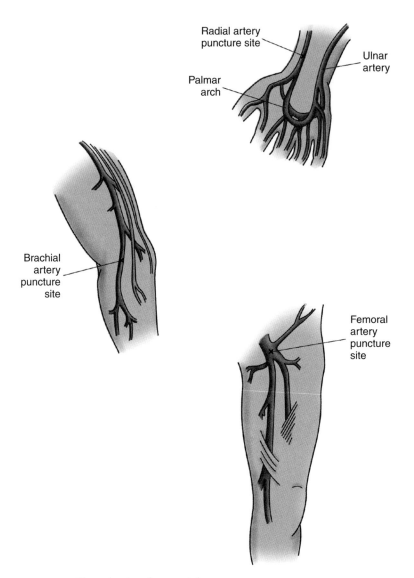

Figure 89.1 Site selection for arterial puncture.

Procedure

- Select the site.
- Position the client with the site easily accessible. If using the radial artery, the wrist should be hyperextended.
- Put on gloves.
- Draw up 1 mL of 1:1,000 heparin into the syringe.
  - Pull the plunger all the way back.
  - Expel all the heparin. The syringe is now coated with heparin.

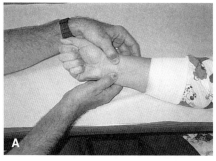
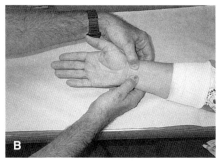
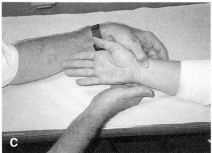

Figure 89.2 Check for collateral circulation using the Allen's test. The client makes a fist while the radial and ulnar arteries are occluded. (A) The thenar surface of the palm becomes pale. (B) The client opens the palm and the pallor remains while the arteries are occluded. (C) When the ulnar occlusion is removed, the palm should return to pink.

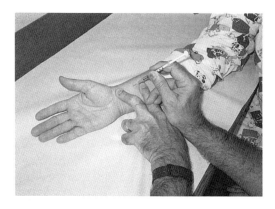

Figure 89.3 Trap the artery between two fingers. After preparing the site, insert the needle at a 90-degree angle into the artery.

- Palpate the artery proximally and distally (Fig. 89.3).
- Cleanse the site with alcohol.
- Apply povidone-iodine to the area in a circular motion, starting where you plan to puncture and working outward.
- Trap the artery between two fingers placed on each side.
- Hold the syringe like a pencil, with the bevel up.
- Using a 90-degree angle, insert the needle.
- The syringe usually fills spontaneously. If it does not fill spontaneously, aspirate gently.
  - If you do not get blood, pull back the needle without coming out of the skin and redirect toward the artery.

- When the specimen is obtained, withdraw the needle.
  - Apply firm pressure to the site for 5 minutes; apply pressure for 10 minutes if the client is on anticoagulants.
  - Expel the air from the syringe.
  - Rotate the syringe to mix the contents.
  - Place the needle tip into a rubber block.
  - Place the syringe into a cup of ice.
- Check the site for bleeding.
- Cleanse the site with alcohol and apply a 2 × 2 pressure dressing.

Client Instructions

- Keep pressure dressing in place for 30 minutes, then remove.
- Observe for signs and symptoms of infection, such as
  - Increase in pain after 24 hours
  - Increase in temperature
  - Redness or swelling
  - Yellow or greenish drainage
  - Foul odor
- If any signs or symptoms of infection are found, return to the office.

BIBLIOGRAPHY

Gomella LG. *Clinician's Pocket Reference.* Norwalk, CT: Appleton & Lange; 2006.
McCall RE, Tankersley CM. *Phlebotomy Essentials.* Philadelphia, PA: Lippincott; 2015.

Chapter **90**

Blood Culture Specimen Collection
Margaret R. Colyar

CPT Code
36415 Blood specimen collection
87040 Blood culture collection

Blood culture specimen collection requires a precise specimen collection procedure to obtain, store, and transport correctly. Culture medium is inoculated with a blood sample and incubated for isolation and identification of pathogens. Many laboratories have their own policy for blood culture specimen collection. Check with the laboratory to determine any special requirements.

OVERVIEW

- Assists in
  - Identification of approximately 70% of pathogens within 24 hours
  - Identification of approximately 90% of pathogens with 72 hours
- Sample collection
  - Types of blood cultures (Table 90.1)
  - Number and timing of blood cultures (Table 90.2)
    - Microorganisms enter bloodstream 30 to 90 minutes before fever spikes.
  - Amount of blood needed (Table 90.3)
- Do *not* use vacutainer needle to draw cultures.
- Do *not* change needle between blood draw and transfer to culture medium (chance of contamination). Some laboratories require change of needle at this step.

Table 90·1	Types of Blood Cultures
Aerobic	
Anaerobic	
Fungal	
Mycobacterial	
Viral	

Table 90·2 Blood Cultures—Number and Timing	
DISEASE PROCESS	**NUMBER/TIMING**
Acute sepsis	Two or three sets from separate sites
Endocarditis	Three sets from three separate sites over
• Acute	1 to 2 hr
• Subacute	Three sets on day 1 (15 min apart)
Fever of unknown origin	Three separate sets 1 hr apart. If negative, redraw in 36 hr
On antimicrobial treatment for 1 to 2 wk	Two separate sets on three successive days

Table 90·3 Blood Cultures—Amount of Blood to Obtain	
AGE	**AMOUNT OF BLOOD**
Neonate	1 mL
Small child	4 mL
Adult	Bacterial—20 mL Fungal—30 mL

RATIONALE

- To confirm bacteremia or septicemia
- To identify causative organisms

INDICATIONS

- Fever/chills
- Sepsis
- Prostration
- Pain/headache
- Nausea/vomiting
- Diarrhea—unexplained
- Signs of shock—drop in blood pressure, increased respirations, tachycardia
- Coma
- Mental confusion/anxiety
- Bacterial pneumonia
- Infectious endocarditis

CONTRAINDICATIONS

- Surveillance of infection before the clinical suspicion of infection exists

PROCEDURE

Blood Culture Specimen Collection

Equipment

- Two inoculated culture media—in bottles (Fig. 90.1)
- Three alcohol swabs
- Three povidone-iodine swabs
- Gloves—nonsterile
- Tourniquet
- Syringes—two to three each—20 mL
- Needles—20 gauge
- 2 × 2 gauze or cotton balls
- Two adhesive bandages (Band-Aids) or tape
- One 4 × 4 gauze

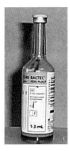

Figure 90.1 Blood culture medium bottle.

Procedure

- Put on gloves.
- Remove outer cap from blood culture medium bottles.
- Cleanse top of bottles with alcohol.
- Vigorously cleanse site with alcohol swab for 1 minute.
- Allow to air-dry.
- Cleanse site with 10% iodine/povidone-iodine swab in circular motion from center outward in concentric circles.
- Let dry for 1 minute.
- Cleanse top of culture medium bottles with povidone-iodine.
- Apply tourniquet to client's arm.
- Do *not* palpate vein after prepared.
- Draw blood specimen.
- Remove the tourniquet from the arm.
- Remove the needle from the arm.
- Apply pressure to the puncture site with a cotton ball or 2 × 2 gauze.
  - Keep pressure to site for 1 minute (if client is on anticoagulant therapy, apply pressure to 3 to 5 minutes).
  - Wipe residual povidone-iodine from site with alcohol prep pads.
- Apply an adhesive bandage or tape to secure.
- Inject appropriate amount of blood in each of two inoculated culture medium bottles.
- Invert bottles four to five times.
- Deposit the needles in a puncture-proof container.
- Label the culture medium bottles with the appropriate information (i.e., client's name, date, time, ID number, and your initials).
- Transport to the laboratory.
  - Do not refrigerate.

Client Instructions

- Adhesive bandage may be removed in 15 minutes.
- Do not rub the site because rubbing increases risk of oozing and results in a bruised appearance.

BIBLIOGRAPHY

Colyar MR. *Well Child Assessment for Health Care Providers*. Philadelphia, PA: F.A. Davis; 2002.

McCall RE, Tankersley CM. *Phlebotomy Essentials*. Philadelphia, PA: Lippincott Williams & Wilkins, 2015.

Myers FE, Reyes C. Blood cultures: 5 steps to doing it right. *Nursing*. 2011:41(3); 62–63.

Springhouse. *Diagnostics, Nurse's Reference Library*. Springhouse, PA: Springhouse; 2000.

Central Venous Catheter Access (Portacath)

Margaret R. Colyar

CPT Code
36540   Collection of blood specimen from venous access device
90798   Intravenous infusion for therapy/diagnosis

Portacaths (ports) or mediports are central vascular access devices, fully implanted under the skin, usually on the patient's chest under general anesthesia. Ports consist of a metal or plastic housing attached to a silicone catheter with a self-sealing silicone gel inside the housing. The tip of the catheter is inserted in the subclavian vein and advanced to the superior vena cava.

OVERVIEW

- When accessing, using, and maintaining the port, the risk of life-threatening complications, such as infection, makes it important to use correct and sterile technique.
- Advantages of the portacath include
  - Nothing external when the port is not in use
  - Little maintenance when the port is not accessed
  - Quick needle-stick venous access versus repeated venipunctures
  - Irritating medicines infused into larger veins without discomfort owing to dilution by rapid blood flow
- Disadvantages of the portacath include
  - Surgical implantation needed
  - Painful access unless topical anesthetic cream used
  - Frequent access may lead to increased infection risk
  - Catheter thrombosis
  - Mechanical problems, such as leaking around the diaphragm
- To be used for continuous infusions, bolus injections, cyclic therapies such as chemotherapy, hypertransfusion with blood products for patients with hemoglobinopathies, and primary/secondary prophylaxis in children with hemophilia

RATIONALE

- To allow irritating medicines to be infused without discomfort

- To provide easy venous access for adults and children with chronic problems who need continuous infusion, bolus injections, cyclic therapies, hypertransfusion, or primary/secondary prophylaxis

INDICATIONS

- Cancer
- Hemophilia
- Sickle cell disease
- Cystic fibrosis
- Other chronic illness with poor intravenous access
- Infections requiring long-term antibiotics

CONTRAINDICATIONS

- Redness, swelling, or tenderness over or around the site of the port
- Unable to get a free-flowing blood return from the port
- Pain or a stinging sensation during infusion

PROCEDURE

Central Venous Access (Portacath)

Equipment

- Topical anesthetic cream (Emla)
- Tegaderm to cover (Emla)
- Alcohol wipes
- Povidone-iodine wipes
- Gloves—sterile
- Huber noncoring needle
- Semipermeable transparent dressing to cover Huber needle
- 2 × 2 sterile gauze
- 0.9% normal saline—10 mL
- Syringe—10 mL
- Heparin 100 U/mL or 10 U/mL/kg

Procedure

- Palpate upper chest to locate port.
- Observe site for redness, swelling, or tenderness.
- To numb the skin, apply Emla cream over port and cover with Tegaderm. Leave Emla on for 30 minutes.
- Remove Tegaderm and wipe off anesthetic cream.
- Set up sterile field.
- Put on sterile gloves.
- Do not touch anything outside the field until the procedure is done.
- Using sterile technique, cleanse the area over the port with alcohol, then with povidone-iodine.
  - Start cleansing in the center of the port, and wipe outward in a circular pattern with a 2-inch radius.

- Leave povidone-iodine to dry for 30 seconds.
- Using your nondominant hand, locate the edge of the port housing and stabilize with the thumb and index finger.
- Insert the Huber needle through the skin and silicone gel until the port's rigid housing is felt (Fig. 91.1).
- Aspirate for blood return to confirm the needle is in the port.
- Flush with 10 mL of 0.9% saline.
- Place sterile gauze under the wings of the Huber needle.
- Cover Huber needle with semipermeable transparent dressing.
- Start infusion.
- Change Huber needle and transparent dressing every 7 days using sterile technique.
- Change administration set using sterile technique every 72 hours if medication or fluid infusing and every 24 hours if total parental nutrition or blood products are infusing.
- To discontinue the Huber needle, first flush with 20 mL of 0.9% saline and 5 mL of heparin. Then remove the transparent dressing and needle, and cover the Portacath with sterile gauze and tape.
- Heparin lock (Heplock) the central venous access port if it is not being used for infusion using sterile technique.
- When port is accessed and not being used for infusion, flush daily with 5 mL of heparin (patients weighing more than 10 kg, use 100 U/mL of heparin; patients weighing less than 10 kg, use 10 U/mL of heparin).

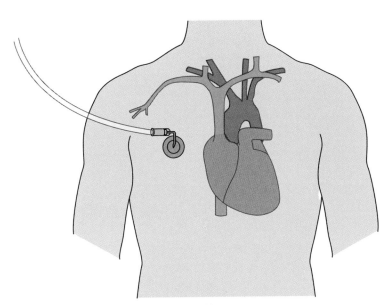

Figure 91.1 Positioning of Huber needle.

Client Instructions

- After portacath needle is removed, sterile gauze is taped to cover the portacath.
  - Gauze and tape should be removed by the next day.
- No dressing is needed when the port is not accessed.
- If the access site becomes red, becomes painful, or has yellow-green drainage, contact your health-care provider immediately.

BIBLIOGRAPHY

Graham AS. Central venous catheterization. *N Engl J Med.* 2007;357:943–945.

92 Chapter

Defibrillation

Margaret R. Colyar

CPT Code
92950 CPR in emergency situation

Defibrillation is a process in which an electrical device is used to send an electric shock to the heart to stop an arrhythmia, resulting in the return of a productive heart rhythm. Defibrillation is performed to correct life-threatening arrhythmias of ventricular fibrillation, pulseless ventricular tachycardia, and cardiac arrest. In cardiac emergencies, it should be performed immediately after identifying that the patient is experiencing an arrhythmia with lack of pulse and unresponsiveness. It is also used to ablate atrial fibrillation and atrial flutter. After defibrillation, the patient's cardiac status, breathing, and vital signs are monitored with a cardiac monitor. Additional tests to measure cardiac damage should be performed, such as a 12-lead electrocardiogram, a chest x-ray, and cardiac catheterization.

OVERVIEW

- Two methods of defibrillation
  - Defibrillator pads
  - Defibrillator paddles
- Different energy settings are required for the two types of defibrillators (Table 92.1)
  - Monophasic—a type of defibrillation waveform in which a shock is delivered to the heart from one direction from one pad or paddle to the other. Does not take into account impedance (patient resistance to flow).

Table 92·1	Monophasic Versus Biphasic Energy Settings			
	FIRST ATTEMPT	**SECOND ATTEMPT**	**THIRD ATTEMPT**	**FOURTH ATTEMPT**
Monophasic				
Adult	200 J	300 J	360 J	360 J
Pediatric	2 J/kg	2 J/kg	2 J/kg	2 J/kg
Biphasic				
Adult	120 J	150 J	200 J	200 J
Pediatric	2 J/kg	2 J/kg	2 J/kg	2 J/kg

Note: J, joules.

- Biphasic—a type of defibrillation waveform in which a shock is delivered to the heart via two pads or paddles. Takes into account impedance (patient resistance to flow).

RATIONALE

- To reestablish a perfusing cardiac rhythm

INDICATIONS

- Cardiac arrest
- Ventricular fibrillation
- Pulseless ventricular tachycardia

CONTRAINDICATIONS

- Patient has a pulse.
- Patient is alert.
- Defibrillator should not be placed over an implanted pacemaker.
- Patient is in asystole.

PROCEDURE

- Check for pulselessness.
- Begin cardiac pulmonary resuscitation (CPR).
- Establish an airway.
- Place pads or paddles
  - One laterally in left midaxillary line at the fourth intercostal space
  - One anteriorly just right of midsternal margin at the second or third intercostal space
- Attach the cables and turn the monitor on.
- Confirm the rhythm.
- Select the appropriate energy level; usually, this is 200 joules.
- Announce, "Charging defibrillator; everybody clear."
- Push the CHARGE button.
- Check to ensure that everyone is clear.

- Push the SHOCK button.
- If the person is still in ventricular fibrillation or pulseless ventricular tachycardia, resume CPR.
- Wait 2 minutes to evaluate rhythm.
- If the person is still in ventricular fibrillation or pulseless ventricular tachycardia, repeat the procedures using the same energy level.

Using Defibrillator Paddles

Procedure

- Apply electrode gel.
- Place paddles on the patient's chest.
  - One laterally in left midaxillary line at the fourth intercostal space
  - One anteriorly just right of midsternal margin at the second or third intercostal space
- Press downward with 25 pounds of pressure.
- Announce, "Charging defibrillator; everybody clear."
- Use the buttons of the paddles to CHARGE and SHOCK.

Atrial Fibrillation and Atrial Flutter Ablation

Procedure

- Place paddles on the patient's chest.
  - One laterally in left midaxillary line at the fourth intercostal space
  - One anteriorly just right of midsternal margin at the second or third intercostal space
- Announce, "Charging defibrillator; everybody clear."
- Program the defibrillator to recognize distinct components of the electrocardiogram.
- Defibrillator will fire the electrical shock only at the correct time.

Treatment options will be determined from the outcome of these procedures. The patient's skin is cleansed to remove gel and, if necessary, electrical burns are treated.

BIBLIOGRAPHY ▬▬▬▬▬▬▬▬▬▬▬▬▬▬▬▬▬▬▬▬▬

Resuscitation Central. http://www.resuscitationcentral.com/

Chapter **93**

Unna's Boot Application
Margaret R. Colyar

CPT Code
29580   Unna's paste boot application
29405   Ankle immobilization

The **Unna's boot** is a compression paste and dressing bandage used mainly for treatment of ulcers arising from venous insufficiency. The Unna's boot is a moist dressing that works to decrease venous hypertension and so diminish the movement of fluids into the interstitium. Moist wound healing prevents the release of moisture, allowing higher collagen production, less **eschar** formation (eschar can diminish wound healing), and an increased rate of **epithelialization**.

OVERVIEW
- Venous ulcers constitute 67% to 90% of all leg ulcers (usually in elderly women).
- The Unna's boot is used to
  - Decrease pain
  - Assist venous return
  - Decrease superficial venous distention
- Venous insufficiency symptoms include
  - Pitting edema in lower legs that responds poorly to diuretics
  - Tenderness
  - Hemosiderin—reddish-brown discoloration of lower calf
  - Scaling
  - **Pruritus**
  - Erythema
- Venous ulceration usually occurs at the medial aspect of the lower leg, especially at the medial malleolus (Fig. 93.1).

RATIONALE
- To increase wound healing in patients with venous insufficiency and venous stasis ulcers
- To promote ankle stabilization

INDICATIONS
- Venous ulcers
- Ankle sprain with severe swelling

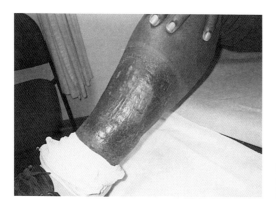

Figure 93.1 Venous ulceration on the medial aspect of the lower leg.

CONTRAINDICATIONS

- Acute pulmonary edema
- Cellulitis
- Deep vein thrombosis
- Arterial insufficiency
- Infected venous ulcers
- Phlebitis

PROCEDURE

Unna's Boot Application

Equipment

- Nonadherent wound dressing (e.g., Telfa)
- Mineral oil
- Paste bandage—impregnated with calamine, gelatin, and zinc oxide
- Soft roll, Kling, or Kerlex
- Elastic wrap (e.g., Ace wrap)
- Gloves—nonsterile
- Tape or metal fasteners

Procedure

- Position the client with the affected leg elevated above the heart and foot flexed at a right angle, promoting venous return and good ankle alignment.
- Apply a nonadherent dressing over any skin lesions.
- Moisturize the rest of the leg with mineral oil to decrease pruritus.
  - Do *not* put mineral oil on any skin lesions.
- Starting at the base of the toes, wrap the paste bandage snugly in an overlapping method to just below the knee.
  - Smooth out any wrinkles.
  - Each layer should overlap the previous wrap by 50% (Fig. 93.2).
- Wrap Kerlex, Kling, or soft roll in the same fashion over the paste bandage (Fig. 93.3).

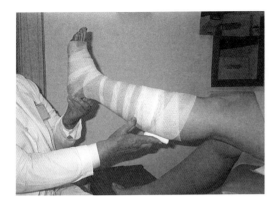

Figure 93.2 Wrap the paste bandage in an overlapping method to just below the knee.

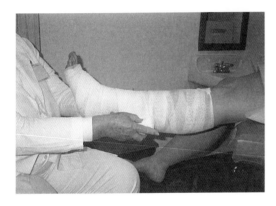

Figure 93.3 Wrap Kerlex, Kling, or soft roll in an overlapping method over the paste bandage.

- Cover with the elastic bandage. Start at the toes and work up until all the previous bandage is covered (Fig. 93.4).
- Secure with metal clips or tape.
- Keep in place 3 to 14 days. Seven days is the average.
  - The length of time the Unna's boot bandage stays on depends on the amount of exudate from the venous ulcer.

Client Instructions

- To decrease swelling and pain, elevate the foot above the heart as much as possible during the day and at bedtime.
- Do *not* get the Unna's boot bandage wet.
  - Wrap the Unna's boot in plastic before bathing and wrap with an elastic bandage up to the knee to prevent seepage of water.
- Check circulatory status frequently.
  - Check for change in color of the toes, numbness, swelling, and pain.
  - Report any changes to the practitioner immediately.
- Report any odor, drainage, or increase in itching to the practitioner.
- Do *not* scratch under the Unna's boot because this may cause wounds.

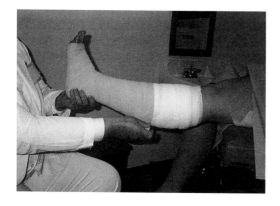

Figure 93.4 Cover the second layer with an elastic bandage in an overlapping method. Secure with metal clips or tape.

BIBLIOGRAPHY

Barr DM. The Unna's boot as a treatment for venous ulcers. *Nurse Pract.* 1996;21(7):55–75.
Colyar MR. Unna boot application. *Adv Nurse Pract.* 2006;14(8):82.
Unna's Boot Application. Rainier Medical Education Programs Web site. https://www.rainiermeded.com/foot-care-unna-boot-application-s/2292.htm

94 Chapter

Venipuncture
Margaret R. Colyar

CPT Code
36415 Routine venipuncture or finger, heel, or ear stick for collection of specimens

Venipuncture is a method used to obtain blood specimens from a vein.

OVERVIEW

- General principles
  - Collect enough of blood specimen to perform the required test.
  - Collect specimen in proper container.
  - Minimize discomfort as much as possible.
  - Minimize inconvenience to client as much as possible.
  - Know proper techniques to obtain specimen.
  - Maintain sterile technique when drawing blood specimen.

- Be aware of state law for informed consent in obtaining blood specimens (i.e., alcohol, HIV, drug screening).
- Know specific requirements for informed consent (i.e., chain-of-command documentation).

RATIONALE

- To obtain information about biochemical and biophysical status of the human organism

INDICATIONS

- Need to obtain biochemical and biophysical information concerning the physiology of a client

CONTRAINDICATIONS

- Inability to stabilize the vein site as required for successful blood drawing

PROCEDURE

Venipuncture

Equipment

- Blood specimen tube (Table 94.1)
- Plastic needle holder
- Needles for plastic needle holder (16, 18, 21 gauge)
- Vacuum butterfly adapters
- Alcohol swabs
- Povidone-iodine swabs
- Cotton balls
- Adhesive tape
- Band-Aids
- Timer
- Blood specimen stacking tray
- Centrifuge
- Blood collection tray
- Transport container
- Labels
- Laboratory order sheets
- Gloves—nonsterile
- 2 × 2 gauze
- Indelible marking pen
- Needle holders
- Tourniquets
- Puncture-resistant sharps box container (biohazard approval and markings)

Procedure

- Equipment preparation
  - Determine the type of needle or butterfly infusion needle required.
  - Attach the unused needle to the plastic needle holder.

Table 94·1	Color of Blood Specimen Tubes and Common Uses
COLOR OF SPECIMEN CONTAINER	**USE**
Red (no coagulation chemicals)	Depakene, digoxin, phenytoin (Dilantin) levels
Speckled or marbled (serum separator)	Chemistry profiles, *Helicobacter pylori* titer, lipid survey, thyroid profile
Purple (EDTA)	Complete blood count, alcohol level, hemoglobin and hematocrit measurements, sedimentation rate
Blue (citrate)	Partial thromboplastin time (INR)
Green (heparin)*	Ammonia, troponin levels
Gray (fluoride-oxalate)	Glucose, lactic acid levels

Note: A catalog of laboratory tests usually is provided by the laboratory facility to assist in choosing the appropriate blood specimen tube for the test ordered.
*Not commonly used.

- Select the appropriate blood specimen tube for test.
- Determine whether the blood sample will need special preparation after collection. Refer to the catalog of tests provided in your laboratory.
- Position the client in a comfortable position.
- Position yourself in a comfortable position with all required equipment within reach.
- Site location
  - Usually the median vein of the antecubital space of the arms is the best site in adults and children older than age 1 year (Fig. 94.1).
  - Avoid thrombosed veins.
  - If no viable antecubital veins, inspect sites distally.
  - Choose a distal site before a proximal site.
- Put on gloves.
- Cleanse the site with antiseptic (povidone-iodine or alcohol prep pads) in a circular pattern beginning at the center and expanding outward.
  - *Alcohol is avoided in cases in which drug and alcohol levels are to be measured. (This should be documented on the record.)*
- Apply a tourniquet approximately 4 to 6 inches above the vein selected firmly enough to obstruct venous flow without obstruction to arterial flow.
- Do not leave the tourniquet on longer than 1 minute.
- When a suitable vein is located, have the client make a fist.
- Palpate the vein. It should be an elastic sensation without pulsation.
- Uncap the needle.
- Stabilize the site.
- Insert the needle bevel side up at a 15-degree angle (Fig. 94.2) in line with the vein in a smooth, clean motion.
- When the needle penetrates the vein, a "give" will be felt.

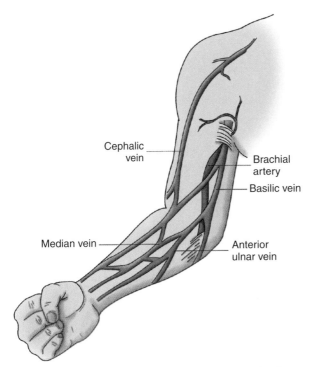

Figure 94.1 Locate the median vein in the antecubital space of the arm.

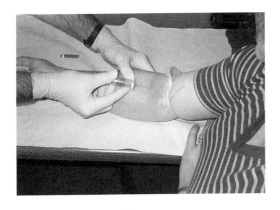

Figure 94.2 Insert the needle bevel up at a 15-degree angle in line with the vein.

- Decrease the angle and slowly insert the needle approximately ⅛ inch more or until the blood flow is adequate.
- Push blood specimen tube onto the needle.
- Allow the blood to flow until the tube is filled.
- Pull back on the blood specimen tube to dislodge it from the needle in the plastic needle holder. This releases the pressure.
- Release the tourniquet.

- Remove the needle.
- Apply pressure to the puncture site with a cotton ball in a smooth motion.
  - *Great care should be taken during this part of the procedure because this has the highest incidence of accidental needle sticks.*
- Have the client apply pressure to the site.
  - Keep pressure to site for 1 minute (if client is on anticoagulant therapy, apply pressure for 3 to 5 minutes).
- Deposit the needle in a puncture-proof container.
- Apply a Band-Aid or cover the cotton ball with tape at the venipuncture site.
- Label the specimen with the appropriate information (i.e., client's name, date, time, ID number, and your initials).
- If the specimen tube containing blood needs to be centrifuged, consult the laboratory manual for time duration.
- Fill out the appropriate laboratory form, and specify what test is to be done.
- On completion, package as directed by the laboratory for transport.

Client Instructions

- You may remove the Band-Aid in 15 minutes.
- Do not rub site because rubbing increases risk of oozing and results in a bruised appearance.

BIBLIOGRAPHY

McCall RE, Tankersley CM. *Phlebotomy Essentials.* Philadelphia, PA: Lippincott; 2015.

Respiratory Procedures

Chapter 95

Aerosol/Inhalation Administration (Nebulizer)

Cynthia R. Ehrhardt

CPT Code
94664 Aerosol inhalation—initial
94665 Aerosol inhalation—subsequent

Inhalation via aerosol administration of medication is used commonly in medical conditions of air flow obstruction, such as bronchospasm and airway hyperresponsiveness. This is considered an effective method of medication administration of drug therapy for the treatment of bronchioli pathway disorders with fewer side effects. Aerosol inhalation is extremely effective in the administration of medication in children younger than age 5 years. Fewer drug interactions and side effects have been associated with aerosol administration. Aerosol inhalation may be used as an episodic or long-term therapy.

OVERVIEW
- Incidence
  - Usage in episodic illnesses is unknown.
  - Use in chronic obstructive disorders, such as asthma and chronic pulmonary obstructive disease, is estimated at 5 million individuals.

RATIONALE
- To facilitate oxygenation in diseases affecting air flow

INDICATIONS
- Presence of medical conditions associated with bronchospasm (air flow obstruction) and hyperresponsiveness that result in compromise of the client's health status

CONTRAINDICATIONS

- None

PROCEDURE

Aerosol/Inhalation Administration

See Figure 95.1.

Equipment

- Pulse oximeter
- Peak flowmeter
- Oxygen with tubing and nebulizer mask
- Aerosol administration kit
- Air compressor (such as Pulmo-Aide or Invacare Passport)
- 0.9% sodium chloride—3 mL
- Medication (commonly used) (Table 95.1)

Procedure

- Position the client in a comfortable upright position.
- Apply the pulse oximeter, and monitor continuously throughout the procedure.
- Perform a peak flow reading and record (see Chapter 97).
- Plug the air compressor in, and open the aerosol administration kit.
- Insert the aerosol medication into the aerosol administration kit at an appropriate dosage and mixture.
- Determine the best method of administration (mask versus mouthpiece). This depends on the age of the client and ability to handle the mouthpiece versus the mask.
- Turn on the machine; a fine mist should form.
- Instruct the client to breathe in until the mist disappears, then slowly exhale.
  - Slow inhalation and exhalation should allow effective administration of medication with fewer side effects.

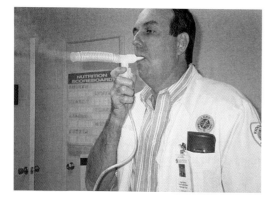

Figure 95.1 Aerosol or inhalation administration.

Table 95·1	Medications Commonly Used in Aerosol Inhalation Administration

β₂-Agonists—Short-Acting Bronchodilators

Albuterol 2.5 mg/mL
- Dosage: 0.2–0.3 mg/3 mL 0.9% sodium chloride every 4 hours
- Precautions with children younger than 2 years of age and preexisting cardiac conditions

Anti-inflammatories
- Corticosteroids
  - Methylprednisolone (Decadron) 0.5 mg
    - 1 mg mixed in 3 mL 0.9% sodium chloride with or without administration of albuterol
    - One-time dosage administration
    - Rapid and direct administration of corticosteroids to the lining of the bronchioles
- Cromoglycates
  - Cromolyn sodium—20 mg per 2-mL ampule
    - Dosage: 1 ampule every 6 hours
    - May be mixed with albuterol and administered simultaneously
    - Slow onset of action; may be several days before significant reduction of airway obstruction occurs
- Anticholinergics
  - Ipratroprium bromide 0.02% (500 mcg/vial)
    - Dosage: 1 vial q 4 hours
    - Use with albuterol to decrease bronchospasm.
  - Atropine 0.1 mg/mL—Rarely used because of potential side effects
    - Use only when reduction in bronchospasm has not occurred with conventional therapy and potential life-threatening situation is occurring.

- Continue the treatment until all the medication is depleted. This is indicated by no further production of aerosol mist.
- Perform posttreatment peak flow and record.

Client Instructions

- Perform home treatments four times a day using medications ordered. Do not perform treatments more than four times a day unless instructed by a health-care provider.
- Breathe slowly in and out to maximize the effectiveness of medication.
- Side effects of the medication may include
  - Nervousness or jittery feeling
  - Fast heart rate or palpitations

- *Seek emergency treatment if any of the following occur*
  - Nasal flaring
  - Intercostal retractions
  - Blueness of fingertips, nailbeds, or around the mouth

BIBLIOGRAPHY ▬▬▬▬

Katzung B, ed. *Basic and Clinical Pharmacology.* 14th ed. Norwalk, CT: Appleton & Lange; 2018.

Smyth HDC, Hickey AJ. *Controlled Pulmonary Drug Delivery.* New York, NY: Springer; 2011.

96 Chapter

Assessing Respiratory Distress

Margaret R. Colyar

CPT Code
  None

When a patient reports shortness of breath, you must be diligent and pay close attention to detail to determine the etiology of the problem and facilitate the right treatment plan. Assessing ventilation, oxygenation, work of breathing, airway resistance, and air flow are all part of assessing respiratory distress.

OVERVIEW

- Shortness of breath can be primary (something wrong with the lungs) or secondary (something wrong elsewhere) (Table 96.1).
- Red flags of imminent respiratory arrest are
  - Decreased level of consciousness
  - Inability to maintain respiratory effort
  - Cyanosis
  - Bradycardia

RATIONALE

- To determine whether the respiratory problem is primary or secondary
- To evaluate the patient in imminent respiratory arrest

CONTRAINDICATIONS

* None

PROCEDURE

Assessing for Respiratory Distress

See Table 96.2.

Table 96·1	Respiratory Distress—Primary or Secondary?
PRIMARY PROBLEMS	**SECONDARY REASONS**
Asthma	Metabolic acidosis
COPD	Stroke
Pulmonary edema	Head trauma
Anaphylaxis	Toxicological overdose
Pneumonia	Sepsis
Pleural effusion	Diabetic ketoacidosis
Pneumothorax	Emphysema

Table 96·2	Assessing for Respiratory Distress
AREA OF ASSESSMENT	**KEY SIGNS**
Ventilation—CO_2 excess or deficit	Anxiety Hyperventilation—fast and deeper breaths
Oxygenation—check for hypoxemia	O_2 saturation: <92% on room air **Red Flag**—cyanosis: CO_2 saturation <67%
Work of breathing	Retractions and use of accessory muscles • Marked chest/abdominal movement • Use of accessory muscles • Intercostal retraction • Sternal retraction • Tracheal tug Inability to speak full sentences Difficulty speaking between breaths Inability to lie flat Extreme diaphoresis Flushed skin Restlessness Agitation **Red Flag**—inability to maintain respiratory effort **Red Flag**—declining level of consciousness

Continued

Table 96·2 | Assessing for Respiratory Distress—cont'd

AREA OF ASSESSMENT	KEY SIGNS
Vital signs	Respiratory rate—tachypnea • Adults: >25 breaths/min • Children: >35 breaths/min • Babies: >50 breaths/min Heart rate—tachycardia • Adults: >100/min • Children: >130/min • Babies: >150/min **Red Flag**—bradycardia • Adults: <60/min • Children: <70/min • Babies: <80/min
Airway resistance	Coughing Coarse breath sounds (rhonchi)—secretions in the airway Wheezing—flow restriction below the trachea Crackles (rales)—presence of fluid or atelectasis at the alveolar level
Air flow	Snoring—obstruction by the tongue Inspiratory stridor—obstruction above the vocal cords (foreign body or epiglottitis) Expiratory stridor—obstruction below the vocal cords (croup, deep foreign body)
Other	Jugular venous distention Ascites Peripheral edema

BIBLIOGRAPHY

McEvoy, M. How to access and treat acute respiratory distress. *J Emergency Medical Services.* 8(38). https://www.jems.com/2013/07/19/how-assess-and-treat-acute-respiratory-d/

Saguil A, Fargo M. Acute respiratory distress syndrome: Diagnosis and management. *Am Fam Physician.* 2012:85(4):352–358.

Chapter **97**

Peak Flowmeter

Cynthia R. Ehrhardt

CPT Code
94160 Vital capacity screening tests; total capacity, with timed forced
expiratory volume

The peak flowmeter is a handheld device that provides an objective assessment of dynamic pulmonary function and response to clinical therapy of pulmonary diseases. This is particularly beneficial for asthmatics because it has been shown that regular monitoring has reduced the frequency, duration, and severity of attacks. Peak flowmeters are relatively inexpensive and easily transported apparatus (Fig. 97.1). The result of the peak flowmeter evaluation is expressed as the peak flow rate.

OVERVIEW
- Limitations of the peak flowmeter
  - Poor user skills
  - Lack of motivation and individual effort
  - Younger than age 5 years
- The normal predicted average peak expiratory flow for males and females is shown in Table 97.1.
- The normal predicted average peak expiratory flow for children and adolescents is shown in Table 97.2.

RATIONALE
- Allows asthmatics to self-monitor their respiratory status objectively
- Permits clinicians treating asthmatics to intervene earlier in therapy
- Reduces the frequency of emergency department visits and/or hospitalizations

INDICATIONS
- Asthma
- Monitor respiratory status

CONTRAINDICATIONS
- None

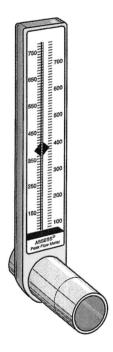

Figure 97.1 Peak flowmeter.

Table 97-1	**Normal Predicted Average Peak Expiratory Flow Rate—Adults***								
AGE (YEARS)	**MALE HEIGHT (INCHES)**					**FEMALE HEIGHT (INCHES)**			
	60	**65**	**70**	**75**	**90**	**55**	**60**	**65**	**70**	**75**
20	554	602	649	693	740	390	423	460	496	529
25	543	590	636	679	725	385	418	454	490	523
30	532	577	622	664	710	380	413	448	483	516
35	521	565	609	651	695	375	408	442	476	509
40	509	552	596	636	680	370	402	436	470	502
45	498	540	583	622	665	365	397	430	464	595
50	486	527	569	607	649	360	391	424	457	488
55	475	515	556	593	634	355	386	418	451	482
60	463	502	542	578	618	350	380	412	445	475
65	452	490	529	564	603	345	375	406	439	468
70	440	477	515	550	587	340	369	432	432	461

*This table shows values at sea level. These are considered averages and may vary widely from individual to individual.

Table 97·2	Normal Predicted Average Peak Expiratory Flow Rate (PFR)—Children and Adolescents*				
HEIGHT (INCHES)	**AVERAGE PFR**	**HEIGHT (INCHES)**	**AVERAGE PFR**	**HEIGHT (INCHES)**	**AVERAGE PFR**
43	147	51	254	59	360
44	160	52	267	60	373
45	173	53	280	61	387
46	187	54	293	62	400
47	200	55	307	63	413
48	214	56	320	64	427
49	227	57	334	65	440
50	240	58	347	66	454

*This table shows values at sea level. These are considered averages and may vary widely from individual to individual.

PROCEDURE

Peak Flowmeter

Equipment

- Peak flowmeter
- Mouthpiece

Procedure

- Place the appropriate-size mouthpiece over the peak flowmeter.
- Check that the indicator is at the bottom of the chamber.
- Hold the peak flowmeter in the proper direction (as recommended by the manufacturer).
- Ask the client to take as deep a breath as possible.
- Ask the client to seal his or her lips over the mouthpiece and blow out as quickly as possible (like blowing out candles) (Fig. 97.2).
- Note the reading on the dial.
- Repeat the procedure three times and record the highest reading.

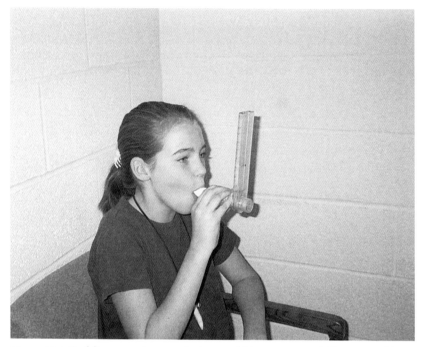

Figure 97.2 Seal lips over the mouthpiece and blow out as quickly as possible.

BIBLIOGRAPHY

Cheever KH. *Brunner & Suddarth's Textbook of Medication-Surgical Nursing.* Philadelphia, PA: Lippincott Williams & Wilkins; 2017.

Hyatt RE. *Interpretation of Pulmonary Function Tests.* Philadelphia, PA: Lippincott Williams & Wilkins; 2014.

Pfenninger JL, Fowler GC. *Procedures of Primary Care Physicians.* St. Louis, MO: Mosby; 2019.

98 Chapter

Pulmonary Function Testing (Spirometry)

Margaret R. Colyar

CPT Code
94010 Spirometry

Pulmonary function testing is a physiological test that measures how well a person inhales and exhales volumes of air based on time. Spirometry is a simple test to measure how much (volume) and how fast (flow) air moves into and out of the lungs. Through routine spirometry, lung diseases can often be diagnosed in the early stages when treatment is most effective. Spirometry is used to establish baseline lung function, evaluate dyspnea, detect pulmonary disease, monitor effects of therapies used to treat respiratory disease, evaluate respiratory impairment, evaluate operative risk, and perform surveillance for occupational-related lung disease.

OVERVIEW

- The National Health and Nutrition Examination Survey [NHANES] III predicted set is used to provide specific equations for whites, African Americans, and Mexican Americans (see https://www.cdc.gov/nchs/data/nhanes/nhanes_07_08/spirometry.pdf).
- If the patient belongs to another ethnic group, the predicted values and lower limits of what is considered normal provided for whites should be reduced by 12% by multiplying the predicted value by 0.88 before comparison with the patient's results.
- The spirometer calculates and records three results:
  - Forced expiratory volume (FEV1)—a person's air flow rates or the volume exhaled out within the first second after full inspiration
    - This indicates whether or not there is airway obstruction.
    - Normal—3 to 5 L or 80% to 120%
  - Forced vital capacity (FVC)—the total volume of air forced out of the lungs
  - FEV1/FVC—a calculated ratio used to diagnose obstructive versus restrictive lung disease
    - Normal values are approximately 80%.
- Defects in lung capacity include
  - Restrictive defects (Table 98.1)
  - Obstructive defects (Table 98.2)
    - Variable intrathoracic upper airway obstruction
    - Variable extrathoracic upper airway obstruction
    - Fixed upper airway obstruction
- The severity of reductions in the FVC and/or the FEV1 can be characterized by the following scale:
  - Mild—70% to 79% of predicted
  - Moderate—60% to 69% of predicted
  - Moderately severe—50% to 59% of predicted
  - Severe—35% to 49% of predicted
  - Very severe—less than 35% of predicted

RATIONALE
- To determine lung function

Table 98·1	Interpretation of Obstructive/Restrictive Lung Disease			
TYPE	**FEV1**	**FVC**	**FEV1/FVC**	**CAUSES**
Obstructive	Low	Normal	Low	Bronchial spasm, airway inflammation, increased intraluminal secretions, and/or reduction in parenchymal support of the airways due to loss of lung elastic recoil Asthma, acute and chronic bronchitis, emphysema, bronchiectasis, cystic fibrosis, pneumonia, alpha-1 antitrypsin deficiency, and bronchiolitis
Restrictive	Low	Low	Normal/high	Obesity, cardiomegaly, ascites, pregnancy, pleural effusion, pleural tumors, kyphoscoliosis, pulmonary fibrosis, neuromuscular disease, diaphragm weakness or paralysis, space-occupying lesions, lung resection, congestive heart failure, inadequate inspiration or expiration secondary to pain, and severe obstructive lung disease

CONTRAINDICATIONS

- Relative contraindications for spirometry include
  - Hemoptysis of unknown origin
  - Pneumothorax
  - Unstable angina pectoris
  - Recent myocardial infarction
  - Thoracic aneurysms
  - Abdominal aneurysms
  - Cerebral aneurysms
  - Recent eye surgery (increased intraocular pressure during forced expiration)
  - Recent abdominal or thoracic surgical procedures
  - History of syncope associated with forced exhalation
▶ *Informed consent required*

PROCEDURE

Spirometry

Equipment

- Computer
- Spirometry device
- Mouthpiece
- Nose clips
- Tissues
- Chair

Table 98·2	Configuration of the Flow-Volume Curve for Different Upper Airway Obstructions	
TYPE	**CAUSES**	**FIGURE**
Variable Intrathoracic Obstructions Reduction of air flow during forced expirations with preservation of a normal inspiratory flow configuration	Localized tumors of the lower trachea or mainstem bronchus, tracheomalacia, and airway changes associated with polychondritis	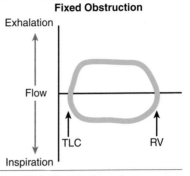
Variable Extrathoracic Obstructions Narrowing of the airway inside the thorax, in part because of a narrowing or collapse of the airway secondary to extraluminal pressures exceeding intraluminal pressures during expiration	Unilateral and bilateral vocal cord paralysis, vocal cord adhesions, vocal cord constriction, laryngeal edema, and upper airway narrowing associated with obstructive sleep apnea	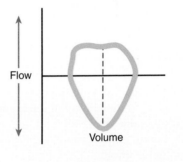
Fixed Upper Airway Obstructions Reduction of inspired flows during forced inspirations with preservation of expiratory flows	Goiters, endotracheal neoplasms, stenosis of both main bronchi, postintubation stenosis, and performance of the test through a tracheostomy tube or other fixed orifice device	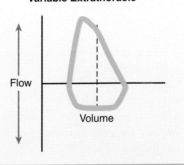

Note: Upper airway obstructions include various abnormalities of the larger central airways (larynx, trachea, right and left mainstem bronchi).

Table 98-3	**American Thoracic Society Guidelines for Spirometry Effort**

- Number of acceptable efforts
- Hesitation or false start
- Delayed time to peak expiration of flow rate
- Coughing
- Glottic closure
- Mouthpiece obstruction
- Air leak around mouthpiece
- Exhalation less than 6 seconds
- Inconsistent effort
- Extrapolated volume greater than FVC or 150 mL, whichever is greater
- Highest two FEV1 rates varying from each other by more than 150 mL
- Highest two FVC rates varying from each other by more than 150 mL

Figures for each of these problems can be seen at http://www.youtube.com/watch?v=FZJ5DmpuPi0.

Procedure

- Calibrate the spirometry device based on the manufacturer's instructions.
- Explain the test to the patient.
- Attach the mouthpiece to the spirometry device.
- Instruct the patient to
  - Loosen any restrictive clothing.
  - Sit up straight.
  - Place feet flat on the floor.
  - Apply the nose clip.
  - Take a big deep breath in.
  - Place his or her mouth around the mouthpiece and the patient blows out as hard and fast as possible and for as long as possible—6 seconds are needed for a good effort.
  - Remove the nose clip.
- Repeat the test at least twice.
  - Two consistent blows are needed.
- Evaluate the person's effort based on the American Thoracic Society's guidelines (see Table 98.3).

BIBLIOGRAPHY

https://www.cdc.gov/nchs/data/nhanes/nhanes_07_08/spirometry.pdf
Miller MR, Hankinson J, Brusaco V, et al. Standardisation of spirometry. *Eur Respir J.* 2005;26:319–338. http://www.thoracic.org/statements/resources/pfet/PFT2.pdf
Spirometry. YouTube. http://www.youtube.com/watch?v=FZJ5DmpuPi0. February 12, 2013.

Chapter **99**

Pulmonary Stress Test
Margaret R. Colyar

CPT Code
94620   Pulmonary Stress Test—Simple

A pulmonary stress test is a 6-minute walk or stationary bicycle test that is useful to evaluate a patient with symptoms of shortness of breath, stridor, and/or wheezing that occurs only when exercising. If paradoxical vocal cord motion or some other pathology such as tracheomalacia or laryngomalacia is suspected, an ear, nose, and throat (ENT) evaluation would be warranted.

OVERVIEW
- Most 6-minute walk tests will be done twice.
  - Once during the initial evaluation, then once following therapeutic intervention to determine whether the patient has experienced significant improvement in functional status

RATIONALE
- To measure the response to medical intervention in a patient with moderate to severe heart or lung disease
- To evaluate dyspnea or shortness of breath
- To determine functional status in congestive heart failure
- To perform a preoperative risk assessment
- To evaluate for disability determination
- To assess response to therapeutic interventions
- To develop exercise prescriptions

CONTRAINDICATIONS
- Absolute contraindications include
  - Unstable angina during the month prior to the test
  - Heart attack the month prior to the test
  - Resting heart rate of >120 beats/min
  - Aortic stenosis
  - Uncontrolled hypertension
    - Systolic blood pressure of >188 mm Hg
    - Diastolic blood pressure of >100 mm Hg
  - Uncontrolled asthma

- Hypoxemia (SaO_2 <85% at rest)
- Febrile illness
- Relative contraindications include
  - Hypertension
  - Cardiac disease
  - Epilepsy
  - Inability to exercise

▶ *Informed consent required*

PROCEDURE

Pulmonary Stress Test

Equipment

- Blood pressure cuff/stethoscope or automatic blood pressure machine
- Pulse oximeter
- EKG machine
- EKG electrodes
- Tape
- Oxygen tank
- Documentation sheet (Table 99.1)
- Stationary bicycle or treadmill

Table 99·1	Documentation Sheet						
Date_____ Using O_2? Y or N							
Name_____ Date of Birth_____							
Diagnosis: _____							
Medications: _____							
Minutes	B/P	O_2 Sat	Pulse	Respirations	Borg Scale	Other*	
Before test							
Minute 1							
Minute 2							
Minute 3							
Minute 4							
Minute 5							
Minute 6 End of test							
Distance Traveled:_____							
Signature							

*Under Other column, document and stop the test if significant EKG abnormalities develop, the patient becomes pale or ashen in appearance, or experiences chest pain, intolerable dyspnea, leg cramps, staggering, excessive sweating, a fall in systolic or diastolic blood pressure (BP) greater than 20 mm Hg below resting value, a rise in systolic BP to greater than 250 mm Hg, a rise in diastolic BP to greater than 120 mm Hg, severe oxygen desaturation (<80%), or achievement of maximum predicted heart rate. Attach EKG strips for each minute to this sheet.

Procedure

- Inform the patient about the testing procedure.
- Fill in information about the EKG machine.
- Apply EKG electrodes.
- Apply blood pressure cuff.
- Apply the pulse oximeter and tape it on.
- Instruct the patient to walk or pedal at a comfortable speed.
- Every minute, document blood pressure, heart rate, respiratory rate, oxygen saturation, EKG rhythm, and the patient's perception of his or her breathing status on a 0 to 10 scale (Table 99.2).
- When the 6 minutes have elapsed, document how far the patient has walked or pedaled.
- Stop the test if significant EKG abnormalities develop, the patient becomes pale or ashen in appearance, or experiences
  - Chest pain
  - Intolerable dyspnea
  - Leg cramps
  - Staggering
  - Excessive sweating
  - A fall in systolic or diastolic blood pressure (BP) greater than 20 mm Hg below resting value
  - A rise in systolic BP to greater than 250 mm Hg
  - A rise in diastolic BP to greater than 120 mm Hg
  - Severe oxygen desaturation (<80%), or achievement of maximum predicted heart rate

Table 99·2	Modified Borg Scale—Perception of Breathing Status
0 No breathlessness, nothing at all	
0.5 Very, very slight (just noticeable)	
1 Very slight	
2 Slight breathlessness	
3 Moderate	
4 Somewhat severe	
5 Severe breathlessness	
6	
7 Very severe breathlessness	
8	
9 Very, very severe breathlessness	
10 Maximum breathlessness	

Source: Borg GA (1982). Psychophysical bases of perceived exertion. *Med Sci Sports Exerc.* 1982;14(5):377381.

INTERPRETATION

- A lower score (reflecting less distance covered in 6 minutes) indicates worse function.
- A higher score (reflecting more distance covered in 6 minutes) indicates improved function.

Client Instructions

- Before your procedure
  - Come at least 30 minutes before the test.
  - Do not smoke for 12 hours before the test.
  - Do not eat or drink for 3 hours before the test.
  - If you have diabetes, ask your primary care provider what you may eat or drink before the test.
  - Wear comfortable clothing and walking shoes such as sneakers.
- During your procedure
  - Body hair may be shaved to place EKG pads on your upper body to monitor an electrocardiogram of your heart.
  - A sensor will be placed on your finger to monitor oxygen in your blood.
  - You will be asked to wear a nose clip and breathe through a mouthpiece.
- During the exercise
  - Your blood pressure, breathing, and heart rate will be monitored several times during the test.
  - You will be asked to exercise as long as you can.
  - You will be asked to rate your breathing during the test on a scale of 0 to 10, with 0 being no breathlessness and 10 being maximum breathlessness.
  - Blood samples may be taken to measure oxygen and carbon dioxide during the exercise.
- After the procedure
  - You can resume your normal activity.
  - You can resume your normal medications.

BIBLIOGRAPHY

Albouaini K, Egred M, Alahmar A, Wright DJ. Cardiopulmonary exercise testing and its application. *Postgrad Med J.* 2007;83(985):675–682. https://www.ncbi.nlm.nih.gov/pmc/articles/PMC2734442/

Pulmonary Exercise Stress Test. Mount Nittany Health Web site. https://www.mountnittany.org/articles/healthsheets/5735. December 12, 1016.

Chapter **100**

X-Ray Interpretation
Chest
Margaret R. Colyar

CPT Code
Usually included as part of the office visit charge. Actual x-ray films are billed according to the views taken. The chest x-ray should be correlated with clinical history, physical examination, and additional diagnostic tool results.

A chest x-ray (radiograph) is considered the best radiological screening and diagnostic tool for most lung disease because of its ability to generate high spatial resolution and to visualize various densities within the thoracic cavity.

OVERVIEW

- Densities
  - Air—DARK
  - Muscles—GRAY
  - Fat—Light GRAY
  - Muscle—Very light GRAY
  - Bones—WHITE
  - Foreign body—varies based on density
    - Coin—DARK
    - Wood splinter—difficult to see
- Inspect the posteroanterior (PA) view to determine whether the x-ray is adequate by using **RIPE.**
  - **R**otation—Do the clavicles and vertebrae form a cross?
  - **I**nspiration—Are there a minimum of eight ribs visible?
  - **P**enetration—Are the interspaces visible and the thoracic vertebral bodies well defined?
  - **E**xposure—Too much or too little?
- General principles
  - Use an orderly and systematic approach to interpret the chest film.
  - Order PA and lateral views. When a portable chest x-ray is taken, you get an anteroposterior (AP) view, which makes the heart look artificially large.
  - Order an expiratory view if a pneumothorax is suspected.

RATIONALE

- To diagnose diseases and disorders of the chest

INDICATIONS

- Trauma to the chest area
- Chronic cough
- Chest pain
- Suspicion of lung infection
- Suspicion of lung carcinoma

CONTRAINDICATION

- Pregnancy (unless shielded)

PROCEDURE

X-Ray Interpretation—Chest

Equipment

- X-ray view box or digital viewing program

Procedure

- Inspect for the presence of any foreign bodies in the thoracic cavity.
- Systematically inspect the skeletal system of the thoracic region.
  - Identify anatomical skeletal landmarks within the thoracic cavity and occurrence of any aberration (Figs. 100.1 and 100.2).
  - Identify any demineralization in the skeleton structure.
  - Determine the lack of continuity and symmetry of skeletal structure (including clavicles, scapulae, humeri, and sternum).
  - Note the appearance of the ribs, beginning with identification of the posterior segments of the first rib on the right and proceeding through the 12th rib. Repeat this process on the opposite side of the thoracic cavity.
  - Note any widening of the rib spaces.
- Systematically inspect for the presence of soft tissue masses.
  - Note the contour of the neck.
  - Look for asymmetry and shadow density changes in
    - Breast shadows
    - Hepatic and splenic shadows
  - Check for the presence of a gas bubble in the stomach shadow (Fig. 100.3).
  - Note any evidence of changes in or shifting of the mediastinal shadows.
- Systematically inspect cardiac system.
  - Note the shape of the cardiac silhouette, which is easily visible.
  - Measure the intrathoracic diameter. Note the width of inside of the rib cage at level of the diaphragm's right side plus the left side.
  - Divide the width of the rib cage by one-half. This should equal the cardiac size. Normal cardiac size is less than half the thoracic size (Fig. 100.4).

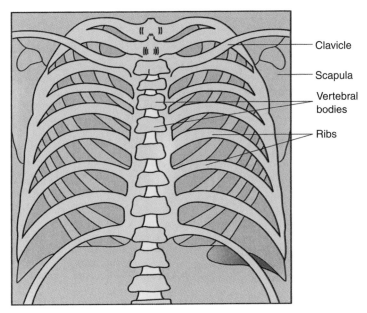

Figure 100.1 Anatomical skeletal landmarks as seen on the posteroanterior view of the chest.

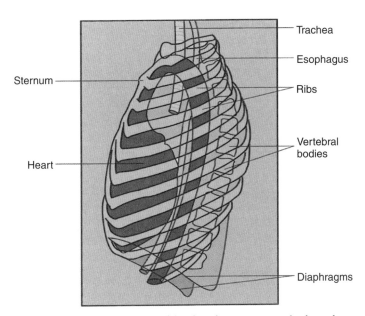

Figure 100.2 Anatomical skeletal landmarks as seen on the lateral view of the chest.

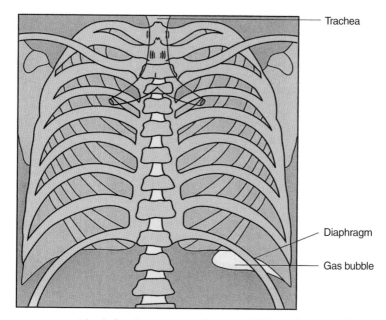

Figure 100.3 Check for the presence of a gas bubble in the stomach.

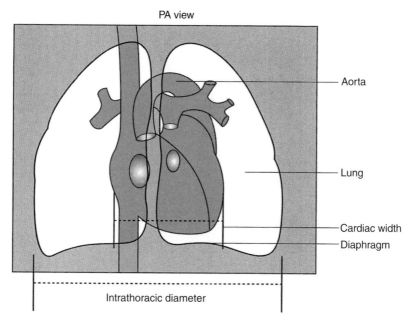

Figure 100.4 Inspect the cardiac system. Measure the intrathoracic diameter. Divide the intrathoracic diameter by 2. Measure the cardiac width. Normal cardiac size is less than half the intrathoracic diameter.

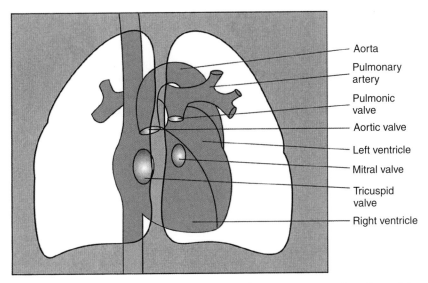

Figure 100.5 Calcifications within the cardiac silhouette represent the valves of the heart.

- Note the clarity of the cardiac borders. The cardiac borders should be well defined.
- Note increased calcification of silhouette of the heart.
  - Calcifications within the silhouette represent the valvular structures of the heart (Fig. 100.5).
- Systematically inspect the presentation of the vascular system.
  - Note any anatomical shift or calcifications in the pulmonary arteries and aorta.
    - The main pulmonary arterial branches should be equal in size, shape, and contour.
    - Inspect the size and shape of thoracic aorta.
    - Locate the base of the aorta as it extends from cardiac silhouette.
    - Note the presence of
      - Aortic dilation
      - Straightening or coarctation of the aortic arch
      - Aortic calcifications
- Systematically inspect the diaphragm—should be slightly higher on the right than on the left.
  - Note the presence or absence of flattening.
  - Note the integrity and symmetry of the anatomical location.
  - Note the absence or presence of ipsilateral hemidiaphragm (abnormal elevation).

- Systematically inspect the lung silhouette for
  - Cohesiveness to the pleural borders
  - Lucency of air within the lungs
  - Presence of pleural lines within the confines of the ribs
  - Calcifications or densities within the lung field—appear whiter
  - Accentuated areas of white within the pulmonary black background. This represents pleural thickening or pleural fluid and can prevent clear demarcation of the anatomical borders.
  - Blunting of the costophrenic borders
- Some common abnormalities include
  - Abscesses, fungus, and lymphomas
    - Appearance of "balls" in the chest
    - Diaphragm may be pulled up
  - Acute asthma flair
    - Hyperinflated lungs
    - Flat diaphragm
  - COPD
    - Blunting of the costophrenic angles
    - Increases AP diameter
  - Congestive heart failure
    - Presence of Kerley B lines (small horizontal lines found in the very periphery of the lung near the rib cage). Kerley B lines represent fluid in the interlobular septa.
  - Cystic fibrosis
    - Low, flat diaphragm
    - Small heart
    - Large lungs
  - Infiltrates
    - Patchy areas
  - Pneumonia
    - More white and less black in whichever lobe is affected (Fig. 100.6)
  - Pneumothorax
    - Lobe of lung decreased in size or absent
  - Sarcoidosis
    - Masses in hylar area
  - Tuberculosis
    - Infiltrates and ball-like scarring in apices

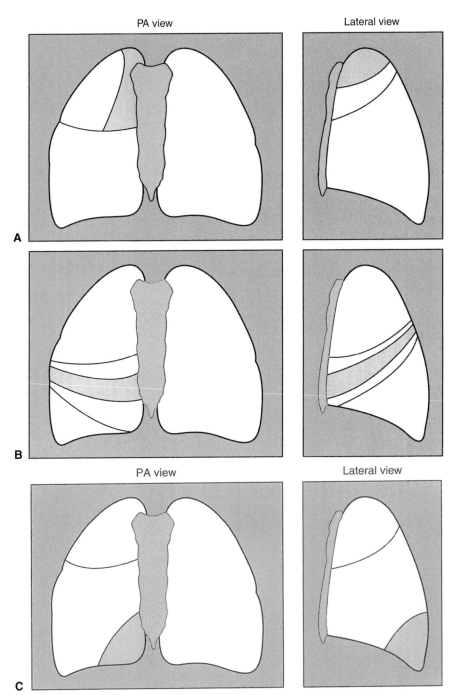

Figure 100.6 Pneumonia—more white and less black in whichever lobe is affected. (A) Right upper lobe pneumonia; (B) right middle lobe pneumonia; (C) right lower lobe pneumonia; and (D) left upper lobe pneumonia.   *Continued*

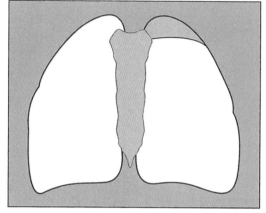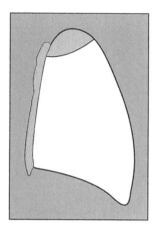

D

Figure 100.6 cont'd

BIBLIOGRAPHY

Jameson J, Fauci A, Kasper D, Hauser S, Longo D, Loscalzo J. *Harrison's Principles of Internal Medicine*. 20th ed. New York, NY: McGraw-Hill; 2018.

Stimac G. *Introduction to Diagnostic Imaging*. Philadelphia, PA: Saunders; 1992.

Vine D. Congestive heart failure. *Am Fam Physician*. 1990;42(3):739.

101

Chapter

Chest Tubes for Emergency Transport

Margaret R. Colyar

CPT Code
32020   Chest tubes (thoracotomy)

The Heimlich valve, a plastic portable one-way valve used for chest drainage, allows evacuation of the lung during coughing and breathing while preventing return of secretions to the lung. It was introduced in the late 1960s to drain the pleural space, avoiding the need for an underwater seal during wartime. Insertion of a portable one-way chest tube is an important procedure for managing life-threatening respiratory situations and stabilizing the patient for emergency transport.

OVERVIEW

- Allows freedom of movement
- Used to drain blood, fluid, or air from the space between inner and outer linings of the lung
- Placement for different types of chest trauma (Table 101.1)

RATIONALE

- To relieve pain due to pressure exerted by excess fluid in the chest cavity
- To drain excess air and fluid from the chest cavity
- To prevent collapse of the lung caused by increased pressure
- To allow lungs to reinflate

INDICATIONS

- Pleural effusion
- Empyema
- Spontaneous pneumothorax
- Sucking chest wound from penetrating trauma
- Hemothorax

CONTRAINDICATIONS

- Clinically stable patients with a small pneumothorax

▶ *Informed consent required*

PROCEDURE

Chest Tube Insertion for Emergency Transport

Equipment

- Heimlich valve (Fig. 101.1)
- Vented drainage bag—urinary or ostomy bag
- Mask
- Scalpel

Table 101·1	Placement of Chest Tubes	
TYPE OF CHEST TRAUMA	**PLACEMENT OF CHEST TUBES**
Hemothorax	4th–5th intercostal spaces midaxillary line
Pneumothorax	2nd–3rd intercostal spaces anterior chest at midclavicular line

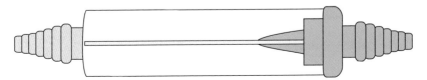

Figure 101.1 Heimlich valve.

- Kelly clamp—two, rubber tipped
- Forceps—sterile
- Syringe—10 mL
- Needle—22 gauge, 1 inch
- Local anesthetic—10 mL
- Tape—2-inch cloth/elastic
- Scissors
- Gloves—nonsterile
- Gloves—sterile
- Povidone-iodine (Betadine)
- Drape—fenestrated
- Alcohol swabs
- 4 × 4 gauze—sterile
- Vaseline gauze or clear plastic that clings (i.e., Saran Wrap)
- Suture—large filament—optional

Procedure

- Position client according to type of chest tube placement needed (Table 101.2; Fig. 101.2).
- Put on nonsterile gloves.
- Place rubber-tipped Kelly clamps in opposite directions on proximal end of the urinary/ostomy bag tube.
- Attach the urinary/ostomy bag tube to blue end of the Heimlich valve.
- Attach the Heimlich valve connecting tube to other end of the Heimlich valve.
- Tape connection site at both ends of the valve.
- Cleanse site with povidone-iodine starting at insertion site and moving in concentric circles three times in outward motion.
- Administer local anesthetic to skin between ribs identified as insertion site.
- Drape the chest tube insertion site.
- Remove nonsterile gloves and put on sterile gloves.
- Palpate intercostal space.
- Stabilize surrounding tissue with nondominant hand.
- Make a small incision where the catheter is to be inserted.
- Insert catheter through the skin, intercostal space, and parietal pleura and into pleural space. A "pop" may be heard or felt.
- Remove the inner blunt-tipped obturator and advance the catheter.
- Attach the radiopaque catheter to the Heimlich valve connecting tube.
- Suture tube to skin or tape securely.
- Place Vaseline gauze or cling film over chest tube insertion site.

Table 101·2 **Positioning of Client for Chest Tube Placement**	
TYPE OF CHEST TRAUMA	**POSITION FOR CHEST TUBE PLACEMENT**
Hemothorax	Orthopneic
Pneumothorax	Supine, high Fowler's, semi-Fowler's

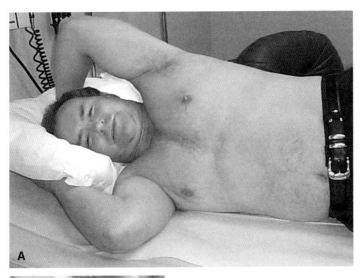

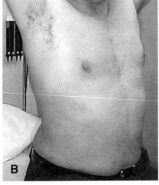

Figure 101.2 Positioning of client for chest tube placement. (A) Supine; (B) orthopneic.

- Apply sterile 4 × 4 gauze on top of Vaseline gauze.
- Tape with 2-inch cloth or elastic tape making an occlusive dressing.
- If available, obtain chest radiograph to ensure proper placement.

Client Instructions

- Transport to emergency department.
- Chest tube is removed when lung has reinflated.

BIBLIOGRAPHY

Gogokos A, Barbetakis N, Lazaridis G, et al. Heimlich valve and pneumothorax. *Ann Transl Med.* 2015:3(4):54.

McDuff A, Arnold A, Harvey J. Management of spontaneous pneumothorax. *Thorax.* 2010;65(10):18–31.

102

Chapter

Flail Chest Stabilization
With or Without Open Chest Wound

Cynthia R. Ehrhardt

CPT Code
None

Flail chest is the consequence of blunt or penetrating (open chest wound) trauma in which there are multiple fractures to the ribs (usually more than three consecutive ribs on the same side), resulting in instability to the chest wall. Flail chest with or without open chest wounds is a potentially life-threatening situation. In an ambulatory setting, the focus is on stabilizing the injury, providing adequate ventilation, and transporting to an appropriately equipped emergency department.

Prevention is focused on eliminating situations that can result in the incidence of blunt trauma and penetration wounds. This includes properly worn seat belts in automobiles with or without airbags, gun and hunting safety, high-rise safety (ladders and roofs), and protection against and avoidance of situations that produce projectile objects.

OVERVIEW

- Incidence
  - Accounts for 25% to 30% of the automobile deaths in the United States each year
  - Three times as likely to occur in individuals not wearing seat belts
- Complications
  - Pneumothorax
  - Hemothorax
  - Hemopneumothorax
  - Cardiac contusions, including cardiac tamponade and thoracic aortic trauma
  - Cardiac arrhythmias
  - Systemic/cardiogenic shock
  - Death
- General principles
  - Activate emergency medical system (EMS).
  - Maintain ABCs (airway, breathing, circulation) of basic life support.
  - Apply oxygen in as high a concentration as possible.
  - Establish monitoring with pulse oximetry and cardiac monitoring.
  - Seal as quickly as possible if an open chest wound.

- Establish intravenous lines (two) as quickly as permitted.
- Treat for cardiogenic shock.
- Transport as quickly as possible.
- Physical examination
  - Observe for signs and symptoms of systemic cardiogenic shock.
  - Inspection
    - Presence or absence of chest wall motion
    - Paradoxical chest wall motion
    - Presence or absence of air-movement noise
    - Cyanosis of the face and neck
    - Subcutaneous emphysema (crepitus skin)
    - Excessive abdominal muscular movement
  - Palpation
    - Crepitus anywhere in the chest wall region with particular attention at the location of blunt trauma
    - Palpable rib or sternal fractures
    - Movable sternum
    - Decrease in intensity of point of maximal impulse, which can be associated with cardiac tamponade, or shift in point of maximal impulse if mediastinal shift occurs and congestive heart failure can be excluded
  - Percussion
    - Dullness suggests hemothorax or pneumothorax
    - Hyperresonance suggests pneumothorax
  - Auscultation
    - Unilateral decreased breath sounds

OPTIONS

- *Method 1*—Flail chest stabilization without open chest wound
- *Method 2*—Flail chest stabilization with open chest wound

RATIONALE

- To prevent life-threatening complications

INDICATIONS

- Blunt trauma
- Penetrating chest wound
- Rib injuries

CONTRAINDICATIONS

- None

PROCEDURE

Flail Chest Stabilization

Equipment

- Pulse oximeter
- Oxygen with nasal cannula, mask, or rebreather mask

- Cardiac monitoring if available
- Intravenous solution kits of Ringer's lactate or 0.9% sodium chloride
- Large-bore intravenous catheters (16- to 18-gauge for adults; 18- to 21-gauge for children)
- 0.9% sodium chloride irrigation solution—500 mL—sterile
- Abdominal dressings (6 inch to 12 inch or larger)—sterile
- Gloves—sterile
- 4 × 4 gauze—sterile
- Occlusive dressing (petroleum or polytetrafluoroethylene [Teflon] base)—sterile
- 4-0 Ethicon suture material
- Adhesive tape rolls (1, 2, 4, or 6 inches)
- Pillow or sandbag
- Sterile dressing or suture tray including
  - Straight and curved hemostats
  - Needle holder
  - Forceps with teeth
  - Iris scissors
  - Emesis basin
  - Sterile towels (fenestrated and nonfenestrated)
- 1% or 2% lidocaine without epinephrine
- 5-mL syringe—sterile
- 22-gauge, 1½-inch needle—sterile
- Intubation tray—optional

Procedure

METHOD 1—FLAIL CHEST STABILIZATION WITHOUT OPEN CHEST WOUND

- Activate the EMS system.
- Maintain ABCs of basic life support.
- Apply oxygen in as high a concentration as possible.
- Establish monitoring with pulse oximetry and cardiac monitoring.
- Locate the edges of the flail section with gentle palpation.
- When located, establish that there is no evidence of open chest injury.
- Apply a thick dressing of at least 3 inches over the site. A small pillow or small sandbag (5 lb or less) can be used.
- Use large strips of tape across the dressing or pad to secure (Fig. 102.1)
- Ensure that the tape tension causes the dressing to support the flail region.
  - Strips of cloth may be used to anchor if tape is not available.
- Initiate two intravenous sites and run intravenous solution to keep patent stable.
- *Monitor and transport to the nearest emergency department equipped to handle the potential secondary complications that can occur with flail chest.*

METHOD 2—FLAIL CHEST STABILIZATION WITH OPEN CHEST WOUND

- Activate the EMS system.
- Maintain ABCs of basic life support.

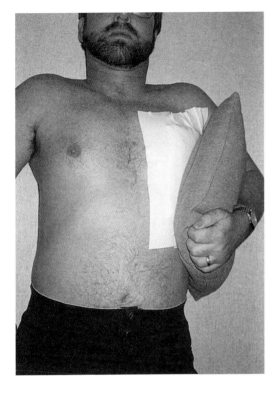

Figure 102.1 Secure the dressing with tape and stabilize with a pillow or sandbag.

- Apply oxygen in as high a concentration as possible.
- Establish monitoring with pulse oximetry and cardiac monitoring.
- With gentle palpation, locate the edges of the flail section.
- Note the presence or absence of sucking sound of air movement each time the individual inhales.
- Locate the open chest wound.
- Put on gloves.
- Seal the open chest wound as quickly as possible.
  - Clean the area around the wound with sterile 0.9% sodium chloride, ensuring that none of the solution enters the wound.
  - Dry with sterile 4 × 4 gauze.
  - Apply petroleum-impregnated dressing or occlusive dressing over the open wound and extending 2 to 3 inches beyond the site.
  - Anchor securely with tape, then proceed with method 1—flail chest stabilization without chest wound dressing.
- If wound is gaping, or dressing does not hold well, apply temporary sutures (see Chapter 22) to the wound, then reapply the occlusive dressing.
- *Monitor and transport to the nearest emergency department equipped to handle the potential secondary complications that can occur with flail chest.*

Client Instructions

- Transport to appropriately staffed emergency department.

BIBLIOGRAPHY

Limmer DJ, O'Keefe MF. *Emergency Care*. 13th ed. Englewood Cliffs, NJ: Prentice-Hall; 2015.

Marx J, Hockberger R, Walls R. *Rosen's Emergency Medicine: Concepts and Clinical Practice*. 13th ed. St. Louis, MO: Saunders; 2013.

103 Chapter

Stab/Penetrating Wound Stabilization

Margaret R. Colyar

CPT Code
20100 Exploration—neck
20101 Exploration—chest
20102 Exploration—abdomen, flank, or back
20103 Exploration—extremity

All stab/penetrating wounds (large or small) have the potential to precipitate a life-threatening situation. The size of the wound does not reflect proportionally the severity of the wound. Small penetrations sometimes are more lethal than are large penetrations. In an ambulatory setting, the focus is on evaluation and stabilization of the injury, providing adequate ventilation if required, and transporting to an appropriately equipped emergency department as quickly as possible when deep injuries and/or involvement of body structures beyond basic lacerations are suspected.

Prevention is focused on eliminating situations that can result in the incidence of penetration wounds. This includes properly worn seat belts in automobiles with or without airbags, gun and hunting safety, avoidance of situations that produce projectile objects, and knowledge of personal safety rules to avoid assault situations.

OVERVIEW

- Incidence
  - Accounts for 35% of injuries seen in the emergency department
  - Estimated to cause permanent disability in 500,000 individuals in the United States each year
- Complications
  - Severance of ligaments, tendons, nerves, muscles, or blood vessels can lead to loss of function.

- Penetrating trauma in thoracic and abdominal cavities can increase risk of trauma and temporary and/or permanent loss of an organ or its function.
- Cardiogenic shock
- Death

OPTIONS

- *Method 1*—Penetrating wound without involvement of major body organ
- *Method 2*—Penetrating wound with involvement of major body organ

RATIONALE

- To stabilize the client
- To prevent life-threatening complications

INDICATIONS

- Penetrating trauma not involving major body organs

CONTRAINDICATIONS

- Penetration of major internal organ is suspected. Stabilize and transfer to the emergency department.

PROCEDURE

Stab/Penetrating Wound Stabilization

Equipment

- Method 1 only
  - Basin—sterile
  - Povidone-iodine soak—povidone-iodine solution and 0.9% sterile saline mixed 50/50
  - Syringe—20 to 60 mL
  - Two needles—27 to 30 gauge and 18 to 20 gauge
  - 1% lidocaine
  - Scissors—sterile
  - Curved hemostats—sterile
  - Forceps—sterile
  - Suture—3-0 to 5-0 nylon
  - Culture swab
  - Topical antibiotic—Bactroban or Polysporin
  - Iodoform gauze—¼ to 1 inch
- Method 2 only
  - Pulse oximeter
  - Oxygen with nasal cannula, mask, or rebreather mask
  - Cardiac monitoring, if available
  - Intravenous solution kits of Ringer's lactate or 0.9% sodium chloride
  - Large-bore intravenous catheters (16 to 18 gauge for adults and 18 to 21 gauge for children)

- 0.9% sodium chloride irrigation solution—500 mL—sterile
- Large abdominal dressings (6-inch to 12-inch or larger)—sterile
- Intubation tray—optional but highly recommended
- Methods 1 and 2
  - Gloves—sterile
  - 4 × 4 gauze—sterile
  - Adhesive tape rolls (1-, 2-, 4-, and/or 6-inch)

Procedure

METHOD 1—PENETRATING WOUND WITHOUT INVOLVEMENT OF MAJOR BODY ORGANS

- If the penetrating wound appears not to involve major organ structures, nerves, tendons, or major blood vessels and appears to meet criteria of deep puncture wound, then see Chapters 6 and 22.

METHOD 2—PENETRATING WOUND WITH INVOLVEMENT OF MAJOR BODY ORGANS

- Activate the EMS system.
- Maintain ABCs of basic life support.
- Apply oxygen in as high a concentration as possible.
- Monitor oxygen saturation with pulse oximetry and cardiac monitoring.
- Establish intravenous lines (two) as quickly as permitted.
- If *open chest wound*
  - Seal as quickly as possible (see Chapter 102).
- If *abdominal injuries*
  - Cover the wound with sterile dressings to prevent further contamination of the wound.
- If an *extremity wound* with suspected derangement of ligaments, tendons, and/or severed nerves
  - Cover the wound with a sterile dressing.
  - Splint in functional position.
- If time allows and major organ trauma is suspected, insert a nasogastric tube and Foley urinary catheter.
- Transport as soon as possible.

Client Instructions

- Transport to appropriately staffed emergency department as indicated.

BIBLIOGRAPHY

Marx J, Hockberger R, Walls R. *Rosen's Emergency Medicine: Concepts and Clinical Practice.* 13th ed. St. Louis, MO: Saunders; 2015.

Gastrointestinal Procedures

104

Anoscopy
Margaret R. Colyar

CPT Code
46600 Anoscopy, diagnostic with or without collection of specimen
46606 Anoscopy with biopsy, single or multiple
46608 Anoscopy with removal of foreign body
46614 Anoscopy with control of bleeding, any method

Anoscopy is the direct visualization of the anus using a **speculum**. It is used to screen, diagnose, and evaluate perianal and anal problems.

OVERVIEW
- Used in
  - Emergency departments
  - Primary care settings

RATIONALE
- To screen, diagnose, and evaluate perianal and anal problems

INDICATIONS
- Rectal or anal bleeding or unusual discharge
- Perianal or anal pain
- Hemorrhoids
- Rectal prolapse
- Digital examination that reveals a mass
- Perianal abscess and condyloma

CONTRAINDICATIONS
- Acute cardiovascular problems—may stimulate the vasovagal reaction
- Acute abdominal problems

- Unwilling patient
- Stenosis of the anal canal
▶ *Informed consent required*

PROCEDURE

Anoscopy

Equipment

- Anoscope (Fig. 104.1)
- Light source
- Gloves—nonsterile
- Drape—nonsterile
- Water-soluble lubricant (K-Y jelly)
- Large cotton-tipped applicators—nonsterile
- Monsel's solution—to control bleeding (ferric subsulfate)
- 4 × 4 gauze—nonsterile
- Biopsy forceps
- Container with 10% formalin

Procedure

- Position the client in the left lateral decubitus position.
- Drape the client.
- Put on gloves.
- Tell the client you are going to touch him or her by the rectum.
- Spread the gluteal fold and examine visually.
- Have the client bear down and observe for hemorrhoids or prolapse.
- Lubricate your second digit with K-Y jelly and perform a digital examination.

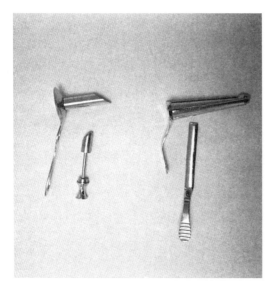

Figure 104.1 Anoscopes.

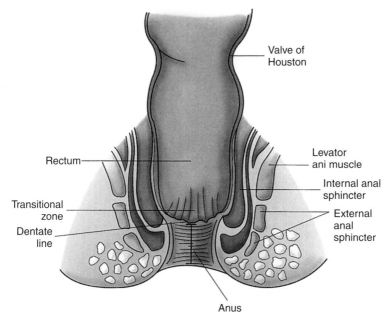

Figure 104.2 Anatomy of the anus and rectum.

- Lubricate the anoscope with K-Y jelly.
- Have the client take slow, deep breaths to relax the sphincter.
- Insert the anoscope slowly and gently into the anus toward the umbilicus.
- Remove the obturator.
- Visualize the rectal mucosa, noting the vasculature, pectinate line, transitional zone (Fig. 104.2), and drainage.
- Remove fecal matter and drainage with a large cotton swab if necessary.
- Obtain a biopsy specimen if needed using the biopsy forceps. Place the tissue specimen in a container with 10% formalin.
- If bleeding is present, apply Monsel's solution and pressure.
- Remove anoscope gently and observe the mucosa for any injury.

Client Instructions

- Slight bleeding is normal after this procedure because of the possibility of an abrasion, tearing of the mucosa or anus, or hemorrhoids.
  - If slight bleeding persists for more than 2 days, notify your health-care provider.
- To decrease pain and swelling, sit in a tub of warm water for 10 to 15 minutes three times per day.

BIBLIOGRAPHY

Pfenninger JL, Fowler GC. *Procedures for Primary Care Physicians.* St. Louis, MO: Mosby; 2019.

105 Chapter

Hemoccult

Margaret R. Colyar

CPT Code
82270 Blood, occult, by peroxidase activity (e.g., guaiac), qualitative;
feces, consecutive collected specimens with single
determination, for colorectal neoplasm screening

The fecal occult blood test (Hemoccult; guaiac) is a very sensitive test and can detect a small trace of blood in the patient's stool even before it is visible to the naked eye. The Hemoccult test can detect bleeding from almost anywhere along the length of the digestive tract. Several conditions can cause the result to be positive: esophagitis, gastritis, peptic ulcer disease, stomach cancer, ulcerative colitis, colorectal cancer or polyps, and hemorrhoids. The result also can be positive when someone has been taking aspirin or other medications that irritate the digestive tract.

The Hemoccult test is part of colon cancer prevention, but must be supplemented with more accurate examinations of the colon, such as a screening sigmoidoscopy, a screening colonoscopy, or a barium enema.

OVERVIEW

- Using Hemoccult annual screening tests, you can reduce the risk of death from cancer-related causes by up to 33%.
- Most colon cancers and polyps bleed intermittently. Some don't bleed at all—especially in early curable stages. Therefore, a negative stool Hemoccult test misses about 60% of colon polyps and 40% of colon cancers.
- False-positive results can occur after ingestion of
  - Vitamin C
  - Aspirin
  - Digestive-irritating medications such as NSAIDs
  - Iron supplements
  - Red meat (the blood it contains can turn the test positive)
  - Cucumber, cauliflower, turnips, broccoli, cantaloupe, artichokes, mushrooms, and horseradish

RATIONALE

- To detect blood in the feces
- To detect colorectal cancer symptoms

CONTRAINDICATIONS

- None

PROCEDURE

Hemoccult

Equipment

- Gloves
- Hemoccult card

Procedure

SINGLE HEMOCCULT SAMPLE

- Put on gloves.
- Using a tongue blade, scoop a small portion of stool onto the indented boxes on the Hemoccult card and close the flap.
- Turn the card over and instill one drop of developer onto each area and the two circles at the bottom of the card.
- Compare the results of the stool samples with the circles at the bottom.
- If the sample turns blue, then the test is positive for blood in the stool sample.
- If the sample does not turn blue, then the test is negative for blood in the stool sample.

Procedure

SERIAL/CONSECUTIVE HEMOCCULT SAMPLES

- Collect stool specimens from three consecutive bowel movements on three different days.
  - Place a collection container under the seat of the toilet to collect the stool.
  - Fill in the information on the front cover of each slide.
  - Open the first flap (with the information area toward you) and proceed as follows:
    - Collect a small amount of stool specimen on applicator.
    - Apply a very thin smear inside box A.
    - Use the other end of the applicator to obtain another sample from a different part of the stool and apply to box B.
    - Close cover and label slide with date and time collected.
    - Repeat all the above steps on the two remaining slides for your next two bowel movements.
  - Keep slide away from heat and light.
  - Return slides to the lab by mailing them or dropping them off in person.

Client Instructions

- For 3 days before and during collection, avoid
  - Red or rare meats (beef, lamb, and liver)
  - Vitamin C in excess of 250 mg a day

- Eliminate 2 days before the test
  - Horseradish, turnips, cauliflower, broccoli, cantaloupe, artichokes, and mushrooms
  - Iron supplements
- For 48 hours before and during collection
  - Have high fiber and roughage in your diet
- For 7 days before and during collection, avoid
  - NSAIDs such as ibuprofen (Motrin, Advil), naproxen (Aleve), or aspirin (more than one adult aspirin a day)
- Do not take the test during a menstrual cycle or if hemorrhoidal bleeding is occurring.

BIBLIOGRAPHY

Stool guaiac test. MedlinePlus Web site. http://www.nlm.nih.gov/medlineplus/ency/article/003393.htm
https://www.cliawaived.com/web/items/pdf/beckman_coulter_hemoccult_sensa_test
~4342file2.pdf

106 Chapter

Flexible Sigmoidoscopy
Margaret R. Colyar

CPT Code
45330 Sigmoidoscopy, flexible; diagnostic, with or without collection of specimens by brushing or washing
45331 Sigmoidoscopy, flexible; with biopsy, single or multiple
45332 Sigmoidoscopy, flexible; with removal of foreign body

Flexible **sigmoidoscopy** is a colorectal cancer screening technique that detects 50% to 60% of colon cancers. With flexible sigmoidoscopy, the inner lining of the rectum and the last 2 feet of the distal colon can be visualized; 60-cm sigmoidoscopy is preferred.

OVERVIEW

- Screening indications
  - Normal clients age older than 50—every 3 to 5 years
  - Annually
    - High-risk clients—age older than 35

- History of polyps
- Inflammatory bowel disease
- Rectal bleeding
- Constipation or diarrhea—change in bowel habits
- Abdominal pain
- Unexplained weight loss
- Anemia
- Family history
- Colorectal cancer
  - Second most common cause of cancer death in the United States
  - Appears to be age related
  - 50% survival rate
  - Causes
    - Inherited
    - Environmental factors (i.e., diet high in fats and low in fiber)
    - Suspicious symptoms
    - Persistent abdominal pain
    - Change in bowel habits
    - Rectal bleeding
    - Positive Hemoccult test
    - Unexplained weight loss or fevers
    - Anemia
- Normal versus abnormal findings and when to **biopsy** (Table 106.1)

HEALTH PROMOTION/PREVENTION

- Healthy diet—high fiber—20 to 35 g per day
- Aspirin 325 mg every day if in high-risk group
  - Contraindicated with aspirin gastritis and gastric ulcers

RATIONALE

- To screen for colorectal cancer

INDICATIONS

- Rectal bleeding
- Positive Hemoccult test
- Mass on digital examination
- Lower abdominal pain and cramping
- Change in bowel habits
- Foreign body in the rectum
- Itching—anal or perianal
- Pain—anal or perianal

CONTRAINDICATIONS

- Acute abdomen
- Diverticulitis

Table 106·1	Normal Versus Abnormal Findings and When to Perform a Biopsy			
DESCRIPTION	NORMAL	ABNORMAL	YES	NO
Adenocarcinoma	X		X	
Crohn's colitis		X	X	
Diverticula	X			X
Diverticulitis		X		X
Hyperplastic polyp, rectum	X		X	
Lipoma	X		X	
Melanosis coli	X			X
Multiple colonic polyps		X	X	
Proctitis		X	X	
Pseudomembranous colitis		X	X	
Rectum, first valve of Houston	X			X
Rectum, dentate line	X			X
Sigmoid colon, valves of Houston	X			X
Transverse colon	X			X
Tubulovillose adenoma		X	X	
Tubular adenoma		X	X	
Ulcerative colitis		X	X	
Vascular ectasia		X	X	
Villose adenoma		X	X	

- Cardiovascular or pulmonary disease
- Ileus
- Suspected perforation
- Megacolon
- Pregnancy
- Recent pelvic or abdominal surgery
- Coagulation disorders

▶ *Informed consent required*

- Bowel preparation needed
  - Clear liquid diet the night before the procedure
    - May take medications
  - Fleet enemas until clear 30 to 60 minutes before the procedure
  - Laxative (bisacodyl) the evening before the procedure

PROCEDURE

Flexible Sigmoidoscopy

Equipment

- Flexible sigmoidoscope—60 cm (Fig. 106.1)
- Light source

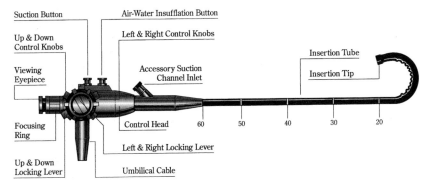

Figure 106.1 Flexible sigmoidoscope.
(Reproduced with permission from Glaxo Wellcome Inc. and the University of Arizona School of Medicine.)

- Two pairs of gloves—nonsterile
- Suction
- K-Y jelly or 2% lidocaine jelly
- 4 × 4 gauze—nonsterile
- Absorbent pads—nonsterile
- Drape—nonsterile
- Culture tubes
- Emesis basin
- Sigmoidoscopy report sheet (Fig. 106.2)

Procedure

- Position the client in the left lateral decubitus position.
  - Right leg flexed at the hip and knee
- Put on two pairs of gloves.
- Lubricate the second or third digit of the dominant hand.
- Perform a digital examination to dilate the sphincter.
- Lubricate the anus and the tip of the sigmoidoscope.
- Lubricate the distal half of the sigmoidoscope but not the lens.
- Remove the top pair of gloves and dispose of them.
- Separate the gluteal folds.
- Insert the scope gently 8 to 10 cm.
- Activate the light, suction, and air.
- With the right hand—advance the scope.
- With the left hand—work the controls on the scope.
- Open the colon by insufflating with a small amount of air, and advance the scope gently.
  - Do not use too much air—this causes discomfort.
- Advance the scope using one of the following techniques
  - Hook and pullout—used to straighten the colon (Fig. 106.3)
    - Hook mucosal fold, and pull back to straighten the colon.

Office
Flexible Sigmoidoscopy

Date: _____ Chart #/ID #: _____

Patient Name: _____

Race: _____ Age: _____ Sex: ____

History Abdominal/Gyn surgery? Yes No

Bowel Prep Used: Dulcolax Tabs Golytely Fleets Other

Reason for procedure: (circle all that apply)

1. Screening	4. Rectal bleeding	8. Anemia
2. Abdominal pain	5. Guaiac-positive stools	9. Weight loss
3. Change in bowel habits	6. Constipation	10. Abnormal x-ray
	7. Diarrhea	11. Other: _____

Distance scope inserted: _____ cm

Findings: (circle and diagram)

1. Normal	4. Mucosal abnormality
2. Hemorrhoids	5. Polyp(s) (describe) _____
3. Diverticuli	6. Mass/lesion
	7. Other: _____

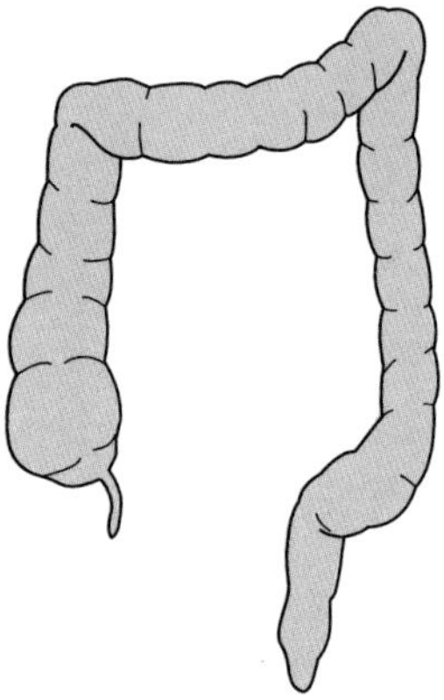

Insertion depth(s) at which abnormality was found: _____ cm

Biopsy performed? Yes No

Additional testing needed: Colonoscopy? GI consult? Barium enema?

Comments and/or pathology report: _____

_____

_____
Signature - Provider

Figure 106.2 Sigmoidoscopy report sheet.

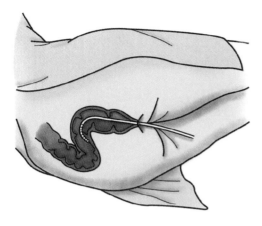

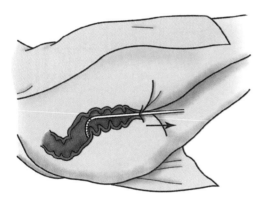

Figure 106.3 Hook and pullout. Hook the mucosal fold, and pull back to straighten the colon.

- **Dither** and **torque**—used to shorten the colon (Fig. 106.4)
  - Alternate insertion with slow partial withdrawal to pleat the colon.
  - Twist the sigmoid shaft clockwise or counterclockwise with a forward and/or backward motion.
  - Observe for natural landmarks (Fig. 106.5) and abnormalities (Fig. 106.6).
  - Take a biopsy specimen of all abnormal areas and put in culture tube for biopsy.
  - Withdraw the sigmoidoscope slowly, reinspecting the mucosa.
  - When in the rectal vault, retroflex the tip of the scope to visualize the distal rectum.
  - Straighten the tip, and gently withdraw the scope.
  - Cleanse, sterilize, and store per manufacturer's instructions.

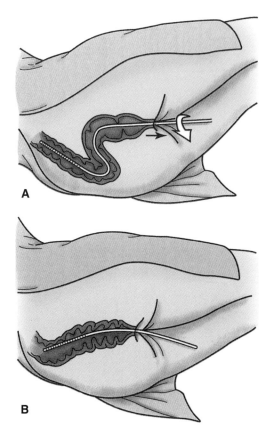

A

B

Figure 106.4 Dither and torque. (A) Pleat the colon by alternating insertion with slow partial withdrawal of the sigmoidoscope. (B) Next, twist the sigmoid shaft clockwise or counterclockwise with a forward and/or backward motion.

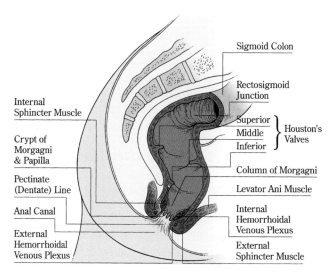

Sigmoid Colon

Internal Sphincter Muscle

Rectosigmoid Junction

Superior
Middle } Houston's
Inferior } Valves

Crypt of Morgagni & Papilla

Pectinate (Dentate) Line

Column of Morgagni

Levator Ani Muscle

Anal Canal

Internal Hemorrhoidal Venous Plexus

External Hemorrhoidal Venous Plexus

External Sphincter Muscle

Figure 106.5 Normal rectal findings. *(Reproduced with permission of Glaxo Wellcome Inc. and the University of Arizona School of Medicine.)*

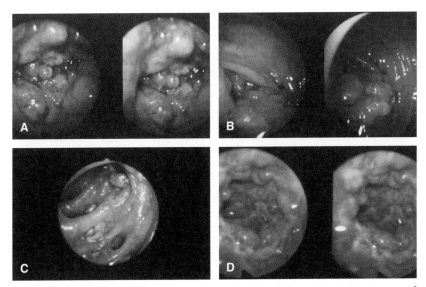

Figure 106.6 Abnormal rectal findings. (A) Cancer of the rectum. (B) Cancer of the sigmoid colon. (C) Diverticulosis of the sigmoid colon. (D) Crohn's disease of the sigmoid colon. *(Reproduced with permission of Glaxo Wellcome Inc. and the University of Arizona School of Medicine.)*

Client Instructions

- The following may be expected but will resolve quickly.
  - Abdominal cramping if a biopsy specimen was obtained
  - Feeling of fullness, distention, or flatus
  - No bowel movement for several days
  - Minor bleeding
- No special diet is recommended after the procedure.
- Watch for signs of infections, such as
  - Elevated temperature
  - Increased or prolonged rectal pain
  - Green or yellow drainage

BIBLIOGRAPHY

Colodny CS. Procedures for your practice. *Patient Care*, April 1996:151–157.
Dominitz JA, McCormick LH, Rex DK. Latest approaches to prevention and screening. *Patient Care*, April 1996:124–142.
Flexible sigmoidoscopy. Diagnostic Tests. National Institute of Diabetes and Digestive Kidney Diseases Web site. https://www.niddk.nih.gov/health-information/diagnostic-tests/flexible-sigmoidoscopy. June, 2016.
Flexible sigmoidoscopy. My Doctor. Kaiser Permanente. YouTube. https://www.youtube.com/watch?v=qGwgWKVbfi4. August 21, 2013.
Reilly HF. Primary care use of the flexible sigmoidoscope to detect colorectal cancer and its precursors. *Primary Care Cancer*, 1994;14(5):41–45.

107

Urea Breath Test

Margaret R. Colyar

CPT Code
83014 Test administration
83013 Test analysis

Helicobacter pylori (H. pylori) is a type of bacterium commonly associated with dyspepsia, gastritis, gastric ulcers, duodenal ulcers, and peptic ulcers. It colonizes the stomach, and this indirectly leads to gastric inflammation, which if left untreated will lead to chronic gastritis and ulceration. The urea breath test (UBT) is based on the *H. pylori* bacteria's ability to break down urea into carbon dioxide. This carbon dioxide then is absorbed by the stomach's lining and passes into the blood. From the blood, it passes into the lungs and is eliminated in the breath.

The UBT method is recommended by the American College of Gastroenterology as an appropriate test for both initial diagnosis and posttreatment testing for active *H. pylori* infection. Patients prefer to be tested for *H. pylori* using a UBT rather than a stool sample. The UBT has excellent sensitivity (95.5%) and specificity (96.0%) for confirming eradication.

OVERVIEW

- Urea breath test (UBT):
  - Most reliable nonendoscopic test to confirm eradication
  - Accurately detects active gastrointestinal colonization by *H. pylori*
  - Preferred alternative when endoscopic follow-up is unnecessary
  - May avoid multiple gastric biopsies due to the variable prevalence and density of the infection throughout the stomach

PATIENT PREPARATION

- Two weeks before the test, stop any antibiotics, proton pump inhibitors, or bismuth.
  - May continue on H2 blocker therapy (see Table 107.1)
  - Fast at least 1 hour before samples are collected.

RATIONALE

- To detect the presence of *H. pylori* in the GI system
- To test for eradication of *H. pylori* posttreatment

Table 107-1	List of H2 Blockers and Proton Pump Inhibitors
H2 Blockers	
Brand Name	**Generic Name**
Axid	nizatidine
Pepcid	famotidine
Tagamet	cimetidine
Zantac	ranitidine
Proton Pump Inhibitors	
Brand Name	**Generic Name**
Aciphex	rabeprazole
Dexilent	dexlansoprazole
Nexium	esomeprazole
Prevacid	lansoprazole
Prilosec	omeprazole
Protonix	pantoprazole
Vimovo	esomeprazole/magnesium
Yosprala	aspirin/omeprazole
Zegerid	omeprazole/sodium bicarbonate

INDICATIONS

- Avoids unnecessary treatments that could make the bacteria resistant to antibiotics
- Best test to confirm that the treatment was successful

CONTRAINDICATIONS

- Use of bismuth preparations within 2 weeks of testing, such as Maalox, Mylanta, Gaviscon
- Use of proton pump inhibitors (see Table 107.1) within 2 weeks of testing
- Use of antimicrobials within 2 weeks of testing

PROCEDURE

Urea Breath Test

Procedure

- Have the patient collect a sample of his or her breath before the test starts by blowing into a balloon or by blowing bubbles into a bottle containing liquid.
- Give the patient a dose of urea labeled with either radioactive carbon-14 or nonradioactive carbon-13.
- Collect samples after administering the urea.
- Compare samples before and after the urea dosage to determine the presence of the bacteria. This difference is compared with the cutoff value to check for infection. Samples are collected at different times, and the test itself takes about 1.5 hours to complete.

- The ratio of $^{13}CO^2$ to $^{12}CO^2$ in breath samples is determined by infrared spectrophotometry.

Note: A positive result is associated with the presence of *H. pylori* infection.

Client Instructions

- Posttherapeutic testing should be done 4 weeks after *H. pylori* treatment to determine whether eradication has been completed and to avoid false-negative results.

BIBLIOGRAPHY

Chey WD, Wong BCY. Practice Parameters Committee of the American College of Gastroenterology. American College of Gastroenterology guideline on the management of *Helicobacter pylori* infection. *Am J Gastroenterol.* 2007;102:1808–1825.
Talley NJ, Vakil NB, Moayyedi P. American Gastroenterological Association technical review on the evaluation of dyspepsia. *Gastroenterology.* 2005;129:1756–1780. https://www.metsol.com/hydrogen-breath-test/healthcare-providers/ubt/.

108 Chapter

X-Ray Interpretation
Abdominal

Margaret R. Colyar

CPT Code
Multiple listings based on view ordered

An abdominal x-ray (radiograph) is considered a basic radiological screening tool when evaluating abdominal disorders. It can be ordered as a kidneys, ureters, and bladder (KUB) flat plate, or 1-view abdomen. If suspicious for free air, order a left lateral decubitus view and chest posteroanterior view. Other, higher technology tools used to evaluate abdominal disorders include computed tomography (CT) and magnetic resonance imaging (MRI). The ability of the abdominal x-ray to generate high spatial resolution and to visualize various densities within the abdominal cavity can aid in diagnostic evaluation of abdominal disorders but should not be the sole basis for diagnosis. The abdominal x-ray should be correlated with clinical history, physical examination, and additional diagnostic tool results.

OVERVIEW

- Densities
  - Air—DARK
  - Muscles—GRAY
  - Fat—Light GRAY
  - Muscle—Very light GRAY
  - Bones—WHITE
  - Foreign Body—Varies based on density
    - Coin—DARK
    - Wood splinter—difficult to see
- Inspect the PA view to determine if the x-ray is adequate using **RIPE**
  - **R**otation—Do the clavicles and vertebrae form a cross?
  - **I**nspiration—Are there a minimum of eight ribs visible?
  - **P**enetration—Are the interspaces visible and the thoracic vertebral bodies well defined?
  - **E**xposure—Too much or too little?
- General principles
  - Adequate knowledge of basic anatomy and physiology is necessary for proper interpretation of the abdominal film.
  - An orderly and systematic approach to interpretation of the abdominal film should be used.
  - Small bowel looks like stacked coins and is typically NOT visible on a normal film.
  - Abdominal x-ray red flags (Table 108.1)

RATIONALE

- To obtain visual information about physical anatomy of the abdominal region
- To obtain a visual overview of basic pathophysiology of gastrointestinal, vascular, renal, and skeletal systems of the human organism

INDICATIONS

- Abdominal trauma
- Abdominal pain
- Suspicion of abdominal pathophysiology
- Ingested foreign body

CONTRAINDICATIONS

- Pregnancy (unless shielded)

Table 108·1 **Abdominal X-Ray Red Flags**
Free air under the diaphragm
Free air on supine films
Small focal bubbles may be abscess

PROCEDURE

X-Ray Interpretation—Abdominal

Equipment

• X-ray view box or digital viewing program

Procedure

• Place the flat and upright films and left lateral decubitus and chest film (if ordered) on the view box with adequate illumination.
• Inspect for the presence of any foreign bodies in the abdominal cavity.
• Systematically inspect the abdominal region skeletal system.
  • Identify anatomical skeletal landmarks within the abdominal cavity (lumbar, sacrum, and pelvis) (Fig. 108.1).
    • Determine any aberration.
  • Note the absence or presence of demineralization.
  • Note the lack of continuity or symmetry of skeletal structures that may represent fracture, dislocation, metastases (lytic—low density; sclerotic—high density; and mixed), and calcifications of the lumbosacral spine, iliosacral region, pelvis, acetabulum, and femur region.
  • Note the presence of pathological calcifications.

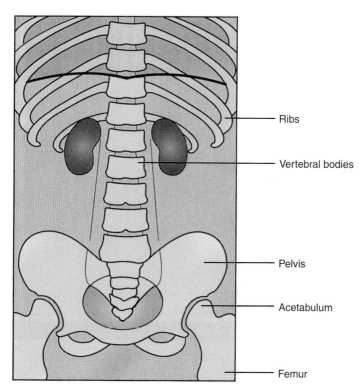

Ribs

Vertebral bodies

Pelvis

Acetabulum

Femur

Figure 108.1 Identify anatomical skeletal landmarks of the abdomen.

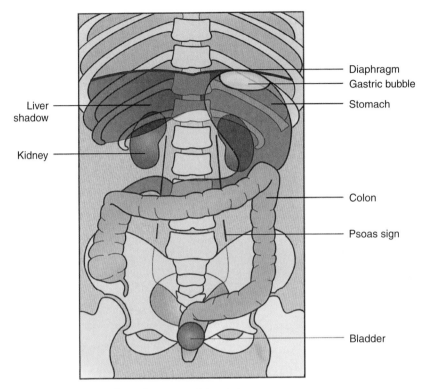

Figure 108.2 Inspect the soft tissues of the abdomen.

- Systematically inspect the soft tissues (Fig. 108.2).
  - Note the presence or absence of the psoas sign.
  - *Diaphragm*—Note the presence or absence of an air and/or fluid pattern under the diaphragm; may indicate abscess.
  - *Liver*
    - Note the homogeneous uniform density of the hepatic shadow.
    - Note the presence or absence of full visualization of hepatic edge.
  - *Spleen*—The splenic shadow generally is hidden by the gastric bubble and splenic flexure of the colon unless splenomegaly is present.
  - *Pancreas*—Usually not visible
  - *Renal*—The entire renal shadow outlines generally are not clearly demarcated. It may be difficult to estimate the overall size of the organs.
  - *Bladder*—If filled, appears as a round homogeneous mass
  - *Uterus*—Usually not visible; however, can present as an irregular mass if fibroids are present.
  - *Vascular*—Note the presence of any calcifications, widening, or tortuosity of the aorta or renal arteries.
  - *Gastrointestinal evaluation*
    - *Stomach*—Note that the gastric shadow with presence of gastric bubble usually is located midline to left upper quadrant region (Fig. 108.3).

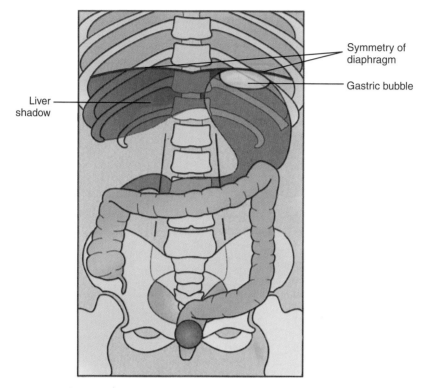

Symmetry of
diaphragm

Gastric bubble

Liver
shadow

Figure 108.3 Inspect the stomach for location and presence of gastric bubble.

- *Intestines*—Air shadow location is scattered in a random, nonspecific pattern throughout the abdominal cavity.
  - Variables, such as age, amount of air ingested, length of small or large intestine, stool concentration, and pathology can cause normal presentations to appear abnormal and vice versa.
  - Abdominal gas pattern location is generally nonspecific (Fig. 108.4).
  - Abnormal concentration of abdominal gas in one location and/or unilateral appearance of the air gas pattern on one side with the absence of any air on the opposite side may suggest *bowel displacement*.
  - Location and concentration of air with accompanying dilated bowel proximally and decreased air shadows distally suggest paralytic ileus (Fig. 108.5).
  - Localization with the presence of dilated bowel with or without air and/or fluid levels proximally and absence of air shadows distally suggests local obstruction.
- *Peritoneum*
  - Note free air in the peritoneal cavity (pneumoperitoneum) (Fig. 108.6). This is usually caused by the disruption of the abdominal wall.

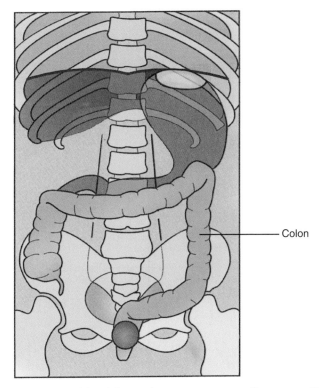

Figure 108.4 The abdominal gas pattern is usually nonspecific in distribution.

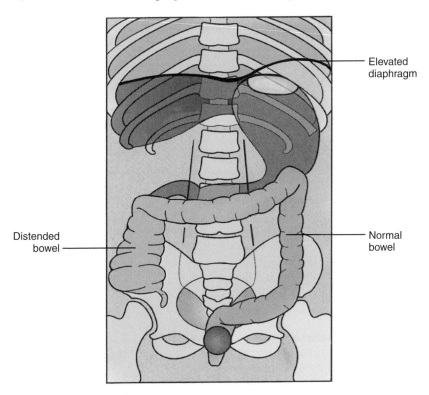

Figure 108.5 Paralytic ileus.

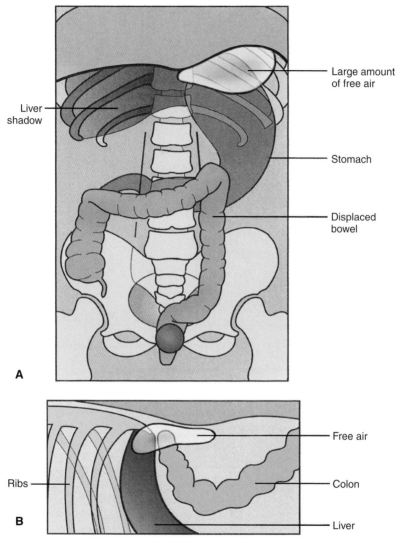

Figure 108.6 Pneumoperitoneum. (A) Upright view; (B) left lateral decubitus view.

- Usually seen with left lateral decubitus and chest posteroanterior views; dark air shadows can be visualized in the diaphragm and against the inferior hepatic margin.
- Inspect for intraperitoneal fluid.
- Usually obscures hepatic edges.
- Displaces abdominal gas pattern.

BIBLIOGRAPHY

Barloon T, Weissman A. Diagnostic imaging in the evaluation of blunt abdominal trauma. *Am Fam Physician.* 1996;54(1):205–211.

Smith WL, Farrell TA. *Radiology 101: The Basics and Fundamentals of Imaging.* Philadelphia, PA: Lippincott Williams & Wilkins; 2013.

Chapter

109

Gastric Lavage
Margaret R. Colyar

CPT Code
91105 Gastric Lavage

Gastric lavage is a procedure used to aspirate gastric contents and irrigate the stomach. Gastric lavage also is used to assist in the evacuation of toxic substances that are only partially digested. Toxic substances usually are ingested in suicide attempts or accidents (children).

OVERVIEW
- Use small-gauge tube (nasogastric route) if
  - The tube will be left in place after gastric lavage
- Use large-gauge Ewald tube (orogastric route) to
  - Evacuate large particles, such as partially digested pills

OPTIONS
- Method 1—Gastric lavage for specimen collection
- Method 2—Gastric lavage for hemorrhage
- Method 3—Gastric lavage for overdose

RATIONALE
- To aspirate gastric contents
- To collect specimens
- To irrigate the stomach
- To evacuate toxic substances
- To stop gastric hemorrhage

INDICATIONS
- Ingested poisons—liquid or solid
- Drug overdose
- Gastric bleeding
- Stomach cleansing before endoscopic testing
- Gastric washings for cytology

CONTRAINDICATIONS
- Alkali or acids ingested that may perforate the stomach
- Convulsions

- Ingestion of petroleum products
- Cardiac dysrhythmias

PROCEDURE

Gastric Lavage

Equipment

- Method 1 only
  - No. 16 Salem sump nasal gastric tube (NGT)
- Methods 1, 2, and 3
  - 60-mL syringe with catheter tip
  - Water-soluble lubricant
  - Gloves—nonsterile
  - Towels or absorbent drapes
  - Wash basin—to empty gastric contents into
  - Emesis basin
  - Ice water
  - 0.9% sodium chloride
  - Containers for specimens
- Methods 2 and 3
  - Large-bore Ewald orogastric tube
  - Suction machine—optional
- Method 3 only
  - Antidote—if needed
  - Call poison control center for appropriate antidote.

Procedure

METHOD 1—GASTRIC LAVAGE FOR SPECIMEN COLLECTION

- Position the client in a Fowler's position (if alert) or left lateral position (if comatose).
- Remove dentures if applicable.
- Measure from the bridge of the nose to earlobe to xiphoid process and mark with tape.
- Drape the client.
- Put on gloves.
- Lubricate the tip of the tube.
- Instruct the client to tilt the head back when the tube is introduced into the nose.
  - *Optional*—Place the NGT in a basin of ice water to stiffen it so that it is easier to insert and does not get coiled on its way to the stomach.
  - *Optional*—If there is a problem inserting because of nose sensitivity, use a topical anesthetic in the nostril.
- Pass the tube through the mouth (Ewald tube) or nose (smaller NGT) into the stomach.
- Have the client sip water through the straw to facilitate passage of the NGT.
  - If drinking water is contraindicated, instruct the client to swallow as the tube is advanced.

- Insert the tube slowly and gently.
  - If any symptoms of respiratory difficulty are observed (cough, dyspnea, cyanosis), the NGT is probably being inserted into the lung. Withdraw immediately and reinsert.
- Tape the tube in place.
- Check position of the tube with an air bubble and aspiration of gastric contents.
- Obtain a specimen of the gastric contents.

METHOD 2—GASTRIC LAVAGE FOR HEMORRHAGE

- Position the client in a Fowler's position (if alert) or left lateral position (if comatose).
- Remove dentures if applicable.
- Measure from the bridge of the nose to earlobe to xiphoid process and mark with tape.
- Drape the client.
- Put on gloves.
- Lubricate the tip of the tube.
- Instruct the client to tilt the head back when the tube is introduced into the nose.
  - *Optional*—Place the NGT in a basin of ice water to stiffen it so that it is easier to insert and does not get coiled on its way to the stomach.
  - *Optional*—If there is a problem inserting because of nose sensitivity, use a topical anesthetic in the nostril.
- Pass the tube through the mouth (Ewald tube) or nose (smaller NGT) into the stomach.
- Have the client sip water through the straw to facilitate passage of the NGT.
  - If drinking water is contraindicated, instruct the client to swallow as the tube is advanced.
- Insert the tube slowly and gently.
  - If any symptoms of respiratory difficulty are observed (cough, dyspnea, cyanosis), the NGT is probably being inserted into the lung. Withdraw immediately and reinsert.
- Tape the tube in place.
- Check position of the tube with an air bubble and aspiration of gastric contents.
- Raise the tube above the client's head.
- Take the plunger out of the 60-mL syringe, and use the syringe as a funnel.
- Attach the syringe funnel to the tubing and instill 100 to 200 mL 0.9% sodium chloride (Fig. 109.1).
- Lower the funnel and allow the sodium chloride to flow out into the washbasin, or detach the funnel and attach the tubing to low suction.
- Continue this procedure of irrigation and suction until the gastric contents change from red to clear.
- Remove the tube if indicated.

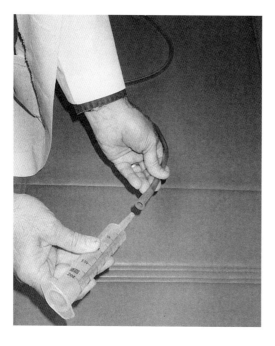

Figure 109.1 Attach the syringe funnel to the tubing and instill the sodium chloride.

METHOD 3—GASTRIC LAVAGE FOR OVERDOSE

- Position the client in a Fowler's position (if alert) or left lateral position (if comatose).
- Remove dentures if applicable.
- Measure from the bridge of the nose to earlobe to xiphoid process and mark with tape.
- Drape the client.
- Put on gloves.
- Lubricate the tip of the tube.
- Instruct the client to tilt the head back when the tube is introduced into the nose.
  - *Optional*—Place the NGT in a basin of ice water to stiffen it so that it is easier to insert and does not get coiled on its way to the stomach.
  - *Optional*—If there is a problem inserting because of nose sensitivity, use a topical anesthetic in the nostril.
- Pass the tube through the mouth (Ewald tube).
- Have the client sip water through the straw to facilitate passage of the NGT.
  - If drinking water is contraindicated, instruct the client to swallow as the tube is advanced.
- Insert the tube slowly and gently.
  - If any symptoms of respiratory difficulty are observed (cough, dyspnea, cyanosis), the NGT is probably being inserted into the lung. Withdraw immediately and reinsert.
- Tape the tube in place.

- Check position of the tube with an air bubble and aspiration of gastric contents.
- Raise the tube above the client's head.
- Take the plunger out of the 60-mL syringe and use the syringe as a funnel.
- Attach the syringe funnel to the tubing.
  - If the poison ingested was liquid, follow the directions of the poison control center for irrigation and instillation of antidote.
  - If the poison ingested was solid, instill 100 to 200 mL 0.9% sodium chloride unless contraindicated.
    - Lower the funnel and allow the sodium chloride to flow out into the washbasin, or detach the funnel and attach the tubing to low suction.
    - Irrigate with sodium chloride until the gastric contents are clear and no particles are seen.
- Instill the appropriate antidote and follow instructions of poison control center.
- Obtain several specimens of gastric contents throughout this procedure.
- Remove the tube if indicated.

Client Instructions

- Throat may be sore for 1 to 3 days. Suck on ice chips or throat lozenges.
- If the procedure was done to treat overdose or poison ingestion, return to the office in 24 hours for recheck.

BIBLIOGRAPHY

Hinkle JL, Cheever KH. *Brunner and Suddarth's Textbook of Medical-Surgical Nursing.* 14th ed. Philadelphia, PA: Lippincott Williams & Wilkins; 2017.
Kellerman RD, Bope ET. *Conn's Current Therapy.* Philadelphia, PA: Elsevier; 2018.

Chapter **110**

Inguinal Hernia Reduction
Margaret R. Colyar

CPT Code
49500 Repair initial inguinal hernia, age 6 months to 5 years; reducible
49505 Repair initial inguinal hernia, age older than 5 years; reducible
49505 Repair recurrent inguinal hernia, any age; reducible

A hernia is a result of weakness in the abdominal muscle wall through which a bowel segment or peritoneal structure protrudes. Types of hernias include (Fig. 110.1)

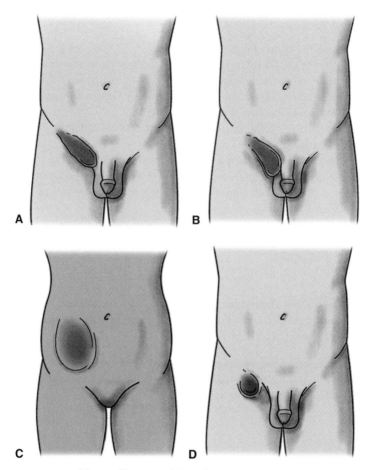

Figure 110.1 Types of hernias. (A) Indirect inguinal hernia; (B) direct inguinal hernia; (C) direct abdominal hernia; and (D) femoral hernia.

- Indirect—protrusion of a bowel segment or peritoneal contents through the inguinal ring and down the spermatic cord through the inguinal canal
  - Often descend into the scrotal area
  - Most common; usually found in men and children
  - Usually **incarcerated** and require surgery
- Direct—protrusion of a bowel segment or peritoneal contents through the abdominal wall in an area of muscle weakness
  - More common in elderly

OVERVIEW

- Causes
  - Intra-abdominal pressure, such as
    - Pregnancy
    - Obesity

- Ascites
- Heavy lifting
- Coughing
- Abdominal wall weakness, such as
  - Inherited
  - Acquired
- Terminology
  - Reducible—can be replaced into the abdominal wall with gentle pressure
  - Incarcerated or irreducible—trapped bowel that cannot be replaced into the abdominal wall with gentle pressure
  - Strangulated—blood supply to herniated bowel is cut off. Signs and symptoms include
    - Abdominal distention
    - Pain
    - Nausea
    - Vomiting
    - Tachycardia

HEALTH PROMOTION/PREVENTION

- Maintain normal body weight.
- Maintain good physical fitness.
- Use proper lifting techniques.
- Avoid straining and lifting.
- Wear a truss to hold the organs in place if the abdominal wall is sagging.

RATIONALE

- To prevent strangulation and incarceration of the hernia

INDICATIONS

- Palpable bulging in the abdomen or groin
- Discomfort

CONTRAINDICATIONS

- If strangulation is suspected, REFER to a surgeon immediately.

PROCEDURE

Abdominal Hernia Reduction

Equipment

- Gloves—nonsterile

Procedure

- Position the client in a recumbent position or Trendelenburg position with knees flexed to decrease intra-abdominal pressure.
- Wait 30 minutes to see whether passive reduction occurs.

- If passive reduction does not occur, guide the herniated bowel gently through the opening, using fingers flat on the abdomen.
- If the client is a child, *follow-up* with a surgeon is necessary for surgical repair.

Client Instructions

- If protrusion recurs, lie down on your back to allow passive reduction to occur. If the hernia does not reduce, return to the office.
- Bowel obstruction is a possibility with any hernia and can be life threatening. Symptoms are
  - Abdominal distention
  - Pain
  - Nausea
  - Vomiting
  - Tachycardia
- If any of these symptoms occur, return to the office or go to the emergency department immediately.

BIBLIOGRAPHY

Ignatavicius DD, Workman ML. *Medical-Surgical Nursing*. 8th ed. Philadelphia, PA: Saunders; 2016.

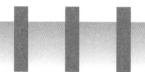

Chapter

Percutaneous Endoscopic Gastrostomy (PEG) Tube Reinsertion

Margaret R. Colyar

CPT Code
43750 Percutaneous placement of gastrostomy tube
43760 Change of gastrostomy tube

A **percutaneous** endoscopic gastrostomy (PEG) tube usually is used to administer feedings and medications and extends from the external abdomen directly into the stomach. Reinsertion of the tube is necessary when the client or caregiver inadvertently dislodges it.

OVERVIEW

* Two types of surgery are used (Fig. 111.1).
  * Permanent gastrostomy with stoma
  * Percutaneous endoscopic gastrostomy

RATIONALE

* To promote continuous nutrition and medication to the client

INDICATIONS

* PEG tube is dislodged.

CONTRAINDICATIONS

* Newly inserted tube—within 4 to 5 days
* No obvious **fistula** opening
▶ *Informed consent required*

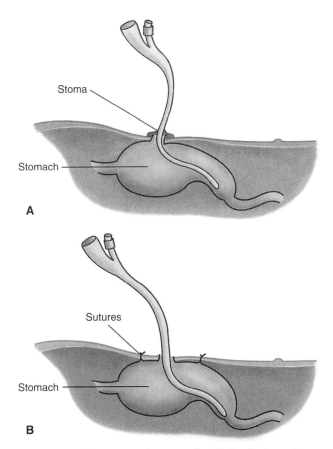

Figure 111.1 Two types of surgery for PEG tube insertion are permanent gastrostomy with (A) stoma and (B) percutaneous endoscopic gastrostomy.

PROCEDURE

PEG Tube Reinsertion

Equipment

- Foley catheter tube—same size as tube dislodged with one size larger balloon
- Topical skin cleanser
- Drape—sterile
- K-Y jelly
- Gloves—sterile
- Scissors—sterile
- 10-mL syringe with Luer-Lok
- 50- to 60-mL syringe with catheter tip
- 0.9% sodium chloride—enough to fill the balloon
- 4 × 4 gauze—sterile
- Tape catheter plug

Procedure

- Position the client in the supine position.
- Cleanse the stoma or insertion site with topical skin cleanser.
- Open the Foley catheter on the sterile drape.
- Put on gloves.
- Check the balloon by inflating with the Luer-Lok syringe filled with sterile saline; then deflate.
- Lubricate the tip of the catheter tube with K-Y jelly.
- Insert the tube 3 to 6 inches into the previous tube site (Fig. 111.2), using sterile technique.
  - Watch the client's face for signs of pain.
  - Stop if unable to advance the tube or the client is in pain.

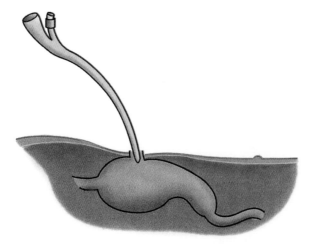

Figure 111.2 Insert 3 to 6 inches of the catheter into the old PEG tube site.

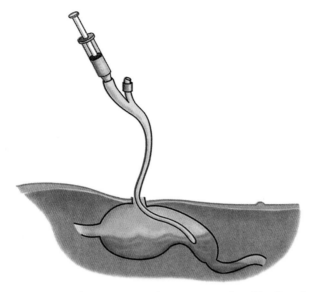

Figure 111.3 Aspirate stomach contents with a 60-mL catheter-tipped syringe to ensure proper placement.

- Aspirate stomach contents with 60-mL catheter-tipped syringe through big port of the tube (Fig. 111.3)
- If gastric contents are obtained, inflate the balloon with the appropriate amount of sterile saline.
- Pull back the tube gently until resistance is met (Fig. 111.4).
- Insert a catheter plug into the large port of the PEG tube.
- Cut a slit halfway through the 4 × 4 gauze.
- Apply the slit 4 × 4 gauze dressing around the newly inserted tube (Fig. 111.5).
- Tape the tube securely to the abdomen.

Client Instructions

- Keep the tube taped securely to the abdomen to prevent the tube from becoming dislodged.
- Observe for signs and symptoms of infection, such as
  - Increase in pain after 24 hours
  - Increase in temperature
  - Redness or swelling
  - Yellow or greenish drainage
  - Foul odor
- If any signs or symptoms of infection are found, return to the office.
- Take acetaminophen (Tylenol) every 4 to 6 hours as needed for pain.
- Return to the office if complications occur.

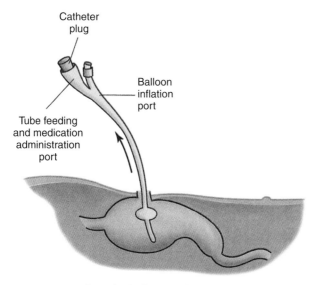

Figure 111.4 Inflate the balloon and gently pull back on the PEG tube until resistance is met. Plug the large port with a catheter plug.

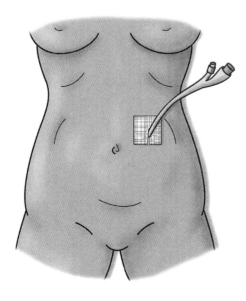

Figure 111.5 Cut a slit in the 4 × 4 gauze and secure it around the PEG tube.

BIBLIOGRAPHY

Arora G, Lukens FJ. Percutaneous endoscopic gastronomy (PEG) tube placement technique. *Medscape*. https://emedicine.medscape.com/article/149665-technique. Updated December 13, 2018.

Gutt CN, Held S, Paolucci V, Encke A. Experiences with percutaneous endoscopic gastrostomy. *World J Surg*. 1996:8:1006–1008, 1108–1109.

Taheri MR, Singh H, Duerksen DR. Peritonitis after gastrostomy tube replacement: A case series and review of literature. *J Parenter Enteral Nutr.* 2011:35(1):56–60.
Zacherl A, Love B, McCorvey R. Office laparoscopy under local anesthesia. *Minim Invasive Surg Nurs.* 1997;11(2):73–78.

Chapter

112

Perianal Skin Tags/External Hemorrhoidal Skin Tags

Margaret R. Colyar

CPT Code
11200 Removal of skin tags, any area, up to and including 15 lesions
11201 Removal of skin tags, any area, each additional 10 lesions
46220 Excision of single external papilla or tag, anus
46230 Excision of multiple external papilla or tag, anus

A skin tag is a tiny, benign, out-pouching of the skin that is typically connected to the underlying skin by a thin stalk. There may be skin left behind after treatment for hemorrhoids. They develop because of friction between clothing and skin or friction between adjacent areas of skin. Perianal skin tags are commonly seen in overweight or obese patients and in those with Crohn's disease.

OVERVIEW
• Perianal skin tags are not contagious or cancerous.
• Perianal skin tags may pose a problem maintaining cleanliness because of trapped moisture and irritation.

RATIONALE
• To remove unsightly skin tags
• To remove skin tags that pose a cleanliness problem
• To prevent infections from skin tags irritated by clothing

INDICATIONS
• Clothing rubbing on skin tags
• Tags that are hard to keep clean

CONTRAINDICATIONS

* On blood thinners

PROCEDURE

Perianal Skin Tag Removal/External Hemorrhoidal Skin Tag Removal

Equipment

* Antiseptic skin cleanser
* Cotton-tipped applicators—sterile
* Topical antibiotic (Bactroban, Bacitracin, or Polysporin)—optional
* Band-Aids
* Drape—sterile
* Tape—optional
* Gloves—sterile
* Sterile surgical kit that includes
  * 2 × 2 or 4 × 4 gauze
  * Forceps with teeth
  * Iris scissors
  * No. 11 or 15 scalpel
* 1% lidocaine
* 5-mL syringe
* 27-gauge, ½- to 1-inch needle
* Hemostatic agent—aluminum chloride, ferric subsulfate, or silver nitrate
* Container with 10% **formalin**

Procedure

* Position the client for comfort.
* Put on gloves.
* Apply antiseptic skin cleanser to the skin tag and surrounding area.
* Infiltrate the base of the skin tag with 1% lidocaine.
* Grasp the skin tag at the largest part with forceps.
* Gently pull the skin tag until the stalk base is visible.
* Using the iris scissors or scalpel, cut or slice the stalk as close to the base of the stalk as possible.
* Apply a hemostatic agent with cotton-tipped applicator. Hold to the area until the bleeding stops.
* Place the skin tags in the container with 10% formalin for laboratory pathology.
* Apply topical antibiotic—optional.
* Apply a Band-Aid or dressing.

Client Instructions

* Keep the wound clean and dry.
* Antibiotics are usually not required.

- Observe for signs and symptoms of infection, such as
  - Increase in pain after 24 hours
  - Increase in temperature
  - Redness or swelling
  - Yellow or greenish drainage
  - Foul odor
- If any signs and symptoms of infection are found, return to the office.
- For pain, take acetaminophen with codeine (Tylenol No. 3) every 4 hours as needed for mild pain for the first 24 to 48 hours. After 24 hours, ibuprofen or naproxen may be used.
- Take sitz baths in warm water for 10 to 15 minutes three times a day or as needed.
- Take laxatives or stool softeners for 2 weeks posttreatment.
- Increase fiber in your diet and increase fluid intake.
- Redness to the site is common and lessens with time.

BIBLIOGRAPHY

Habif T. *Clinical Dermatology: A Color Guide to Diagnosis and Therapy.* 6th ed. St. Louis, MO: Mosby; 2015.
Lang RS, Hensrud DD. *Clinical Preventive Medicine.* St. Louis, MO: Mosby; 2004.
Murtagh J. *Practice Tips.* 7th ed. New York, NY: McGraw-Hill; 2017.
Pfenninger JL, Fowler GC. *Procedures for Primary Care Physicians.* St. Louis, MO: Mosby; 2019.

Chapter 113

Pilonidal Cyst/Abscess Incision and Drainage (I&D)

Margaret R. Colyar

CPT Code
11770   Excision of pilonidal cyst or sinus, simple
11771   Excision of pilonidal cyst or sinus, extensive
11772   Excision of pilonidal cyst or sinus, complicated

A pilonidal cyst is a closed sac or capsule, usually filled with fluid, semisolid material, hair, and skin debris near the natal cleft of the buttocks. It is also referred to as a pilonidal abscess, pilonidal sinus, or sacrococcygeal fistula.

OVERVIEW

- Incidence—26 per 100,000 people
- More common in Caucasians
- More common in men than in women
- Usually occurs between 15 and 24 years of age and is rare after 40 years of age.
- Causes (Table 113.1)
- Signs and symptoms can be found in Table 113.2.
- Prevention (Table 113.3)

COMPLICATIONS

- Abscess formation
- Recurrence—40% to 50%
- Systemic infection
- Development of squamous cell carcinoma (rare)

CONTRAINDICATIONS

- If the patient is taking blood thinners, REFER to a surgeon.

Table 113·1	Causes of Pilonidal Cysts

- Ingrown hair
- Occupation that requires prolonged sitting
- Hirsutism
- Deep cleft between buttocks

Table 113·2	Signs and Symptoms of Pilonidal Cysts

Over the lower spine
- Pain
- Redness of skin
- Warmth of skin
- Localized swelling
- Drainage of pus from an opening in the skin
- Fever (uncommon)

Table 113·3	Suggested Prevention of Pilonidal Cyst Formation

- Good hygiene in the sacrococcygeal area
- Shave or remove hair with depilatory cream
- Avoid prolonged sitting
- Avoid excessive pressure to the area of the tailbone
- Weight loss if obese

PROCEDURE

Pilonidal Cyst/Abscess Incision and Drainage (I&D)

Equipment

- Antiseptic skin cleanser
- 1% to 2% lidocaine with or without epinephrine
- 3- to 10-mL syringe
- 27- to 30-gauge, ½-inch needle
- 4 × 4 gauze—sterile
- No. 11 scalpel
- Drape—sterile
- Gloves—sterile
- Curved **hemostats**—sterile
- **Iodoform** gauze—¼ to ½ inch
- Culture swab
- Scissors—sterile
- Tape

Procedure

- Position the client with the pilonidal cyst prone.
- Cleanse the cyst and a 3-inch-diameter area surrounding the cyst with antiseptic skin cleanser.
- Drape the cyst with a sterile drape.
- Put on gloves.
- Perform a field block by anesthetizing the perimeter around the cyst with 1% or 2% lidocaine with or without epinephrine. Do *not* inject lidocaine into the abscess because it does not work well in an acidic medium. If the client cannot tolerate a field block, topical anesthesia can be used to freeze the top of the abscess if desired.
- Using the no. 11 scalpel, incise the cyst deeply enough and long enough to allow easy drainage of the purulent material and to prevent premature closure of the wound.
- Obtain a culture by inserting the culturette deeply into the wound cavity or by withdrawing purulent drainage with a syringe and 18-gauge needle.
- Probe sinus tracts with curved hemostats and break up any septa. If deep, REFER to a surgeon.
  - If superficial (less than 5 mm), perform an elliptical excision to remove the pilonidal sinus.
- After expressing all purulent material, pack with iodoform gauze, leaving a small amount protruding from the wound.
  - Leaving the wound open lowers the risk of a recurring pilonidal cyst infection.
  - You could also close the wound with stitches. While the healing time is shorter, there is a greater incidence of recurrence.
- Dress with sterile gauze.

Client Instructions

- Return to the office in 2 days to have dressing changed.
- Observe for signs and symptoms of infection, such as
  - Yellow or green drainage
  - Red streaks
  - Increasing pain
  - Elevated temperature
- If symptoms of infection occur, return to the office.
- Prevent recurrence of the abscess by taking an antibiotic—dicloxacillin 250 mg four times a day or cephalexin 500 mg three times a day.
- For pain relief, take Tylenol No. 3 every 4 to 6 hours for the first 24 hours; then take ibuprofen.
- If the abscess recurs, return to the office for evaluation.

BIBLIOGRAPHY

Armstrong JH, Barcia PJ. Pilonidal sinus disease: the conservative approach. *Arch Surg.* 1994;129:914–917.

Koyfman A. Pilonidal cyst and sinus. *Medscape.* https://emedicine.medscape.com/article/788127-overview. Updated May 20, 2019.

Pfenninger JL, Fowler GC. *Procedures for Primary Care Physicians.* St. Louis, MO: Mosby; 2019.

114

Chapter

Prostate Massage

Margaret R. Colyar

CPT Code
None

Prostate massage is a technique used to extract prostatic secretions as a screening for prostatitis and is part of the digital rectal examination routinely performed on men to check for nodules of prostate cancer.

OVERVIEW

- Prostrate massage increases PSA levels immediately after the procedure. Wait 2 weeks to draw a PSA.
- Symptoms of prostatitis are found in Table 114.1.
- The differential diagnosis of prostatitis is found in Table 114.2.

Table 114·1	**Symptoms of Prostatitis**

Pain
- Back
- Genitourinary
- Ejaculation
- Suprapubic

UTI symptoms
- Dysuria
- Frequency
- Urgency

Erectile dysfunction

Table 114·2	**Differential Diagnoses of Prostatitis**

- Cystitis/urethritis
- Hematuria
- Inflammatory bowel disease
- Inflammation—perirectal
- Inflammation—perivesical
- Interstitial cystitis
- Stone—bladder
- Tumor—genitourinary
- Stricture—urethral

RATIONALE

- To express prostatic secretions
- To diagnose prostatitis
- To aid in diagnosis of prostatic cancer
- To aid in increasing the amount of PCA-3 in urine—specific for prostate cancer

CONTRAINDICATIONS

- None

▶ *Informed consent required*

PROCEDURE

Prostatic Massage

Equipment

- Gloves—nonsterile
- Lubricant—K-Y jelly
- Sterile specimen bottle

Procedure

- Position the patient forward over the examining table or in the knee-chest position.
- Put on gloves.
- Apply lubricant to the examining finger.
- Spread the patient's buttocks.
- Advance the index finger into the anus.
- Palpate the prostate for lumps.
- Stroke the prostate from the periphery toward the midline several times on each side.
- Collect expressed prostate secretions in a sterile bottle and send to the laboratory for evaluation.

Interpretation—usually 4 drops to 1 teaspoon of expressed prostate secretions
- Normal—Clear as water
- Infected—opaque, milky, or yellowish purulent fluid with jelly, wormlike material, and precipitates (calculi)
- No drainage—obstructed ducts

Client Instructions

- You may have the urge to urinate and feel rectal pressure for 15 to 60 minutes after prostatic massage.
- Notify primary care provided if you experience
  - Chills
  - Myalgia
  - Rigors
  - Temperature greater than 101°F

BIBLIOGRAPHY

Ateya A, Fayez A, Hani R, Zohdy W, Gabbar MA, Shamloul R. Evaluation of prostatic massage in treatment of chronic prostatitis. *Urology.* 2006;67(4):674–678.

Feliciano AN. Learning the technique of prostatic massage by Dr Antonio Novak Feliciano. CureZone.org Web site. http://curezone.com/art/read.asp?ID=61&db=5&CO=74

Pfenninger JL, Fowler GC. *Procedures for Primary Care Physicians.* St. Louis, MO: Mosby; 2019.

Chapter

115

Rectal Prolapse Reduction

Margaret R. Colyar

CPT Code
45900   Reduction of rectal prolapse

Rectal prolapse is an uncommon condition and usually occurs in children younger than 1 year and most commonly in older adults, predominantly female. It happens when part or the entire rectum slides out of place.

OVERVIEW

- There are two types
  - Full-thickness—has circular folds in the prolapsed mucosa. All three layers of the rectum are prolapsed.
  - Mucosal—mucous membrane alone is prolapsed and may look like hemorrhoids.
- Predisposing factors for rectal prolapse are listed in Table 115.1.

RATIONALE

- To return prolapsed rectum internally
- To restore bowel function

CONTRAINDICATIONS

- Strangulated rectal prolapse
- Perforation

PROCEDURE

Manual Reduction of a Rectal Prolapse

Equipment

- Gloves—nonsterile
- 1% or 2% lidocaine
- 3-mL syringe
- 25-gauge needle
- Antiseptic soap
- 4 × 4 gauze

Table 115·1	**Predisposing Factors for Rectal Prolapse**

- Pressure
  - Benign prostatic hypertrophy
  - Diarrhea
  - Stool withholding
  - Pregnancy
  - Previous abdominal or rectal surgery
  - Weakened muscles
  - Weakened ligaments
- Excessive coughing
  - Pertussis
  - COPD
- Neurological disorders
  - Pelvic/lumbar trauma
  - Lumbar disk disease
  - Cauda equina syndrome
  - Spinal tumors
  - Multiple sclerosis

Procedure

- Place patient in the dorsal lithotomy or knee-chest position.
- Put on gloves.
- Cleanse external anal sphincter with antiseptic soap.
- Inject external anal sphincter with lidocaine.
- Using two fingers, gently, slowly, and with steady pressure push the distal end of the prolapse into the lumen and through the anal sphincter.
- If you experience excessive mucosal edema, sprinkle the prolapsed rectum with table sugar or table salt to osmotically reduce the swelling.

Client Instructions

- Avoid straining to have a bowel movement.
- Keep bowel movements soft—eat a high-fiber diet and consider stool softeners.
- Consider physical therapy to strengthen muscles.

BIBLIOGRAPHY ▰▰▰▰▰▰▰▰▰▰▰▰▰▰▰▰

Krause RS. Reduction of rectal prolapse. Medscape Web site. http://emedicine.medscape
.com/article/80982-Overview#a30. May 21, 2019.
O'Neill T. How to reduce your prolapse. Michigan Medicine, University of
Michigan Bowel Control Program. http://www.med.umich.edu/1libr/MBCP/
ReduceYourRectalProlapse.pdf. March 2017.

Chapter 6

Thrombosed Hemorrhoid Removal

Margaret R. Colyar

CPT Code
46221 Hemorrhoidectomy, by simple ligature
46230 Excision of external hemorrhoid tags and/or multiple papillae
46320 Enucleation or excision of external thrombotic hemorrhoid
46935 Anoscopy destruction of hemorrhoids; any method, external

---

External hemorrhoids that have **thrombosed** (formed a clot), usually after defecatory straining, may or may not need removal. If pain is not severe and the clot is small, removal is not necessary.

OVERVIEW

- Recurrence rate—2% to 5%
- Signs and symptoms include
- Constant anal pain
- Sensation of sitting on a marble
- Itching
- Purple mass at the anus (Fig. 116.1)

RATIONALE

- To prevent necrosis, pain, and infection

INDICATIONS

- Thrombosed hemorrhoid that is painful

CONTRAINDICATIONS

- Small thrombosed hemorrhoid that is not causing pain
- Immunocompromised client
- Bleeding disorders
- Pregnancy
- Rectal prolapse

▶ *Informed consent required*

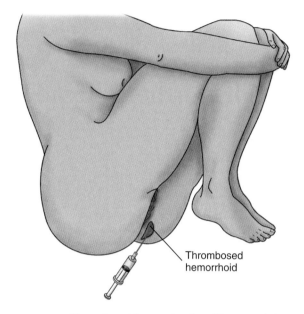

Figure 116.1 Thrombosed hemorrhoid. Infiltrate with lidocaine around the hemorrhoid.

PROCEDURE

Removal of Thrombosed Hemorrhoid

Equipment

- Antiseptic skin cleanser
- Gloves—sterile
- 27-gauge, 1½-inch needle
- 1% or 2% lidocaine with epinephrine
- No. 11 scalpel
- Curved scissors—sterile
- Hemostats—sterile
- Cautery, silver nitrate sticks, or Monsel's solution
- 4 × 4 gauze—sterile
- Tape—3 inch
- Tape—1 inch

Procedure

- Position the client side lying with thrombosed side down.
- Separate buttocks, and tape (using 3-inch tape) to side of table to keep area exposed.
- Cleanse the area with antiseptic skin cleanser.
- Drape the client.
- Put on gloves.

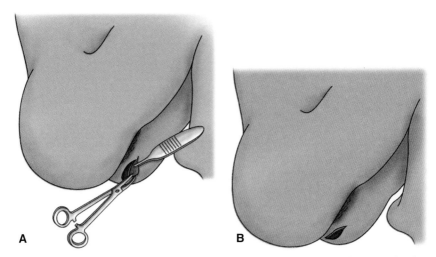

Figure 116.2 (A) Make an elliptical incision around the thrombosed hemorrhoid and (B) remove.

- Infiltrate around the hemorrhoid with 1% or 2% lidocaine with epinephrine.
- Using the no. 11 scalpel, make an elliptical incision around the vein (Fig. 116.2).
- Evacuate all of the clot.
- Explore the cavity for clots, and break down any septa (pockets) with the hemostats.
- Leave the cavity open.
- Pack with dry gauze and secure with 1-inch tape.

Client Instructions

- To decrease pain, do the following:
  - Apply ice packs to wound intermittently for 24 hours.
  - Take acetaminophen every 4 to 6 hours as needed.
- Leave packing in for 24 hours, then remove gently.
  - Minor bleeding is expected.
- To promote healing
  - Soak wound in pan or tub of warm water for 20 to 30 minutes three to four times per day for 1 week.
- To prevent recurrence
  - Avoid prolonged sitting and straining to stool.
  - Include in your daily diet
    - Fruits, vegetables, and bran
    - Four to five glasses of water
- Return to the office in 4 weeks.

BIBLIOGRAPHY

Kellerman RD, Bope ET. *Conn's Current Therapy*. Philadelphia, PA: Saunders; 2017.
Pfenninger JL, Fowler GC. *Procedures for Primary Care Physicians*. St. Louis, MO: Mosby; 2019.

Glossary

A

Acetone A colorless, volatile, inflammable liquid, miscible in water, useful as a solvent, and having a characteristic sweet, fruity, ethereal odor

Acrochordon A small outgrowth of epidermal and dermal tissue. SYN: skin tag

Actinic keratoses Horny, keratotic, premalignant lesions of the skin caused by excess exposure to sunlight

Alignment To put in a straight line

Allen's test Objective test to assure patency of the ulnar artery

Amblyopia Reduction or dimness of vision, especially where there is no apparent pathological condition of the eye

Angioma Form of tumor, usually benign, consisting principally of blood vessels or lymph vessels

Ankyloglossia Abnormal shortness of the frenulum of the tongue. SYN: tongue-tie

Anoscope Tool used to directly visualize the anus

Antecubital In front of the elbow; at the bend of the elbow

Antidote A substance that neutralizes poisons or their effects

Approximate To place or bring objects close together

Arrhythmia Irregularity or loss of rhythm, especially of the heartbeat. SYN: dysrhythmia

Arthrocentesis Puncture of a joint space by using a needle

Arthropods Crustaceans, insects, myriapods, arachnids

Asymmetrical Lack of symmetry

Atrioventricular (AV) node A tangled mass of Purkinje fibers located in the lower part of the interatrial septum from which the AV bundle (bundle of His) arises

Atrophy A decrease in size of an organ or tissue

Audiogram An objective measuring tool for the detection of hearing problems or hearing loss

Auricular Relating to the auricle of the ear

Avulsion A tearing away forcibly of a part or structure

B

Bartholinitis Inflammation of one or both of the Bartholin's glands at the opening to the vagina

Basal cell carcinoma A malignancy of the skin that rarely metastasizes. A lesion with whitish borders around a central depression

Benzoin   A solution applied to the skin to prepare the site for application of adhesives

Biochemical   Chemical changes accompanying the vital functions of plants and animals

Biopsy   Excision of a lesion or small piece of living tissue for microscopic evaluation by punch, shave, curettage, or elliptical excision

Bradycardia   Slow heartbeat less than 60 beats per minute

Bronchospasm   Abnormal narrowing with obstruction of the lumen of the bronchi due to spasm of the peribronchial smooth muscle

Bundle branches   Part of the ventricular conducting system that carries current down the right and left sides of the interventricular septum

Bundle of His   The uppermost portion of the ventricular conducting system. It emerges from the AV node and divides into the right and left bundle branches.

C

Cautery   A means of destroying tissue by electricity, freezing, heat, or corrosive chemicals

Cellulitis   A spreading inflammation of cellular or connective tissue

Cervical cap   Helmet-shaped rubber device that fits over the cervix to provide nonsystemic, nonhormonal, and reversible method of contraception

Cervicovaginal   Pertaining to the cervix and the vagina

Chemosis   Edema of the conjunctiva about the cornea

Coagulopathies   A defect in the blood-clotting mechanisms

Collateral circulation   Circulation of small anastomosing vessels, especially when a main artery is obstructed

Colposcopy   Examination of the vaginal and cervical tissues by using a colposcope

Condyloma acuminatum   Wart in the genital and perianal areas. The virus that causes the wart is usually sexually transmitted.

Confrontation   A method employed in determining the extent of visual fields in which the patient is compared with that of the examiner

Costophrenic   Pertaining to the ribs and diaphragm

Crepitus/crepitation   A crackling sound heard in certain diseases

Cryogenic   Producing or pertaining to low temperatures

Cryoglobulinemia   Presence in the blood of an abnormal protein that forms gels with low temperatures. Found in association with pathological conditions such as multiple myeloma, leukemia, and certain forms of pneumonia.

Cryoprobe   Device for applying cold to a tissue

Cryosurgery   Technique of exposing tissues to extreme cold in order to produce well-demarcated areas of cell injury and destruction. The tissue is usually cooled to below 20°C

Curettage   Scraping of a cavity

Curette   A spoon-shaped scooping and scraping instrument for removing foreign matter from a cavity

Cutaneous   Pertaining to the skin
Cyanosis   Slightly bluish, grayish, slatelike, or dark purple discoloration of the skin caused by the presence of abnormal amounts of reduced hemoglobin in the blood
Cycloplegics   Medium that produces paralysis of the ciliary muscles
Cystocele   A bladder hernia that protrudes into the vagina

D

Decubitus view   Lying down, flat
Defecatory   Evacuation of the bowels
Deflection   The deviation from zero shown by the indicator of a measuring instrument
Depolarization   Electrical stimulus of the heart muscle causing heart cells to contract
Dermabond   Skin closure adhesives used over flat areas of the body that do not require increased potential for tension to the repair site (i.e., over joints)
Dermatofibroma   A nonmalignant skin fibroma (a fibrous, encapsulated, connective tissue tumor)
Dermis   The skin
Desiccation   The process of drying up
Diaphragm   Contraceptive barrier device of various sizes that consists of a soft latex rubber dome supported by a round metal spring on the outside
Digital block   Nerve block accomplished by injecting anesthetic agents between the web of the fingers or toes
Diphasic   Having two phases
Disseminate   Scatter or distribute over a considerable area
Dither   A technique during the sigmoidoscopy procedure
Doppler   Ultrasound instrument used to detect arterial blood flow
Dorsal   Pertaining to the back
Dysmenorrhea   Pain in association with menstruation
Dyspareunia   Occurrence of pain in the labial, vaginal, or pelvic areas during or after sexual intercourse
Dysplasia   Abnormal development of tissue
Dysrhythmias   Abnormal, disordered, or disturbed cardiac rhythms

E

Edema   A local or generalized condition in which the body tissues contain an excessive amount of tissue fluid
Effusion   Escape of fluid into a part
Electrocardiogram (EKG)   Tool to assist with diagnosis or ruling out a myocardial infarction, potentially life-threatening arrhythmias, and many other heart problems
Electrode   A medium intervening between an electric conductor and the object to which the current is to be applied
Endocervix   The lining of the canal of the cervix uteri
Endoscopy   Inspection of the body organs or cavity by use of the endoscope

Enucleation   To remove the eyeball surgically

Epistaxis   Onset of nasal hemorrhage with or without trauma

Epithelialization   The growth of skin over a wound

Erythema migrans   An annular erythema following an insect bite, especially that of the tick infected with the spirochete that causes Lyme disease

Eschar   A slough, especially one following a cauterization or burn

Exarticulation   Amputation of a limb through a joint; excision of a part of a joint

Exocervix   Outside the cervix

Extra-articular   Outside a joint

F

Fascia   A fibrous membrane covering, supporting, and separating muscles

Fasciitis   Inflammation of any fascia

Felon   Infection or abscess of soft tissue of the terminal joint of a finger

Fenestrated   Having openings

Fibrillation   Irregular heartbeat from multiple foci

Field block   Method of anesthetizing a small area by injecting anesthetic solution around the lesion to block the nerves supplying the operative field

Fistula   An abnormal tubelike passage from a normal cavity or tube to a free surface or to another cavity

Flail chest   A condition of the chest wall resulting from two or more fractures on each affected rib resulting in a segment of ribs that is not attached on either end; the flail segment moves paradoxically in with inspiration and out during expiration

Fluoresce   To emit light when exposed to ultraviolet rays

Fluorescein   A red, crystalline powder, used for diagnostic purposes and for detecting foreign bodies in or lesions of the cornea of the eye

Fluorescence   The emission of light of one wavelength, usually ultraviolet

Flutter   Regular saw-toothed beat from single ectopic focus

Foci   Locations

Forceps   Pincers for holding, seizing, or extracting

Formalin   Aqueous solution of 37% formaldehyde

Fornix   Any body with vaultlike or arched shape

Fossa   A furrow or shallow depression

Frenotomy   Division of any frenum, especially for tongue-tie

Frenulum   A small fold of tissue that limits the movement of an organ or part

Frenulum linguae   Fold of mucous membrane that extends from the floor of the mouth to the inferior surface of the tongue along its midline

Furuncle   Abscess of hair follicle or sweat gland; a boil

G

Ganglion cyst   Cystic tumor developing on a tendon or aponeurosis; sometimes occurs on the back of the wrist

Gluteal   Pertaining to the buttocks

Granuloma   A granular tumor or growth, usually of lymphoid and epithelial cells

H

Heimlich valve   Plastic one-way valve used for chest drainage

Hemoccult   Hidden blood

Hemolysis   The destruction of red blood cells with the liberation of hemoglobin, which diffuses into the surrounding fluid

Hemolytic   Pertaining to the breaking down of red blood cells

Hemopneumothorax   Blood and air in the pleural cavity

Hemosiderin   An iron-containing pigment derived from hemoglobin from disintegration of red blood cells

Hemostatic agent   Any drug, medication, or blood component that serves to stop bleeding, for example, ferrous subsulfate or aluminum chloride

Hemostats   Devices that arrest the flow of blood

Hemothorax   Blood or bloody fluid in the pleural cavity caused by rupture of blood vessels as a result of inflammation of the lungs in pneumonia or pulmonary tuberculosis, malignant growth, or trauma

Hemotympanum   Blood in the middle ear

Herniated   Having a protrusion or projection of an organ or a part of an organ through the wall of the cavity that normally contains it

Hidradenitis   Inflammation of a sweat gland

Holter monitor   Portable EKG machine with a memory

Hyperpnea   An increased respiratory rate or breathing that is deeper than that usually experienced during normal activity

Hyperresonance   Increased resonance produced when the area is percussed

Hypertrophy   Increase in size of an organ or structure that does not involve tumor formation

Hypospadias   Placement of the penile os on the underside of the penis

I

Iatrogenic   Caused by treatment or diagnostic procedures

Impregnated   Saturated

Incarcerated   Imprisoned, confined, constricted, as an irreducible hernia

Indurated   Hardened

Infarction   Formation of an area of tissue in an organ or part that undergoes necrosis following cessation of blood supply

Infiltrate   To pass into or through a substance or a space

Inspissated   Thickened by evaporation or absorption of fluid

Intercostal   Between the ribs

Interphalangeal   In a joint between two phalanges (bones of the toes or fingers)

Introitus   An opening or entrance into a canal or cavity, as the vagina

Inverted   Turned inside out or upside down

Iodoform   Gauze

Irreducible   Not capable of being reduced or made smaller, as a fracture or dislocation

Ischemic   Local and temporary deficiency of blood supply arising from obstruction of the circulation to a part

Ischiorectal   Pertaining to the ischium and rectum

IUD   Intrauterine device. Inserted through the cervix and retained in the uterus to prevent pregnancy

K

Keloid   Scar formation in the skin following trauma or surgical incision

Keratoacanthoma   A papular lesion filled with a keratin plug that can resemble squamous cell carcinoma

L

Laceration   An injury to the integument system usually associated with trauma and resulting in the disruption of integrity

Latrodectism   The toxic reaction to the bite of spiders of the genus *Latrodectus,* that is, black widows

Lavage   Washing out of a cavity

Lentigo   Small, brown macules or yellow-brown pigmented areas on the skin sometimes caused by exposure to sun and weather

Leukoplakia   Formation of white spots or patches on the tongue or cheek. May become malignant

Ligament   A band or sheet of strong fibrous connective tissue connecting the articular ends of bones, serving to bind them together to facilitate or limit motion

Limb leads   On EKG, these measure electrical waves of depolarization and repolarization, moving up and down and left and right in a vertical or frontal plane. The electrodes for these measurements are placed on the arms and legs

Loculated   Divided into cavities

Lordotic   Abnormal anterior convexity of the spine

Lumbar puncture   Diagnostic procedure involving introduction of a hollow needle in the subarachnoid space of the lumbar portion of the spinal column

M

Maceration   Process of softening a solid by steeping in a fluid

Macroglobulinemia   Presence of globulins of high molecular weight in serum

Manubrium (sterni)   The upper segment of the sternum articulating with the clavicle and first pair of costal cartilages

Melanoma   A malignant, darkly pigmented mole or tumor of the skin

Menorrhagia   Excessive bleeding at the time of a menstrual period, in number of days, amount of blood, or both

Metacarpophalangeal   Concerning the metacarpus and the phalanges

Metaplasia   Conversion of one kind of tissue into a form that is not normal for the tissue, characterized by small, waxy, globular epithelial tumors that are umbilicated and contain semifluid caseous matter or solid masses

Midclavicular line   Vertical line extending from the midpoint of the clavicle

Molluscum contagiosum The usual mildly contagious form of molluscum that affects mainly children and younger adults
Mosaicism Abnormal chicken wire, cobblestone, or tile floor pattern
Multifocal Concerning many foci
Mydriatic Any drug that dilates the pupil

N

Nebulizer An apparatus for producing a fine spray or mist
Necrotic Pertaining to death of areas of tissue or bone surrounded by healthy parts
Nevi Congenital discoloration of circumscribed areas of the skin from pigmentation
Nulliparous Woman who has never been pregnant

O

Oblique view Slanting, diagonal
Obturator Anything that obstructs or closes a cavity or opening; two muscles on each side of the pelvic region that rotate the thighs outward
Orbiculus oris Circular muscle surrounding the mouth
Organomegaly Enlargement of visceral organs
Orogastric Concerning the mouth and stomach
Orthopnea Respiration condition in which there is discomfort in breathing in any but erect sitting or standing position
Ossicular Pertaining to one of the bones of the inner ear
Osteomyelitis Inflammation of bones, especially the marrow, caused by a pathogenic organism
Oximetry Method of determining the amount of oxygen in the blood

P

P wave On EKG, represents atrial depolarization and contraction. Usually occurs prior to the QRS complex.
PMI Point of maximal impulse
PR interval On EKG, includes the P wave and the straight line connecting it to the QRS complex. It measures the time from the beginning of atrial depolarization to the start of ventricular depolarization.
Papanicolaou (Pap) smear A study for early detection of cancer cells
Paracervical Pertaining to tissues adjacent to the cervix
Paronychia Acute or chronic infection of marginal structures about the nail
Parous Woman who has been pregnant
Patency The state of being freely open
Percutaneous Effected through the skin
Perforate To puncture or to make holes
Perforation The act of making a hole, such as that caused by ulceration
Perianal cyst A cyst located around or close to the anus
Perichondrium Membranes of fibrous connective tissue around the surface of cartilage

Peritoneal   Concerning the peritoneum

Phalanx   Any one of the bones of the fingers or toes

Pilonidal cyst   A cyst in the sacrococcygeal region, usually at the upper end of the intergluteal cleft

Pneumothorax   Collapsed lung

Polychromatic   Multicolored

Porokeratosis plantaris discreta   A rare skin disease marked by thickening of the stratum corneum in linear arrangement, followed by its atrophy

Porphyria   A group of disorders that result from a disturbance in porphyrin metabolism, causing increased formation and excretion of porphyrin or its precursors

Prolapse   A falling or dropping down of an organ or internal part, such as the uterus or rectum

Properitoneal   In front of the peritoneum

Proteolytic   Hastening the hydrolysis of proteins

Pruritus   Severe itching

Punctation   Abnormal stippled appearance

Purkinje fibers   Atypical muscle fibers lying beneath the endocardium. They form the electrical impulse–conducting system of the heart

Pyoderma gangrenosum   A purulent skin disease

Q

Q wave   On EKG, first downward stroke of the QRS complex

QRS complex   On EKG, represents beginning of ventricular contraction; usually lasts less than 0.12 sec

R

R wave   On EKG, first upward stroke of the QRS complex

Reducible   Able to be restored to the original position

Repolarization   Resting or relaxation phase of the heart muscle

S

S wave   On EKG, downward deflection of the QRS complex after the R wave

ST segment   On EKG, flat piece of baseline between the QRS complex and the beginning of the T wave. It measures the time from the end of ventricular depolarization to the start of ventricular repolarization

Sebaceous cyst   A cyst filled with sebum from a distended oil-secreting gland

Seborrheic keratoses   Pigmented, raised, warty, and slightly greasy lesions, usually on the trunk, hands, and face

Septa   Tissue pockets

Septicemia   Presence of pathogenic bacteria in the blood

Sigmoidoscopy   Colorectal anal screening technique using lighted tube to visualize the inner lining of the rectum and the distal colon

Sinoatrial nodes   Dominant pacemaker cells in the heart located high up in the right atrium

Slough   To shed or cast off dead tissue cells

Speculum   A retractor used to separate the walls of a cavity to allow for visual examination

Spicule   A sharp body with a needle-like point

Squamous cell carcinoma   A form of epidermoid carcinoma, principally of squamous cells

Stenosis   Constriction or narrowing of a passage or orifice

Steri-Strip   Noninvasive skin closure device

Stoma   A mouth, small opening, or pore

Strabismus   Disorder of the eye in which the optic axes cannot be directed to the same object

Strangulated   Constricted so that air or blood supply is cut off, as a strangulated hernia

Subcutaneous emphysema   Pathological distention by gas or air beneath the skin

Subungual   Situated beneath the nail of the finger or toe

Suturing   A procedure used to repair lacerations of the skin. Suturing may involve the use of suturing material or use of Dermabond.

Syncope   A transient loss of consciousness caused by inadequate blood flow to the brain

T

T wave   On EKG, repolarization of the ventricles

Tachycardia   Abnormal rapidity of heart action, usually defined as a heart rate more than 100 beats per minute in adults

Tamponade   Pathological condition resulting from accumulation of excess fluid in the pericardium

Telangiectasia   A vascular lesion formed by dilation of a group of small blood vessels

Tenaculum   Sharp, hooklike pointed instrument with slender shank for grasping and holding a part, as an artery

Tendon   Fibrous connective tissue serving for the attachment of muscles to bones and other parts

Tensile   Strong

Thrombosed   Coagulated; clotted

Torque   A force producing rotary motion

Transformation zone   Area of columnar epithelium and squamous metaplasia in the vagina or on the cervix

Tympanometry   Procedure for objective evaluation of the mobility and patency of the eardrum and for detection of middle ear disorders and patency of the eustachian tubes

Tympanostomy   Incision of the tympanic membrane

U

Ulceration   Suppuration occurring on a free surface, as on the skin or on a mucous membrane, to form an ulcer

Unifocal   Having one focus

Unna's boot   Compression and paste bandage used to treat ulcers caused by venous insufficiency

V

Vasovagal   Concerning the action of stimuli from the vagus nerve on blood vessels

Vector   On EKG, the average direction of electrical flow within the heart

Venipuncture   Puncture of a vein for any purpose

Venous insufficiency   An abnormal circulatory condition characterized by decreased return of the venous blood to the trunk of the body

Verruca vulgaris   Common wart, usually on the back of hands and fingers, but may occur anywhere on the skin

Vitreous humor   Clear, watery gel filling the cavity behind the lens of the eye

Volar   Palm of the hand or sole of the foot

W

Wood's light   Tool that emits ultraviolet rays used to detect fluorescent materials in skin and hair diseases

X

Xiphoid process   Lowest portion of the sternum

INDEX

Page numbers of figures are in *italics*. Page numbers of tables are followed by t.